SKANDIA INTERNATIONAL SYMPOSIA

Trace Elements in Health and Disease

SKANDIA INTERNATIONAL SYMPOSIA

Trace Elements in Health and Disease

SYMPOSIUM, OCTOBER 23–25, 1984

EDITED BY

HARRY BOSTRÖM AND NILS LJUNGSTEDT

SPONSORED BY THE SKANDIA GROUP

ALMQVIST & WIKSELL INTERNATIONAL · STOCKHOLM · SWEDEN

First published by
Almqvist & Wiksell International, Stockholm, Sweden, 1985

ISBN 91-22-00733-4

In this series were earlier published:

Stroke, pp 1–288, Stockholm 1967
Cancer and Aging, pp. 1–280, Stockholm 1968
Aging of Connective and Skeletal Tissue, pp. 1–336, Stockholm 1969
Alcoholic Cirrhosis and Other Toxic Hepatopathias, pp. 1–372, Stockholm 1970
Regional Enteritis (Crohn's Disease), pp. 1–324, Stockholm 1971
Suicide and Attempted Suicide, pp. 1–320, Stockholm 1972
Early Phases of Coronary Heart Disease, pp. 1–362, Stockholm 1973
Rehabilitation after Central Nervous System Trauma, pp. 1–256, Stockholm 1974
Drug Dependence—Treatment and Treatment Evaluation, pp. 1–312, Stockholm 1975
Ärftliga ämnesomsättningsrubbningar (in Swedish), pp. 1–175, Stockholm 1975
Health Control in Detection of Cancer, pp. 1–291, Stockholm 1976
Unexpected Complications in Medical Care, pp. 1–301, Stockholm 1979
Congenital Diseases in Childhood, pp. 1–336, Stockholm 1980
Etiska synpunkter på uppspårande av sjukdomar före födseln (in Swedish), pp. 1–73, Stockholm 1980
Medical Aspects of Mortality Statistics, pp. 1–387, Stockholm 1981
Recent Trends in Diabetes Research, pp. 1–308, Stockholm 1982
Theoretical and Clinical Aspects of Allergic Diseases, pp. 1–302, Stockholm 1983
Detection and Prevention of Adverse Drug Reactions, pp. 1–294, Stockholm 1984

Printed in Sweden
NORSTEDTS TRYCKERI, STOCKHOLM 1985

Preface

DURING the past decades, science has taken more and more interest in trace elements, since new and refined analytical methods have made it possible to measure very low concentrations of them in biological material. Therefore, it came natural to Skandia to arrange a symposium on trace elements.

The meeting was opened by two lectures on trace elements in the diet: need of supplements and marginal deficiences, respectively. After a presentation of trace elements in water supplies, health effects and environmental aspects were discussed.

Analytical problems were elucidated in two lectures: quality assurance considerations on sample collection, treatment, preservation and storage of biomedical specimens, as well as analytical methods.

The main part of the meeting was devoted to the role of trace elements and their effects in certain diseases: diabetes mellitus, connective-tissue diseases, rheumatoid arthritis, cancer, cardiovascular diseases, alcoholic cirrhosis, coeliac disease and renal failure.

The discussions after the lectures are as usual included in the book. We consider them to be very valuable complements to the papers.

We feel honoured that such an eminent and distinguished group of experts accepted the invitation and the Skandia Group wants to thank the authors and the other participants for their valuable contributions to the symposium. We also want to thank Mrs Elizabeth Silins for her most valuable assistance in preparing this book.

Harry Boström *Nils Ljungstedt*

Skandia International Symposia
S-103 50 Stockholm, Sweden

Contents

Participants

AASETH, JAN, M.D.
Department of Clinical Chemistry
Hedmark Central Hospital, N-2400 Elverum, Norway

ABDULLA, MOHAMED, M.D.
Department of Clinical Chemistry
University Hospital, S-221 85 Lund, Sweden

AGGETT, PETER J., M.D., Senior Lecturer
Department of Child Health, University of Aberdeen
Foresterhill, Aberdeen AB9 2ZD, Great Britain

AHLROT-WESTERLUND, BRITT, M.L.
Unit of Neurochemistry and Toxicology
University of Stockholm, Enköpingsvägen 126, S-172 46 Sundbyberg, Sweden

ANDERSON, RICHARD A., Ph.D., Chemist
USDA, Vitamin and Mineral Nutrition Laboratory
Beltsville Human Nutrition Research Center, Beltsville, MD 20705, USA

BERLIN, MATHS, M.D., Professor
Department of Hygiene
University of Lund, P.O. Box 2009, S-220 02 Lund, Sweden

BOSTRÖM, HARRY, M.D., Professor
Medical Adviser to the Skandia Group
Department of Medicine
Akademiska Sjukhuset, S-751 85 Uppsala, Sweden

BRUCE, ÅKE, M.D., Professor
Swedish National Food Administration
P.O. Box 622, S-751 26 Uppsala, Sweden

Christophersen, Olav Albert, M.D.
Norsk Pharmacia A/S, Darresgate 2, Oslo 5, Norway

Danielson, Bo G., M.D., Ass. Professor
Department of Internal Medicine
Akademiska Sjukhuset, S-751 85 Uppsala, Sweden

Ekman, Lars, M.D., Ass. Professor
KabiVitrum AB, P.O. Box 12170, S-102 24 Stockholm, Sweden

Engel, Arthur, M.D., Former Director General of the National Board of Health
Sibyllegatan 77, S-114 43 Stockholm, Sweden

Fellström, Bengt, M.D., Ass. Professor
Department of Internal Medicine
Akademiska Sjukhuset, S-751 85 Uppsala, Sweden

Fjellström, Karl-Erik, M.D., Ass. Professor
Department of Medicine
Akademiska Sjukhuset, S-751 85 Uppsala, Sweden

Frank, Adrian, D.V.M., Ph.D., Assoc. Professor
National Veterinary Institute, S-750 07 Uppsala, Sweden

Grefberg, Nils, M.D.
Department of Internal Medicine
Akademiska Sjukhuset, S-751 85 Uppsala

Hall, Sten, M.D.
Department of Clinical Chemistry
General Hospital, S-721 89 Västerås, Sweden

Hällgren, Roger, M.D., Ass. Professor
Department of Internal Medicine
Akademiska Sjukhuset, S-751 85 Uppsala, Sweden

Hambraeus, Leif, M.D., Professor
Institute of Nutrition, Biomedical Centre
University of Uppsala, P.O. Box 551, S-751 22 Uppsala, Sweden

Hurley, Lucille S., Ph.D., Professor
Department of Nutrition
University of California, Davis, CA 95616, USA

IYENGAR, G. VENKATESH, D.Sc., Ph.D., Visiting Scientist
US Food and Drug Administration
HFF-266, 200 C Street S.W., Washington, DC 20204, USA

JACKS, GUNNAR, D.Eng., Ass. Professor
Department of Cultural Technology
Royal Institute of Technology, S-100 44 Stockholm, Sweden

JAMESON, STEN, M.D., Ass. Professor
Department of Internal Medicine
Akademiska Sjukhuset, S-751 85 Uppsala, Sweden

JOHANSSON, ERLAND, Ph.D., Ass. Professor
The Gustaf Werner Institute
University of Uppsala, P.O. Box 531, S-751 21 Uppsala, Sweden

KIILLERICH, SØREN, M.D.
Department of Clinical Chemistry
Glostrup Hospital, DK-2600 Glostrup, Denmark

LINDH, ULF, Ph.D.
The Gustaf Werner Institute
University of Uppsala, P.O. Box 531, S-751 21 Uppsala, Sweden

LJUNGSTEDT, NILS, B.LL., Manager
Secretary General of the Skandia International Symposia
Skandia Insurance Company Ltd, S-103 50 Stockholm, Sweden

NILSSON, PER, M.D.
Department of Internal Medicine
Akademiska Sjukhuset, S-751 85 Uppsala, Sweden

NORRBY, JOHANNES, B.Sc. (Econ.), M.F., Deputy Managing Director
Skandia Insurance Company Ltd, S-103 50 Stockholm, Sweden

NORRMAN, ERIC, L.S.A.
Research Information Centre
Swedish University of Agricultural Sciences, S-750 07, Uppsala, Sweden

PERRY, ELIZABETH F.
Hypertension Division, Washington University School of Medicine
Box 8048, 660 S. Euclid, St. Louis, MO 631 10, USA

PERRY, H. MITCHELL, JR., M.D., Professor of Medicine and Director Hypertension Division, Washington University School of Medicine, Box 8048, 660 S. Euclid, St. Louis, MO 63110, USA, and
Physician Coordinator for Hypertension, US Veterans Administration, Washington, DC, USA

PLANTIN, LARS-OLOF, Dipl.Eng., Ass. Professor
Research Center
Huddinge University Hospital, S-141 86 Huddinge, Sweden

SALONEN, JUKKA T., M.D., Ph.D., Professor of Epidemiology
Department of Community Health
University of Kuopio, P.O. Box 6, SF-70221 Kuopio 21, Finland

SHAMBERGER, RAYMOND J., Ph.D., Head, Section of Enzymology
Department of Biochemistry, The Cleveland Clinic Foundation
9500 Euclid Avenue, Cleveland, Ohio 44106, USA

STJERNFELDT, MICHAEL, M.D.
Department of Paediatrics
University Hospital, S-581 85 Linköping, Sweden

SVENSON, KARIN, M.D.
Department of Internal Medicine
Akademiska Sjukhuset, S-751 85 Uppsala, Sweden

SÖDERHJELM, LARS, M.D., Professor
Department of Paediatrics
General Hospital, S-851 86 Sundsvall, Sweden

THEORELL, HENNING, M.L.
Linnégatan 67, S-114 60 Stockholm, Sweden

WALDENSTRÖM, JAN G., M.D., D.Sc. h.c., Professor Emer.
Department of Internal Medicine I
Malmö Allmänna Sjukhus, S-214 01 Malmö, Sweden

WEISMANN, KAARE, M.D., Consultant Dermatologist
Department of Dermatology
Bispebjerg Hospital, DK-2400 Copenhagen NV, Danmark

WEISS, LARS, M.D.
Department of Internal Medicine
Akademiska Sjukhuset, S-751 85 Uppsala, Sweden

WENGLE, BO, M.D., Ass. Professor
Department of Internal Medicine
General Hospital, S-801 17 Gävle, Sweden

WESTER, PER O., M.D., Professor
Department of Internal Medicine
University Hospital, S-901 85 Umeå, Sweden

WIKSTRÖM, BJÖRN, M.D.
Department of Internal Medicine
Akademiska Sjukhuset, S-751 85 Uppsala, Sweden

WRETLIND, ARVID, M.D., Professor
Vitrum Institute for Human Nutrition
P.O. Box 12170, S-102 24 Stockholm, Sweden

Opening Adress

By Johannes Norrby

Ladies and Gentlemen,
Participants of the 17th Skandia International Symposium,

It is my honour on behalf of Skandia Group Management and Skandia Life Management to extend to you all a warm welcome to this symposium. We are honoured and happy to see so many prominent scientists and so many representatives of organisations concerned. I also give you the best wishes from Olle Lifvergren, manager of the Life Division and from Björn Wolrath, presently speaking chinese in Peking.

When we select the topics for these symposia we keep to subjects of interest to the insurance industry. A glance at the list of titles shows that this interest ranges over a broad field, covering not only such directly insurance-connected subjects as mortality statistics but also, for example, suicide, drug and rehabilitation problems as well as recent trends in the research of different diseases. Last year the topic was "Detection and Prevention of Adverse Drug Reactions"—a complement to the 1978 symposium on "Unexpected Complications in Medical Care".

During the past decades, new and refined analytical methods have made it possible to measure the very low concentration of trace elements in biological material. In recent years a large number of publications have appeared, dealing with a great variety of biological problems, which have been elucidated by the utilisation of these new techniques.

Studies have shown that some of the trace elements are vital to the maintaining of the life process, for example, by cooperating with different enzyme systems which in their turn control vital biochemical and biological processes. Other trace elements are of interest because they have toxic effects in certain concentrations. As indicated by the various topics which will be dealt with, the balance of trace elements in human beings seems to be related not only to health and well-being in general but also to the development of a variety of specific diseases.

Great attention has also been paid to environmental changes such as acidification of ground and water secondary to air pollution and the possible effects of these changes on the content of trace elements in the food of man and of domestic animals.

It is, therefore, important for our life insurance company to follow and perhaps to stimulate research concerning trace elements. Consequently, we have this year chosen the subject Trace Elements in Health and Disease.

I want to express our gratitude for the valuable assistance several of you have given the Committee when it worked out the programme.

At earlier symposia medical doctors have dominated the panel and the audience. This years topic has, however, been met with great interest also by other professionals. We are happy to have among the participants several representatives for nutrition centres, the Swedish National Food Administration and for pharmaceutical industries. We hope all participants will benefit from the experiences from different parts of the world as presented to you during these three days by the speakers. We also hope you will benefit from the formal discussions and from informal discussions in the social events outside this room.

With these words, dear participants, I hope you all feel most welcome to the 17th Skandia International Symposium.

I now give the floor to professor Harry Boström. He is heading the Symposium Committee and also chairman of this morning session.

Need of Dietary Supplements of Trace Elements

By Åke Bruce

For a long period nutrition scientists were mainly concerned with vitamins. During 1920–1940 new vitamins were discovered, their deficency disorders were described and daily requirements estimated. Today, vitamin intake does not constitute a major nutritional problem in the developed countries. Vitamin deficiencies are rare and more attention has now to be paid to other types of nutrition disorders. During the last decades attention has been focused on the trace elements and the present scientific surge of interest in this topic can be compared to that in vitamins 50 years ago.

DOSE EFFECT

The present recommendations for the daily intake of mineral and trace elements are sometimes based on clinical studies on intakes causing deficiency diseases in humans. More often they are extrapolated from the results of animal studies or balance studies on humans.

Figure 1 shows a dose-response curve for an essential nutrient. At the lowest intake deficiency diseases occur. At present such human disorders have been reported mainly for zinc, copper, iodine and selenium. Occasional cases have also been published for chromium and molybdenum while human deficiency of manganese is still virtually unknown.

With present analytical methods it is possible to determine low serum or intracellular levels of trace elements or low activities of some mineral-dependent enzymes (for example selenium-glutathione peroxidase), indicating subclinical conditions due to marginally low dietary intakes. These intakes do not, however, under normal conditions, have any negative effect on the metabolism or other physiological parameters. But, in certain situations such as physiological stress or other disorders, individuals with bor-

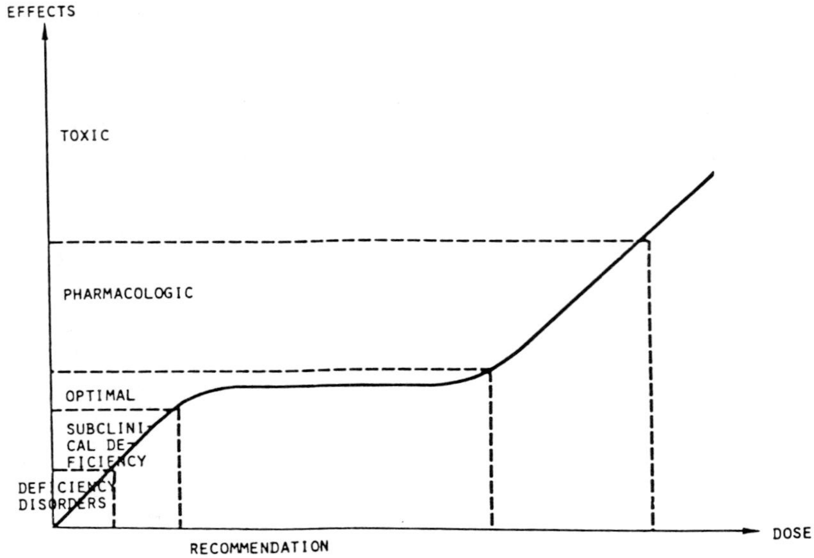

Fig. 1 Various vitamin effects

derline levels may develop an impaired metabolism. With the exception of zinc, there are rather little data on human implications of such conditions.

Usually there is a rather wide range of intakes which provide the human body with sufficient amounts of a nutrient without any signs of under- or overnutrition. This range is very wide for most vitamins while it is rather narrow for some trace elements, e.g., selenium. The dietary recommendations are established somewhere in this range.

Intakes of some nutrients above the optimal level may have a pharmacological effect. Often this aspect is not readily distinguished from nutritional effects. Many anecdotal reports in the scientific literature on positive effects of trace element supplementation may in fact be pharmacological effects.

At high intakes toxic effects may occur. Usually these effects are not caused by intakes through the diet. They may constitute a hygienic problem in some environments or under some working conditions.

INDICATIONS FOR TRACE ELEMENT SUPPLEMENTATION

The proper therapeutic use of trace element supplementation is for treating patients with deficiency diseases due to inadequate intakes, disturbed absorption or increased tissue requirements. Today there is quite a substantial literature available, particularly on the clinical indications for zinc, iodine and copper therapy and on supplementation of trace elements during prolonged total parenteral nutrition.

Clinical use of trace element supplements for treatment of deficiency disorders due to a long period of low intakes, malabsorption or aberrant trace element metabolism is outside the scope of this paper.

For healthy individuals trace elements and minerals should be supplied by the diet. A balanced and varied diet composed according to present dietary guidelines will usually contain sufficient amounts of all nutrients. There are, however, occasions when such a diet cannot be eaten. Minor disorders, such as trauma or infections in the mouth and throat, may limit the possibilities to eat or chew certain types of foods. During convalescence after a period of illness the appetite may be impaired and the dietary intake of nutrients insufficient. Dieting for overweight also makes it difficult to obtain all necessary nutrients in sufficient amount through the diet. Patients with food intolerance may exclude some groups of foodstuffs. Vegetarians excluding food of animal origin may find it difficult to obtain all trace elements and minerals (e.g., selenium and zinc) in appropriate amounts from their ordinary diet.

Occasionally there are other and more social reasons for incomplete diets. Vacations in the mountains or in a small boat with all food dried or canned may also limit the amount of nutrients in the diet. However, if insufficient diets are to be consumed for a longer period, it is advisable to consult a dietitian or nutritionist (Bruce 1984).

TRACE ELEMENT PREPARATIONS

The present Swedish Nutrition Recommendations are based on the latest edition of the American Recommended Dietary Allowances (Food and Nutrition Board 1980, Bruce 1981). Table 1 shows these recommendations for adults. The aim of the recommendations is to provide "the levels of intake of essential nutrients considered, on the basis of available scientific

Table 1 Trace element recommendations for adults
(Food and Nutrition Board 1980)

	Males	Females
Recommended daily dietary allowances		
Iron (mg)	10	18
Zinc (mg)	15	15
Iodine (μg)	150	150
Estimated safe and adequate daily dietary intakes		
Copper (mg)	2.0– 3.0	
Manganese (mg)	2.5– 5.0	
Fluoride (mg)	1.5– 4.0	
Chromium (μg)	50 –200	
Selenium (μg)	50 –200	
Molybdenum (μg)	150 –500	

knowledge, to be adequate to meet the nutritional needs of practically all healthy persons''. The latest edition of the RDA also contains data on ''Estimated safe and adequate daily dietary intakes of selected vitamins and minerals''. Because there is less information on what to base these allowances, the figures are not given in the main table of RDA and are provided in the form of ranges of recommended intakes. Nevertheless, these ranges now seem to have been generally accepted as preliminary recommendations.

The recommendations in Table 1 can also serve as a basis for a suitable trace element formula to be used by healthy individuals consuming an incomplete diet. A multi-trace element tablet ought to contain the essential elements which are normally provided by the diet in amounts equal to the recommendations.

Only a few multi-trace element tablets are sold in Swedish pharmacies and some in health-food shops. The composition of these tablets varies and several do not fulfill the criteria mentioned above. Most of them have a rather uneven profile, e.g., in the same tablet some elements are in doses above the recommendations while other doses are equal to or below the standard.

REGULATIONS

Many new non-prescription drugs have appeared in the pharmacies during the last years. This is particularly relevant for dietary supplements containing minerals, vitamins or dietary fibre.

The basic principle of Swedish legislation on drugs is state control of all products sold for the purpose of preventing, curing and alleviating illness or symptoms of illness. The reason for this control is the wish to prevent harmful and ineffective drugs from reaching the market. The supervision is carried out by the National Board of Health and Welfare which has the right to classify the product as a drug and decide whether it needs a prescription or not. The Board mainly looks at the purpose and the effects of the products and can restrict the sale if the product is not scientifically justified. From its point of view it can be argued that certain trace element preparations are not necessary, since deficiency disorders have hardly been reported in general populations and therefore prevention is unnecessary.

The Swedish Food Administration looks upon these products from another standpoint. Swedes are free to select their diet, although they are advised to eat a varied diet according to present dietary guidelines and nutrition recommendations. However, anybody is free to select a diet with high contents of fat and sugar, i.e., ''empty calories'', and supplement this with vitamin and mineral preparations. As mentioned earlier, there are also occasions when educated consumers will need a supplement. Therefore, in the Administrations's opinion, suitable supplemental preparations should

Table 2 Tentative content of trace elements in supplements

	Recommended dosage (mg/day)	Lowest and highest dosage permitted (mg/day)
Iron	18	10 –25
Zinc	15	7.5 –25
Copper	2	1 – 3
Iodine	0.15	0.075– 0.25
Manganese	2.5	1 – 4
Chromium	0.05	0.025– 0.1
Selenium	0.05	0.025– 0.1
Molybdenum	0.15	0.075– 0.25

be available on the market. However, these supplements should only contain nutrients in doses according to present recommendations.

Recently, the Board of Health and Welfare and the Food Administration have agreed on this matter and have published a draft of preliminary regulations for supplements containing vitamins, minerals and trace elements. Supplements, containing all relevant trace elements according to Table 2 and in doses corresponding to these recommendations, only will need a simple registration before they are offered for sale. Products with other compositions or other doses will need scientific documentation to prove the suitability of their formulations. These regulations will probably be effective early in 1985.

REFERENCES

BRUCE, Å. (1981). Svenska näringsrekommendationer. *Vår föda* 33, 354–372.

— (1984). Nutritional aspects on vitamins and vitamin supplementation. In *Vitamins*. National Board of Health and Welfare, Drug Information Committee, Uppsala, Sweden.

Food and Nutrition Board (1980). *Recommended Dietary Allowances*. National Academy of Sciences, Washington, D.C., U.S.A.

Dietary Intake of Trace Elements

Marginal Deficiences and Their Interactions in Early Development

By Lucille S. Hurley

I. INTRODUCTION: INDUCTION OF TRACE ELEMENT DEFICIENCY

The importance of the essential trace elements in the diet has been amply demonstrated in both animals and man (Underwood 1977). The effect of severe deficiencies of these essential nutrients is well established, especially in experimental animals, and with the recent increase in use of long term parenteral nutrition, has also been demonstrated in humans for certain elements. However, in terms of health and disease in both humans and animals, the effects of long continued *marginal* deprivation of an essential element may be more pertinent than those of acute severe deficiency.

Deficiency of trace elements can occur through primary or secondary means. Primary deficiency results from inadequate intake of an essential nutrient in the diet, including the water consumed. Secondary, or conditioned, deficiencies can result from a number of interactions of trace elements with other factors. These include interactions of trace elements with genetic factors, so that a certain strain is particularly sensitive to a low dietary level of the element or requires exceptionally large amounts in order to overcome a genetic defect in its metabolism. Drugs or other chemicals can also interact with trace elements, resulting in deficiency states which may be more or less severe. Trace elements can also interact with other nutritional factors. For example, binding factors in food can bind trace elements and prevent or inhibit their absorption from the gastrointestinal tract. Trace elements can also interact with other nutrients, so that the effects of marginal deficiencies may be enhanced. Finally, trace elements interact with each other in such a way that a large amount of one may induce a deficiency of another.

Through these interactions of trace elements with other factors, it is possible to induce marginal deficiencies of essential elements even under conditions in which their dietary intake would appear to be adequate. In cases in which the need for essential elements is crucial, such as growth, pregnancy, and the fetal and neonatal periods, marginal deficiencies may have serious deleterious effects. This paper will review briefly the effects of deficiencies of manganese, copper, and zinc in early development, and will use research on this subject to provide examples of the principles described above.

II. PRIMARY DEFICIENCIES: EFFECT OF INADEQUATE INTAKES

A. Manganese

Information on the effects of manganese deficiency is derived almost entirely from animal studies, both in domestic and experimental animals; one case of manganese deficiency has been reported in a human subject, but this has never been confirmed (for reviews see Hurley 1981, Hurley 1984, Keen et al. 1984). The very low concentrations of manganese in animal tissues and fluids and the resulting problem of contamination during analysis have retarded studies of manganese metabolism and biochemistry. With the development of flameless atomic absorption spectrophotometry, analytical difficulties are attenuated, but manganese estimation in animal tissues and fluids remains subject to many sources of error.

1. *Skeleton.* One of the major effects of manganese deficiency, during both prenatal life and postnatal growth, is on the skeleton. Skeletal abnormalities resulting from manganese deficiency include a chondrodystrophic type of disproportionate growth, curvature of the long bones and the spine, and dysplasia of the knee joint. These abnormalities are related to abnormal chondrogenetic bone growth demonstrated by depressed synthesis of mucopolysaccharides, and can be ascribed to the function of manganese as a cofactor for the glycostyltransferase enzymes which are important in catalyzing the first step in the synthesis of glycosaminoglycans and glycoproteins (Leach 1971).

2. *Ataxia.* When manganese deficiency is imposed during the prenatal period, the offspring show congential irreversible ataxia characterized by lack of equilibrium, abnormal body righting reflexes, and retraction of the head. The abnormal body righting reflexes are easily demonstrated by the inability of the animals to swim. The failure of body righting reflexes is caused by abnormal development of the otoliths, the calcified structures essential for balance found in the vestibular portion of the inner ears. Depression of the activity of the glycostyltransferase enzymes can account for the defects of otolith development observed in manganese deficient animals.

3. *Convulsive disorders.* Manganese deficiency also affects brain function. Manganese deficient rats are much more susceptible to convulsions

than are normal rats, with a low threshold for electroshock, and epileptiform electroencephalograms (Hurley et al. 1963). These observations led Tanaka (1977) to measure the manganese in whole blood of children with convulsive disorders. He found that approximately 30% of these children had whole-blood manganese concentrations significantly lower than normal, about 1/3 of the normal value. Papavasiliou et al. (1979) measured whole-blood manganese in adult epileptics and similarly found that the concentration was significantly lower than in controls. The lower manganese levels could not be ascribed to the anticonvulsant drugs taken by these patients, as there was no correlation with blood levels of the drugs. Furthermore, patients who had frequent seizures had lower blood manganese levels than those with infrequent seizures.

In recent studies with manganese deficient and normal rats, we have found that whole-blood manganese concentration correlates very well with the concentration of manganese in the liver (Keen et al. 1983a). This observation suggests that whole-blood manganese is a valid indicator of tissue manganese level and may be useful as a reflection of manganese nutrition. Thus, the reports relating low whole-blood manganese levels to convulsive disorders may indicate defects of manganese metabolism or interacting factors leading to marginal manganese deficiency.

4. *Ultrastructural defects*. Manganese is concentrated in the mitochondrial portion of cells, and in mice that have been given a manganese deficient diet throughout their lives, abnormal mitochondria were observed with electron microscopy (Bell & Hurley 1973). The mitochondria showed evidence of membrane defects; the outer membrane was damaged and in some cases appeared to be missing. The reticuloendothelial system was also abnormal.

One of the biochemical functions of manganese is as a part of the metalloenzyme manganese superoxide dismutase. This enzyme, which is found primarily in mitochondria, is thought to protect cells from damage by superoxide free radicals, as it catalyzes the dismutation of the superoxide anion to hydrogen peroxide; in its absence, hydroxyl radicals, which are very deleterious to cells, are formed (Fridovich 1975). In manganese deficient mice and chickens, the activity of manganese superoxide dismutase is significantly lower than in controls (de Rosa et al. 1980, Paynter 1980). We have recently studied the enzymic development of this enzyme in rats and mice. In rats, the level of manganese superoxide dismutase activity in liver was very low at birth, and increased over 6-fold by day 60 in controls. In manganese deficient rats, enzyme activity was similar to that of controls until about 15 days of age, but by 60 days of age it was only half of the control value. Mice showed a similar developmental curve (Zidenberg-Cherr et al., in press a).

Because of the membrane defects that had been observed in manganese deficient animals, we developed the hypothesis that membrane damage resulted from depressed activity of manganese superoxide dismutase, leading to an increased concentration of superoxide anions or reaction products such as hydroxyl radicals. We therefore estimated lipid peroxidation in these animals by measuring malonaldehyde formation, using the thiobarbituric acid (TBA) technique. In isolated liver mitochondria, lipid peroxidation was significantly higher at day 20 in deficient rats than in controls. Between 20 and 60 days of age, lipid peroxidation increased in deficient rats but not in control rats. The ratio of TBA reaction products to manganese superoxide dismutase activity was also higher in the deficient rats at all time points (Zidenberg-Cherr et al. 1983). Ultrastructural examination of liver showed that membrane damage became apparent in the manganese deficient animals by 60 days of age (Zidenberg-Cherr et al., in press b). These results are consistent with the hypothesis that damage to mitochondrial membranes produced by manganese deficiency may be due ultimately to depressed activity of manganese superoxide dismutase.

5. *Carbohydrate metabolism.* Manganese deficient animals show a diabetic type of glucose tolerance curves (Everson & Shrader 1968, Baly 1984 b). Plasma insulin levels were not commensurate with the high plasma glucose, and manganese concentration in the pancreas was only half the control value. Insulin output was measured in an isolated perfused pancreas preparation. Both the first phase of insulin output, reflecting release of stored hormone, and the second phase of insulin output, representing release of newly synthesized as well as preformed hormone, were significantly lower in the manganese deficient rats than in the controls. Additional studies indicated that synthesis of insulin, as well as release, was impaired by manganese deficiency (Baly et al. 1985).

Manganese also functions as part of the metalloenzyme pyruvate carboxylase. Activity of this enzyme was lower in manganese deficient rat pups at certain stages of development than in controls, and in adult rats, pyruvate carboxylase acitivity, although normal in fed animals, was significantly lower than normal in rats deprived of food for 48 hours (Baly et al., in press).

The third manganese containing metalloenzyme, arginase, is necessary for urea formation, and its activity is also depressed by inadequate dietary intake (Kirchgessner & Heiseke 1978). The functional significance of this low arginase activity is not known.

B. Copper

1. *Neurological abnormalities.* The importance of copper in prenatal development first became apparent from studies of the disease "enzootic ataxia" in newborn lambs in certain parts of western Australia. The disorder was characterized by spastic paralysis, severe incoordination, blindness in some cases, and anemia. The brains of affected animals were small, with

collapsed cerebral hemispheres and shallow convolutions. Myelin was low in quantity in these brains. Ataxic lambs had subnormal levels of copper in liver and blood, and their mothers had low copper concentrations in their blood and milk. The disease could be prevented by supplementing the ewes with copper during early pregnancy. The major biochemical lesion in the brains of affected animals appears to be a reduction in the copper-containing terminal respiratory enzyme, cytochrome oxidase, due to low levels of brain copper. The low level of cytochrome oxidase activity may lead to tissue anoxia (for review see Hurley 1981, Hurley & Keen 1979).

Neonatal ataxia has also been reported in newborn copper deficient goats, swine, guinea pigs, and rats. In rats, newborn pups from copper deficient dams were hyperirritable, with convulsive seizures following stimulation. Gross neural lesions included focal pale areas in the cerebral cortex and corpus striatum, prominent cerebral edema, and cortical necrosis (Carlton & Kelly 1969). Mitochondria isolated from the brains of copper deficient rat pups were enlarged and abnormal in shape, and had low levels of cytochrome oxidase activity (Prohaska & Wells 1975).

2. *Growth retardation*. Growth retardation was one of the earliest effects of copper deficiency to be described. Growth retardation has been reported in copper deficient rats, lambs, foals, calves, puppies, chicks, turkeys, guinea pigs, mice, rabbits, and swine (Hurley & Keen 1979).

3. *Skeletal abnormalities*. Lambs in western Australia affected with enzootic ataxia were found to have poorly developed, light, brittle bones with thin cortices, and rib fractures were common. In contrast, lambs born of dams supplemented with copper during pregnancy did not show skeletal lesions. Skeletal abnormalities have also been found in calves and foals raised on copper deficient soils, including wide epiphyses and beaded ribs. Most puppies born to female dogs fed copper deficient diets became lame within 2 to 4 months of age. The leg bones were usually severely deformed with the foreleg characteristically bowed outward, and the hind legs bowed inward. Wrist joints were often hyperextended, with bony enlargements. The skeletal lesion appears to be associated with an impairment of osteogenesis, with thinning of the cortex and trabeculae of long bones, but with unimpaired growth of epiphyseal cartilage. Copper supplementation can arrest this syndrome, but the damage that occurs before supplementation is irreversible (Baxter & Van Wyk 1953).

The increased fragility of copper deficient bones results from the low number of cross links present in the collagenous matrix, as copper deficiency impairs the cross linking of the connective tissue proteins collagen and elastin.

4. *Cardiovascular lesions*. The most dramatic sign of copper deficiency is sudden death. The high mortality rate of copper deficient rats, chickens, and swine is usually due to internal hemorrhage caused by rupture of the heart, aorta, or other large vessels, with smaller lesions throughout the

cardiovascular system (O'Dell 1976 a, b). Lesions of a similar nature have been reported in copper deficient turkey poults, swine, rabbits, guinea pigs, and cattle afflicted with "falling disease".

Copper deficiency during the fetal period produces retarded and diminished formation of elastin, and the elastin that is made does not undergo the normal maturation steps. Elastin from copper deficient animals may contain as little as half the cross-linking amino acids found in normal elastin (Starcher et al. 1964, Hill et al. 1967). The primary biochemical lesion responsible for the reduction in cross links is thought to be a decrease in lysyl oxidase activity (Rucker & Tinker 1977). Thus, dietary deficiency of copper is related to abnormalities of connective tissue. If the deficiency occurs during the development period, retardation of skeletal growth and development and abnormalities of the cardiovascular system result.

Signs of copper deficiency have been observed in human infants, and in human adults maintained with total parenteral nutrition. Signs of deficiency included skeletal abnormalities (including osteoporosis), neurological disturbances, and depigmentation, anemia, and neutropenia (Hurley & Keen 1979).

5. *Other*. Under certain conditions of copper deficiency, anemia has been observed in a number of species. Serum iron concentration tends to be low, while liver iron levels are higher than normal, and the anemia is of a hypochromic type. The condition presumably results from a role of copper in iron absorption and mobilization. Recent studies suggest that many factors influence the development of anemia in copper deficient animals (Cohen et al., in press).

C. *Zinc*

1. *Severe deficiency*. A severe dietary deficiency of zinc in experimental animals results in prenatal death and malformation (for review see Hurley 1981). These malformations in rats include cleft lip and palate, brain and eye malformations, skeletal deformities, and numerous abnormalities of the heart, lungs, and urogenital system. The brain malformations include neural tube defects, hydrocephaly, exencephaly, and anencephaly predominating. The basic defect responsible for the malformations observed in zinc deficiency appears to be the result of abnormal nucleic acid synthesis. DNA synthesis is depressed and the activities of DNA polymerase and thymidine kinase are significantly lower in zinc deficient embryos than in control embryos early in gestation. Chromosomal aberrations including gaps, fragments, and terminal deletions are also found in both maternal and fetal tissues in zinc deficient rats. In addition, biochemical abnormalities of chromatin have been reported in zinc deficient *Euglena gracilis* (Vallee & Falchuk 1981). Maturational biochemical abnormalities in development of lung and pancreas during prenatal life, and in development of immune

function in the fetus and neonate, also occur in zinc deficiency (Hurley 1981, Beach et al. 1979, 1980, 1982, 1983).

The effects of zinc deficiency in pregnancy occur very rapidly. In rats, plasma zinc concentration falls by 50% in less than 16 hours after the introduction of a zinc deficiency regimen (Hurley et al. 1982). This rapid effect of dietary zinc deficiency on plasma zinc has also been shown to occur in humans, although the time period is somewhat longer, several days rather than several hours (Gordon et al. 1981). As maternal plasma is the only source of zinc for the developing embryo, a zinc deficient diet can have an immediate effect on the developing organism. In the rat, only a few days of zinc deficiency during pregnancy is sufficient to produce congenital malformations (Hurley et al. 1971). Short-term transitory deficiency of zinc also affects prenatal growth and postnatal survival. Offspring of rats given a zinc deficient diet for only a few days during gestation had low birth weights, stillbirths, and high postnatal mortality (Hurley & Mutch 1973).

2. *Marginal deficiency*. Pregnant mice given a diet that was marginally deficient in zinc for only the last 2/3 of their pregnancy produced offspring with abnormal serum immunoglobulin M (IgM) (Beach et al. 1982). At six weeks of age, IgM was not detectable. At six months of age, IgM was present but at significantly lower concentrations than in controls. When these offspring were mated and their offspring were examined, again IgM was significantly lower than in controls at six weeks and ten weeks of age, but not at six months. In the following generation, the F_3 generation, IgM was low at six weeks, but normal at ten weeks and six months. Postnatal survival was also depressed for two generations. Thus, the effect of marginal prenatal zinc deficiency for even a part of pregnancy had a permanent effect on the offspring that persisted through two or three generations.

A link between zinc deficiency and poor pregnancy outcome has been suggested by some human studies (Hambidge et al. 1975, Jameson 1976, Çavdar et al. 1977), but the importance of zinc deficiency as a risk factor in human pregnancy has not been established. We are, therefore, studying the effects of marginal zinc deficiency during pregnancy in Rhesus monkeys. The monkeys were fed a purified diet beginning on day zero of pregnancy that contained 4 ppm zinc, a level that did not affect plasma zinc concentration until after 90 days of gestation (average normal gestation 165 days). Beginning in the third trimester, zinc-deprived monkeys showed low levels of plasma zinc (below 54 μg/100 ml), and late in pregnancy, dermatitis, depressed activity of serum alkaline phosphatase and serum glutamate-pyruvate transaminase, low hematocrit and hemoglobin levels, a change in serum albumin/globulin ratio, and impaired immune response (Golub et al. 1984a). Concentration of plasma vitamin A was low in zinc deficient monkeys, with a positive correlation between plasma vitamin A and plasma zinc concentrations in all monkeys, and between plasma retinol-binding protein (RBP) and plasma zinc in zinc-deprived monkeys at day 135 of pregnancy.

Polynomial regression calculations indicated a curvilinear relationship between plasma zinc, RBP, and vitamin A, suggesting that above a certain threshold level of plasma zinc, vitamin A transport is not dependent primarily on plasma zinc concentration, but that below this level, vitamin A release and transport from the liver seem to be strongly related to plasma zinc concentration (Baly et al. 1984a).

Marginal deprivation of zinc had clear effects on the monkey fetus. As there was no depression of maternal plasma zinc until after day 90 of gestation (past the period of organogenesis), no malformations were expected or observed. However, total pregnancy loss (abortion, stillbirth, and neonatal death) was higher in zinc-deprived dams (33.3%) and in pair-fed controls (30.7%) than in ad libitum-fed controls (11.1%). Complications of delivery were also high. Birthweight, crown rump length (trunk length), and femur length (long-bone growth) were significantly smaller in newborn male but not female infants of zinc deficient monkeys than of control (ad libitum- or pair-fed) monkeys. Newborn infants of zinc-deprived monkeys also showed low levels of plasma zinc and plasma iron, while muscle tonus was low (Golub et al. 1984b). Delayed skeletal maturation and defective mineralization, with features similar to human rachitic syndromes, were observed (Leek et al. 1984).

Behavioral abnormalities from zinc deficiency have also been reported for a number of species, including monkeys (Golub et al. 1984c).

III. SECONDARY (CONDITIONED) DEFICIENCIES: INTERACTIONS

A. *Trace element–gene interactions*

In general, the interactions of trace elements and genetic factors are of two types: one involves mutant genes whose phenotypic expression is similar to the signs of deficiency or toxicity of an element. The essentiality of manganese, copper, and zinc, and their importance in development, can be demonstrated by genetic mutants with errors of trace element metabolism. The second type of trace element–gene interaction involves strain differences within a species. In this paper, we shall present only a few examples without attempting to provide a comprehensive discussion.

1. *Single-gene interactions.* Two analogous genes that affect manganese metabolism have been identified: *pallid* in mice and *screwneck* in mink (Hurley 1981). In both cases, animals show ataxia, head retraction, and abnormal development of the otoliths indistinguishable from the effects observed in the offspring of manganese deficient animals. The prenatal development of abnormal otoliths in these genetic mutants can be prevented by feeding pregnant females high levels of dietary manganese.

Several mutant genes affecting copper metabolism have been reported. The effects of the *crinkled* gene in mice can be ameliorated by high dietary copper during prenatal development (Hurley 1981). The alleles at the *mot-*

tled locus in mice produce a variety of effects, whose similarity to signs of dietary copper deficiency varies according to the defects of copper metabolism that they cause. These mutants are of special interest because of their X-linkage, similar to that of Menkes' syndrome. The lethal human genetic disease Menkes' syndrome has been shown to be related to abnormal copper metabolism, and infants show many of the signs of copper deficiency (for review see Hurley & Keen 1979).

Another example of a genetic mutant in humans related to trace element metabolism is acrodermatitis enteropathica, a disorder in which the phenotypic expression of the gene mimics zinc deficiency. If the disease is not treated, infants with this condition usually die at an early age. All the signs of the disorder can be cured and prevented by zinc supplementation (Moynahan 1974). The Adema disease of Friesian calves resembles that of infants with acrodermatitis enteropathica (Flagstad 1977).

2. *Strain variations*. Strain differences have been demonstrated in the response of mice and rats to manganese deficiency. In mice, the effects of feeding a manganese deficient diet during pregnancy on otolith development in the offspring were quite different depending on the genetic background (Hurley & Bell 1974). Rats also showed strain differences in response to dietary manganese deficiency. Of two widely used strains, Sprague-Dawley rats were much more susceptible to the effects of manganese deficiency than were Wistar rats (Dungan et al. 1984).

Strain differences in copper metabolism have been shown to influence the susceptibility of sheep to copper deficiency. The frequency of enzootic ataxia was quite different among breeds even when they were consuming the same forage, and the difference was due to differences in copper absorption (Wiener 1979).

B. Trace element–drug interactions

Drugs or other chemicals which can interact with an element either as a primary or secondary consequence of the drug's action may also influence the development of a trace element deficiency (Hackman & Hurley 1984a). For example, D-penicillamine and triethylenetetramine, two drugs used in the treatment of Wilson's disease, a genetic disorder in which copper accumulates in body tissues, produce low plasma copper levels and abnormalities of embryonic development in rats (Keen et al. 1983b, c).

The diuretic drug acetazolamide produces certain specific malformations in rats. The level of zinc in the maternal diet had a pronounced effect on the frequency of these malformations. With a zinc deficient diet, rats produced fetuses all of which showed ectrodactyly, while increasing dietary zinc up to the control level reduced the incidence of the acetazolamide syndrome in a dose-response manner (Hackman & Hurley 1983).

Thus, while under normal circumstances the trace element content of a maternal diet may be adequate, the presence of drugs such as acetazolamide or D-penicillamine may result in an increased requirement of the elements such that conditioned deficiency with resulting teratogenicity can occur.

C. Multifactorial interactions: trace elements, genetic factors, and drugs

Trace elements can interact with drugs and with genetic factors in a multifactorial way. In studies assessing the effect of dietary zinc and genetic strain on acetazolamide-induced malformations, the incidence of forelimb ectrodactyly, a characteristic malformation caused by acetazolamide, was much greater in CBA mouse fetuses than in SWV fetuses. SWV fetuses had no ectrodactyly when dams were fed at least 9 ppm zinc, but 5–8% showed the malformation when dams received a zinc deficient diet. The incidence of ectrodactyly in the CBA strain decreased as dietary zinc increased (Hackman & Hurley 1983).

Another example of the interaction of zinc with a drug and with genetic factors is from a study using salicylate. With various levels of dietary zinc, two strains of rats, and four different levels of the drug, the frequency of malformations was influenced by the level of dietary zinc, by the amount of salicylate given, by the interaction of the genetic strain and the dietary zinc level, and the interaction of the dietary zinc concentration and the amount of salicylate given (Hackman & Hurley 1984b).

D. Trace element–nutritional interactions

1. *Dietary binding factors.* Dietary binding factors, such as phytate and fiber, are well established as agents leading to conditioned deficiency of trace elements. The hypogonadal dwarfism of Middle Eastern zinc deficiency is a classical example of this kind of interaction. In these cases, a diet composed largely of phytate-rich whole grain appears to be the major factor leading to zinc deficiency (Underwood 1977). Other binding factors in foods may also influence the availability of trace elements for absorption in the intestinal tract. The subject of bioavailability of trace elements is currently receiving a good deal of attention.

2. *Interactions of trace elements and other nutrients.* Trace elements can interact with other essential nutrients. For example, the effect of marginal zinc deficiency on vitamin A metabolism in pregnant monkeys is discussed above. These data, as well as other studies in rats, suggest that even marginal zinc deficiency may produce some effects on vitamin A deficiency. In addition, studies in rats indicated that high levels of dietary vitamin A may exacerbate the effects of marginal zinc deficiency (Peters et al., in preparation).

3. *Trace element–trace element interactions.* Trace element interactions are of two major types: (1) one of the elements is involved in the metabolism

of the other, and (2) two elements share a common transport site or ligand. Two examples of element–element interactions will be given: manganese–iron and zinc–copper.

Manganese–iron. An interaction between iron and manganese in affecting hemoglobin production was demonstrated in early work by Matrone and coworkers (1959). High concentrations of dietary manganese depressed the formation of hemoglobin in anemic pigs, presumably by decreasing iron absorption. Conversely, iron deficiency increased the intestinal absorption of manganese. Feeding iron-supplemented milk to rats caused an inhibition of manganese transfer after only one day of feeding (Gruden 1977). In recent studies, weanling mice were fed a cow's milk diet with or without added iron. The level of supplementation was the same as that recommended for human infants by the American Academy of Pediatrics. Iron-supplemented mice had higher tissue iron stores and less anemia than controls. However, they also had lower levels of manganese in their tissues than did controls; thus the increase in tissue iron stores was at the expense of manganese stores (Fransson et al. 1982).

Zinc–copper. Interaction of dietary zinc and copper is well established. Feeding high levels of dietary zinc results in lower than normal tissue copper levels and signs of copper deficiency (Fischer et al. 1981, Grant-Forest & Underwood 1958). An interaction between zinc and copper has also been reported when one element is present in the diet at a deficient level and the other at normal levels. Thus, dietary zinc deficiency has been reported to cause slight increases in tissue copper levels in some studies. Similarly, copper deficiency has been reported to result in slight increases in zinc absorption (Hall et al. 1979, Gipp et al. 1973). We have recently investigated the interaction between zinc and copper in the pregnant rat by feeding diets during pregnancy that varied in zinc and copper concentrations. A factorial design was used with diets containing 1, 10, 100, or 1,000 μg zinc/gram and 0.5, 5, 10, or 100 μg copper/gram. Malformations were found only in fetuses from rats fed the zinc deficient diets (1 μg/g) and the frequency of malformed fetuses increased as the concentration of dietary copper increased. An antagonistic effect of dietary zinc on maternal and fetal tissue copper concentration was observed. The concentration of fetal liver zinc from rats fed a copper deficient diet was significantly higher than that from controls. The concentration of iron in maternal and fetal tissues was significantly affected by the level of dietary zinc, with values highest in the zinc deficient groups. Thus, when the concentration of zinc in the diet is deficient, an interaction can occur between dietary zinc and copper such that high levels of copper potentiate the teratogenicity of zinc deficiency (Reinstein et al. 1984).

IV. HUMAN REQUIREMENTS AND DIETARY SOURCES

A. Manganese

Estimations of the human requirement for manganese are based primarily on balance studies. Data from several sources suggest that manganese intakes of 0.035 to 0.070 mg/kg body weight per day would result in a balance of manganese intake with excretion (for review see Hurley & Keen, in press). 1.25 mg of manganese per day has been reported to be the requirement for girls between six and ten years of age, but 3 mg per day was inadequate for adolescent girls. In young women, intakes of 2.5–3.2 mg per day resulted in balance, but some apparently healthy subjects ingested less than 2 mg/day. In adult males, the manganese requirement appears to be between 2 and 4 mg/day. Very little is known of the manganese requirements of infants, and there are conflicting reports of manganese retention in neonates. Daily manganese intakes from human diets vary with the amounts of cereals, nuts, leafy vegetables, and tea consumed. Estimates of the daily manganese intake in adults in various parts of the world varied from 2 to 4 mg.

Foods are highly variable in their manganese content. Major food groups in descending order of their manganese content (on the fresh basis) are nuts, whole cereals, dried fruits, roots, tubers and stalks, fruits, nonleafy vegetables, animal tissues and fluids, poultry and poultry products, and fish and seafoods.

B. Copper

The 1980 Recommended Dietary Allowances of the Food and Nutrition Board of the National Academy of Sciences (U.S.A.) lists a daily intake of 2 to 3 mg of copper as safe and adequate for adults. On the basis of dry solids in the diet, this equals about 3 mg/kg. There is some recent evidence that suggests that some portions of the American population consume less than 2 mg/day (Klevay et al. 1980). The richest food sources of copper include grains, shellfish, organ meats, legumes, dried fruits, fresh fruits, and vegetables. Cow's milk is a very poor source of copper.

C. Zinc

The Recommended Dietary Allowances for zinc are 3 to 5 mg for infants, 10 mg for children and 15 mg for adults, with additional amounts recommended for pregnant and lactating women. These allowances do not, however, take into account differences in bioavailability or other dietary characteristics which may influence the requirement for zinc. The question of food sources of zinc is especially complex because of the important effect of food composition on the bioavailability of this element. In general, the best sources of zinc are meat, seafood, and poultry. Lentils, peas, beans, and other legumes and seeds are important sources when meat, seafood, and poultry are limited, but the problem of bioavailability of zinc from these sources arises because of the phytate and fiber content.

REFERENCES

BALY, D. L., GOLUB, M., GERSHWIN, M. E. & HURLEY, L. S. (1984a). Marginal zinc deficiency and vitamin A metabolism in pregnant rhesus monkeys. *Amer. J. clin. Nutr.* 40, 199–207.

BALY, D. L., CURRY, D. L., KEEN, C. L. & HURLEY, L. S. (1984b). Effect of manganese deficiency on insulin secretion and carbohydrate homeostasis. *J. Nutr.* 114, 1438–1446.

BALY, D. L., CURRY, D. L., KEEN, C. L. & HURLEY, L. S. (1985). Dynamics of insulin and glucagon release in rats: influence of dietary manganese. *Endocrinology.*

BALY, D. L., KEEN, C. L. & HURLEY, L. S. (In press). Pyruvate carboxylase and phosphoenolpyruvate carboxykinase in developing rats: effects of manganese deficiency. *J. Nutr.*

BAXTER, J. H. & VAN WYK, J. J. (1953). A bone disorder associated with copper deficiency. I. Gross morphological, roentgenological, and chemical observation. *Bull. Johns Hopkins Hosp.* 93, 1–23.

BEACH, R. S., GERSHWIN, M. E. & HURLEY, L. S. (1979). Altered thymic structure and mitogen responsiveness in postnatally zinc deprived mice. *Devel. Comp. Immunol.* 3, 725–738.

BEACH, R. S., GERSHWIN, M. E., MAKISHIMA, R. K. & HURLEY, L. S. (1980). Impaired immunologic ontogeny in postnatal zinc deprivation. *J. Nutr.* 110, 805–815.

BEACH, R. S., GERSHWIN, M. E. & HURLEY, L. S. (1982). Gestational zinc deprivation in mice: Persistence of immunodeficiency for three generations. *Science* 218, 469–471.

— (1983). Persistent immunological consequences of gestational zinc deprivation. *Amer. J. clin. Nutr.* 38, 579–590.

BELL, L. T. & HURLEY, L. S. (1973). Ultrastructural effects of manganese deficiency in liver, heart, kidney and pancreas of mice. *Lab. Invest.* 29, 723–736.

CARLTON, W. W. & KELLY, W. A. (1969). Neural lesions in the offspring of female rats fed a copper deficient diet. *J. Nutr. 97,* 42–52.

ÇAVDAR, A. O., ARCASOY, A., BAYCU, T. & HIMMETOGLU, O. (1977). Zinc deficiency and anencephaly in Turkey. *Teratology* 22, 141.

COHEN, N. L., KEEN, C. L., HURLEY, L. S. & LONNERDAL, B. (In press). Determinants of copper deficiency anemia in rats. *J. Nutr.*

DE ROSA, G., KEEN, C. L., LEACH, R. M. & HURLEY, L. S. (1980). Regulation of superoxide dismutase activity by dietary manganese. *J. Nutr.* 110, 795–804.

DUNGAN, D. D., ZIDENBERG-CHERR, S., KEEN, C. L., LONNERDAL, B & HURLEY, L. S. (1984). Comparative aspects of dietary manganese deficiency in Wistar and Sprague-Dawley rats. *Fed. Proc.* 43, 1054.

EVERSON, G. J. & SHRADER, R. E. (1968). Abnormal glucose tolerance in manganese-deficient guinea pigs. *J. Nutr.* 94, 89–94.

FISCHER, P. W. F., GIROUX, A. & L'ABBE, M. R. (1981). The effect of dietary zinc on intestinal copper absorption. *Amer. J. clin. Nutr.* 34, 1670–1675.

FLAGSTAD, T. (1977). Intestinal absorption of ^{65}Zn in A46 (Adema disease) after treatment with oxychinolines. *Nord. Vet. Med.* 29, 96–104.

FRANSSON, G.-B., KEEN, C. L. & LONNERDAL, B. (1982). Iron supplementation of milk through iron-lactoferrin: effect of tissue iron and manganese. *Fed. Proc.* 41, 778 (abstr.).

FRIDOVICH, I. (1975). Superoxide dismutases. *Ann. Rev. Biochem.* 44, 147–159.

GIPP, W. F., POND, W. G., TASKER, J., VAN CAMPEN, D., KROOK, L. & VISEK, W. J. (1973). Influence of level of dietary copper on weight gain, hematology and liver copper and iron storage of young pigs. *J. Nutr.* 103, 713–719.

GOLUB, M. S., GERSHWIN, M. E., HURLEY, L. S., BALY, D. L. & HENDRICKX, A. G. (1984a). Studies on marginal zinc defiency in Rhesus monkeys. I. Influence on pregnant dams. *Amer. J. clin. Nutr.* 39, 265–280.

— (1984b). Studies of marginal zinc deprivation in rhesus monkeys. II. Pregnancy outcome. *Amer. J. clin. Nutr.* 39, 879–887.

GOLUB, M. S., KEEN, C. L., VIJAYAN, V. K., GERSHWIN, M. E. & HURLEY, L. S. (1984c). Early development of brain and behavior in mice fed a marginally deficient diet. In *The Neurobiology of Zinc. Part B: Deficiency, Toxicity, and Pathology,* pp 65–75. Ed. by C. Fredrickson. Alan R. Liss, Inc.

GORDON, P. R., WOODRUFF, C. W., ANDERSON, H. L. & O'DELL, B. L. (1981). Acute zinc deficiency in man impairs platelet aggregation. *Fed. Proc.* 40, 839.

GRANT-FROST, D. R. & UNDERWOOD, E. J. (1958). Zinc toxicity in the rat and its interrelation with copper. *Aust. J. exp. Biol. med. Sci.* 36, 339–346.

GRUDEN, W. (1977). Interrelationship of manganese and iron in rat's duodenum. *Nutr. Rep. Int.* 15, 577–580.

HACKMAN, R. M. & HURLEY, L. S. (1983). Interactions of dietary zinc, genetic strain and acetazolamide in teratogenesis in mice. *Teratology* 28, 355–368.

— (1984a). Drug–nutrient interactions in teratogenesis. In *Drugs and Nutrients: The Interactive Effects,* pp. 299–329. Ed. by D. A. Roe and T. E. Campbell. Marcel-Dekker, Inc., New York.

— (1984b). Interactions of salicylate, dietary zinc, and genetic strain in teratogenesis in rats. *Teratology.* 30, 225–236.

HALL, A. C., YOUNG, B. W. & BREMNER, I. (1979). Intestinal metallothionein and the mutual antagonism between copper and zinc in the rat. *J. inorg. Biochem.* 11, 57–66.

HAMBIDGE, K. M., NELDNER, K. H. & WALRAVENS, P. A. (1975). Zinc, acrodermatitis enteropathica, and congenital malformations. *Lancet* 1, 577.

HILL, C. H., STARCHER, B. & KIM, C. (1967). Role of copper in the formation of elastin. *Fed. Proc.* 26, 129–133.

HURLEY, L. S. (1981). Teratogenic aspects of manganese, zinc, and copper nutrition. *Phys. Rev.* 61, 249–295.

— (1984). Nutritional aspects of manganese. *Third International Workshop: Trace Element Analytical Chemistry in Medicine and Biology,* 3:239. Neuherberg, Federal Republic of Germany, April 16–18, 1984.

HURLEY, L. S. & BELL, L. T. (1974). Genetic influence on response to dietary manganese deficiency in mice. *J. Nutr.* 104, 133–137.

HURLEY, L. S. & KEEN, C. L. (1979). Teratogenic effects of copper. In *Copper in the Environment, Part II. Health Effects,* pp. 33–56. Ed. by Nriagu, John Wiley and Sons, Inc., New York.

— (In press). Manganese. In *Underwood's Trace Elements in Human and Animal Nutrition, 5th Edition.* Ed. by W. Mertz, Academic Press, New York.

HURLEY, L. S., & MUTCH, P. B. (1973). Prenatal and postnatal development after transitory gestational zinc deficiency in rats. *J. Nutr.* 103, 649–656.

HURLEY, L. S., WOOLEY, D. E., ROSENTHAL, E. & TIMIRAS, P. S. (1963). Influence of manganese on susceptibility of rats to convulsions. *Amer. J. Physiol.* 204, 493–496.

HURLEY, L. S., GOWAN, J. & SWENERTON, H. (1971). Teratogenic effects of short-term and transitory zinc deficiency in rats. *Teratology* 4, 199–204.

HURLEY, L. S., GORDON, P., KEEN, C. L. & MERKHOFER, L. (1982). Circadian variation in rat plasma zinc and rapid effect of dietary zinc deficiency. *Proc. Soc. Exp. Biol. Med.* 170, 48–52.

JAMESON, S. (1976). Effects of zinc deficiency in human reproduction. *Acta med. scand.* 593 Suppl., 5–89.

KEEN, C. L., CLEGG, M. S., LONNERDAL, B. & HURLEY, L. S. (1983a). Whole blood manganese as an indicator of body manganese status. *New Engl. J. Med.* (Letter) 308, 1230.

KEEN, C. L., COHEN, N. L., LONNERDAL, B. & HURLEY, L. S. (1983b). Teratogenesis and low copper status resulting from triethylenetetramine in rats. *Proc. Soc. Exp. Biol. Med.* 173, 298–605.

KEEN, C. L., MARK-SAVAGE, P., LONNERDAL, B. & HURLEY, L. S. (1983c). Teratogenic effects of D-penicillamine in rats: Relation to copper deficiency. *Drug–Nutrient Inter.* 2, 17–34.

KEEN, C. L., LONNERDAL, B. & HURLEY, L. S. (1984). Essential ultratrace manganese. In *Biochemistry of the Elements*, pp. 89–132. Ed. by E. Frieden. Plenum Publishing Co., New York.

KIRCHGESSNER, M. & HEISEKE, D. (1978). Arginase-Aktivitat in der Leber wachsender Ratten bei Mn-Mangel. *Int. Z. Vit. Ern. Forschung* 48, 75–78.

KLEVAY, L. M., RECK, S. J., JACOB, R. A., LOGAN, G. M., JR., MUNOZ, J. M. & SANDSTEAD, H. H. (1980). The human requirement for copper. I. Healthy men fed conventional American diets. *Amer. J. clin. Nutr.* 33, 45–50.

LEACH, R. M. (1971). Role of manganese in mucopolysaccharide metabolism. *Fed. Proc.* 30, 991–994.

LEEK, J. C., VOGLER, J. B., GERSHWIN, M. E., GOLUB, M. S., HURLEY, L. S. & HENDRICKX, A. G. (1984). Studies of marginal zinc deprivation in rhesus monkeys. V. Fetal and infant skeletal effects. *Amer. J. clin. Nutr.* 40, 1203–1212.

MATRONE, G., HARTMAN, R. H. & CLAWSON, A. J. (1959). Studies on manganese–iron antagonism in the nutrition of rabbits and baby pigs. *J. Nutr.* 67, 309–317.

MOYNAHAN, E. J. (1974). Acrodermatitis enteropathica: a lethal inherited human zinc-deficiency disorder. *Lancet* 2, 399–400.

O'DELL, B. L. (1976a). In *Trace Elements in Human Health and Disease,* Vol. 1, pp. 391–413. Ed. by A. S. Prasad and D. Oberleas. Academic Press, Inc., New York.

— (1976b). Biochemistry of copper. *Med. Clin. N. Amer.* 60, 687–703.

PAPAVASILIOU, P. S., KUTT, H., MILLER, S. T., ROSAL, V., WANG, Y. Y. & ARONSON, R. B. (1979). Seizure disorders and trace metals: Manganese tissue levels in treated epileptics. *Neurology* 29, 1466–1473.

PAYNTER, D. J. (1980). Changes in activity of the manganese superoxide dismutase enzyme in tissues of the rat with changes in dietary manganese. *J. Nutr.* 110, 437–447.

PETERS, A., KEEN, C. L. & HURLEY, L. S. (In preparation). Effects of high dietary levels of vitamin A in combination with marginal zinc deficiency on reproduction in rats.

PROHASKA, J. R. & WELLS, W. W. (1975). Copper deficiency in the developing rat brain: Evidence for abnormal mitochondria. *J. Neurochem.* 25, 221–228.

REINSTEIN, N. H., LONNERDAL. B., KEEN, C. L. & HURLEY, L. S. (1984). Zinc–copper interactions in the pregnant rat: fetal outcome and maternal and fetal zinc, copper and iron. *J. Nutr.* 114, 1266–1279.

RUCKER, R. B. & TINKER, D. (1977). Structure and metabolism of arterial elastin. *Int. Rev. exp. Pathol.* 17, 1–47.

STARCHER, B. C., HILL, C. H. & MATRONE, G. (1964). Importance of dietary copper in the formation of aortic elastin. *J. Nutr.* 82, 318–322.

TANAKA, Y. (1977). Manganese: its neurological and teratological significance in man. *Nat. Meet. Amer. Chem. Soc.,* Chicago, (abstract). Port City Press, Baltimore.

UNDERWOOD, E. J., Ed. (1977). *Trace Elements in Human and Animal Nutrition,* 4th Edition. Academic Press, New York.

VALLEE, B. L. & FALCHUK, K. H. (1981). Zinc and gene expression. *Phil. Trans.* B 294, 185–197.

WIENER, G. (1979). Review of genetic aspects of mineral metabolism with particular reference to copper in sheep. *Livestock Production Sci.* 6, 223–232.

ZIDENBERG-CHERR, S., KEEN, C. L., LONNERDAL, B. & HURLEY, L. S. (1983). Superoxide dismutase activity and lipid peroxidation in the rat. Developmental correlations affected by manganese deficiency. *J. Nutr.* 113, 2498–2504.

ZIDENBERG-CHERR, S., KEEN, C. L., CASEY, S. M. & HURLEY, L. S. (In press a). Developmental changes affected by manganese deficiency: Mn-superoxide dismutase, Cu Zn-superoxide dismutase, Mn, Cu, Fe, and Zn in mouse tissues. *Biol. Trace Elem. Res.*

ZIDENBERG-CHERR, S., KEEN, C. L. & HURLEY, L. S. (In press b). The effects of manganese deficiency during prenatal and postnatal development on mitochondrial structure and function in the rat. *Biol. Trace Elem. Res.*

Discussion (the papers by Bruce and Hurley)

Chairman: BOSTRÖM

WEISMANN: I have two questions for Dr Hurley. I know you have performed very interesting studies with rats and I want to ask if you have been able to produce copper deficiency in the offspring by giving high zinc levels to the rats? Have you observed that?

HURLEY: We have been doing some studies on copper/zinc interactions and, using a wide range of zinc and copper levels, we have found that the main effects occur when one of the elements is deficient; then high levels of the other element will exacerbate the effects of the deficiency. If the amount of one element is adequate in the diet or high, then there is relatively little effect of the other. But, on a statistical basis with high levels of zinc there were, in pregnant rats, some effects on copper concentrations in the fetal tissues. However, there were no other signs of prenatal copper deficiency such as you'd get with severe copper deficiency.

WEISMANN: Thank you. I have a second question. How do you explain the lack of serum IgM in the zinc-deficient offspring? Is it a genetic adaption or why does it follow the generations? Do you think, for example, that acrodermatitis could be induced by occasional zinc deficiency and then carried on by genetic factors?

HURLEY: Well, I don't think that is too likely for acrodermatitis enteropathica, but we don't know the mechanism of this effect that we have reported. We are working on that now. If it were a straight effect on the genetic constitution, one would not expect the effect to be diminished with each succeeding generation. Perhaps some enzymes or some components of the zinc metabolism machinery are altered during the critical period in prenatal development, so that the normal processes cannot occur, but we don't really have a solid hypothesis at this point.

WEISMANN: Do you think it is because of the change in the absorptive processes in the gastrointestinal tract? Could it be raised through that?

HURLEY: Well, it's really hard to speculate without any more data.

BRUCE: Dr Hurley, when you showed the genetic variation in manganese, your data indicated that one rat needed about 700 times more manganese than the others. Would you consider that strain to have some type of inborn error of metabolism?

HURLEY: Oh yes, that last one was a mutant strain and it is an inborn error of metabolism. In other words, when we produce manganese deficiency, we're producing a phenocopy of that mutant and by giving the mutant mother a very high level of manganese during pregnancy we can prevent the effects of the gene as far as the development of otoliths go.

BRUCE: Are you aware of any human equivalent to that disease?

HURLEY: No.

ANDERSON: I have a question for Dr Bruce. In your tentative content of trace elements in supplements given in Table 2, the tentative recommended amount of the first ones, e.g. iron, zinc, copper and iodine, is about 50% higher than the suggested or recommended RDA, whereas if you look at the values for manganese, chromium, selenium and molybdenum, these tentative amounts are 50% lower than the suggested amounts. How did you come up with these tentative recommendations?

BRUCE: The doses recommended in Table 2 are based on the recommended daily allowances and estimated safe and adequate daily intake values in your last RDA. For iron, zinc and iodine, where proper RDA-values have been established, these figures are the mean of the recommendations for adult males and females, and the suggested permissible lowest and highest dose is approximately 50% below or above that value. For the remaining trace elements, for which estimated safe and adequate daily intakes are presented as a range, the recommended dose is the lower value in these ranges. Also for these values the suggested variation is about +50% of the value. Until more data are available on the nutritional needs of trace elements, we will base the recommended dosage on the lower values in these ranges.

PERRY: Dr Hurley, your examples involved essential interactions between essential trace metals. I'm curious whether you have any information about the possible interaction between cadmium and zinc. Cadmium, of course, is directly above and chemically similar to zinc and there are wide variations, at least in human exposure to cadmium, so that there is at least a potential for having a practical interaction. What I'm really asking you, do you have any information on actual interactions in animals or any feelings about practical interactions in human beings?

HURLEY: We have done a limited number of studies on cadmium and zinc interactions. I'd like to say first that there have been some studies done on the teratogenic effects of cadmium and their prevention by zinc but these have all been done by injection, not by oral intake, and so I think that their relevance to the human situation, except for people who work in cadmium smelters or something like that, is not too significant. In the experiments we have done, we have fed very high levels of cadmium in the diet to pregnant rats and have not found any effects on prenatal development. However, this was only at the gross morphological level and we did not continue these experiments into the postnatal period. So I think that is something that should be done, because it doesn't really answer the question entirely. I don't think that it is really a serious problem although we do need some more information on it.

PERRY: Did you do this in animals that were marginal as far as their zinc intake was?

HURLEY: Well, we did this a long time ago and I'm not sure I can remember.

SALONEN: I was going to comment on the question about glutathione peroxidase. There is at least one additional data set in addition to the well-known New Zealand one. This is published by Levander and co-workers from Finnish subjects and shows that there is a saturation in glutathione peroxidase level at a serum selenium level of about 100 μg/l.

ABDULLA: I have a question to Dr Hurley. We are finding it more and more difficult to interpret the results of animal experiments with relation to human requirements, especially when we are discussing marginal deficiencies. As you know, the intake of trace elements from common diets in affluent countries is far below the recommended values. We do not, however, find any clinical effects in risk groups. So I wonder, how relevant are your data when discussing human requirements?

The second question I want to ask is with regards to your experiment with zinc-deficient mice. Did you measure the IgA and IgG levels?

HURLEY: I'll answer the second question first. Yes, all that was measured and of the serum immune globulins, the IgM was the only one that showed this difference. But there was another immunological test done, the sheep-red-blood-cell-plaque-forming test, and that also showed a similar effect but did not persist for as long a time.

In regard to your first question, I think that there are human data that do suggest that zinc may be a factor in pregnancies with problems such as low birth weight. Dr Jameson has published some studies on this. Dr Çavdar in Turkey has also found correlations between zinc nutrition and zinc status of pregnant women and abnormalities in their infants, but I think that the main problem is that we do not, as yet, have all of the necessary tests available. We don't know what to look for to determine what the zinc status of a person is. Measuring plasma zinc is not always an adequate indication and until we have some functional tests, such as Dr Bruce mentioned in regard to vitamins, we really don't know what to look for. So we may be missing all kinds of things that could make a difference in pregnancy outcome and in early development. If you look at what the range of "normal" is considered for plasma zinc, it's so broad that it's of very little practical use. I think our monkey studies may provide some leads as to what research could be carried out in humans.

Another point is that in many human pregnancy studies it has been found that there is an inverse relationship between the birth weight of the infant and the plasma zinc of the mother. This has been very puzzling and would suggest that zinc has no relationship at all to the outcome of pregnancy. But we found the same thing in our zinc-deficient monkeys, not in the control monkeys but in the zinc-deficient monkeys, and that suggests that possibly, in those human cases, there was a problem of marginal zinc deficiency.

HAMBRAEUS: Well, my comment was also referring to the use of glutathione peroxidase as an indicator of the selenium balance. I think that the curve Dr Bruce showed is completely right, but, on the other hand, it has been shown in many studies that you can rely upon glutathione peroxidase as indicator up to a certain level and that you cannot rely upon it after this plasma level is reached. This has been shown in one and the same population and it is not only a question of different populations. I think it is essential to recognize this as it may be one of the explanations why there is some confusion in the debate in the literature regarding the usefulness of supplements.

FRANK: I have a question to Dr Bruce. Do you have any recommendations for the intake of cobalt, cobalamin, vitamin B_{12}, or supplements of it? I didn't find any in your tables.

BRUCE: No, that's true, since cobalt is only essential in vitamin B_{12}. The tentative dose for this vitamin is 3 μg (range 1.5–4.5 μg).

CHRISTOPHERSEN: I would like to return to this question of glutathione peroxidase. I think that it is very difficult to explain the epidemiological data concerning selenium and cancer unless we assume that the biological effect of selenium is mediated via some enzyme activity. It could very well be glutathione peroxidase. If this interpretation is correct, it means that a plateau is not reached until one reaches an enriched level in the population corresponding to that in the most selenium-rich states in the United States which is much higher than in this case.

BRUCE: Studies on human selenium metabolism are going on very actively all over the world now. There are very many conflicting results which will be clarified in a few years.

FJELLSTRÖM: Dr Bruce, I think there are some major difficulties in the interpretation or application of the list of recommended daily allowances of trace elements. If I understand it correctly, the figures given in the table are the amount of trace elements in the diet but it does not take into account at all the huge variations in gastrointestinal absorption of trace elements depending on in which composition they are presented in the gastrointestinal tract. Wouldn't it be better to have a list with recommendations of the amount of trace elements needed for the organism to be in metabolic balance with respect to that trace element?

BRUCE: Is anyone willing to present such a list today?

FJELLSTRÖM: I don't know for sure but do you agree that there are large difficulties in the application of the daily allowances because of variations in the absorption which may vary 10- or even 50-fold?

BRUCE: I agree. As we have heard from Dr Hurley's presentation, there are various interactions and in particular the interactions between individual trace elements make the situation even more complicated. I am sure that in the future we will know more about various interactions and can adjust the recommendations appropriately.

HURLEY: I think it is certainly true that dietary composition influences absorption, but the RDA's try to take this into acount, so that a factor is allowed for absorption assuming that there is a mixed diet, that is, a diet containing a mixture of different types of food. If somebody eats nothing but whole-wheat bread, then that's going to be different, but I think that the list that Dr Bruce has shown us was very good, because it did contain all the trace elements that are essential and that we think may produce problems, and it didn't just pick out some. The problem of trace element/trace element interaction is diminished if all of them are present. Many of the vitamin-mineral preparations that are available in the United States, for example, do not contain all the essential trace elements. They'll contain some but not others and I think that's where the real danger of deleterious interactions comes in.

Trace Elements in Water Supplies

By Gunnar Jacks

INTRODUCTION

Trace elements in drinking water may be derived either from the water bearing strata or from the distribution system or more commonly from both. In general, trace elements in drinking water make up only a minor fraction of the human intake. Natural waters in general contain small amounts of trace elements, so small that they neither make up an essential supply nor reach toxic levels. This is true with some exceptions, for instance As, which may be high in a water source. However, after passing the distribution system, pipes, joints and taps the pattern may be entirely different. Well known are the incidences of lead poisoning in soft water areas like Scotland and northeastern USA.

A new threat has appeared in areas affected by acid rain, where there are signs that heavy metals have been mobilized in the soil zone. So far, however, there are no reports on water standards having been exceeded in well water. Chemical changes in water brought about by acid rain may, however, bring about increased corrosion in water distribution systems (Environment 82).

MOBILITY OF TRACE ELEMENTS IN SOILS

Trace elements, for instance heavy metals, occur in soils and rocks in different positions. They may be built into rock forming minerals like silicates. In these positions they are released very slowly as weathering affects the minerals. The important and mobilizable pool of trace elements occur as adsorbed on surfaces in soils and rocks. There are three important adsorbants for trace elements (Andersson 1977):

- organic matter
- clay minerals
- iron and manganese oxides and hydroxides.

The organic matter in soils is usually known as humus, degradation products of plant matter. This humic matter may be regarded as polyphenols with some active groups (Steelink 1963). The most important groups are carboxyls and carbonyls.

The carboxyls on a phenol skeleton may form a strong chelate for a heavy metal:

$$R\begin{matrix}COOH\\COOH\end{matrix} + Cu^{2+} \rightleftharpoons R\begin{matrix}COO\\COO\end{matrix}\!\!>Cu^{2+} + 2\,H^{+}$$

Copper is strongly bound to organic matter. Organic soils are not seldom Cu-deficient.

Clay minerals in general have defects in their structure which render them negatively charged on their outer surfaces (Millot 1970). They may thus adsorb cations, for instance lead ions. Lead has a special affinity to clays (Andersson 1977).

The third important adsorbant, the iron and manganese oxides, may also contain heavy metals substituting for iron and manganese. An important property of iron hydroxides is the ZPC, the zero point of charge, which lies at a pH of 5–6. Above that pH they are positively charged, below negatively charged. Thus, in acid soils iron hydroxides become anion adsorbers.

The most forceful replacer of adsorbed cations is the hydrogen ion as is shown above. Thus, in general, when the pH of the soil water or ground water decreases, trace metals tend to increase in water. A threshold value for pH, below which several heavy metals and aluminium show sharply rising concentrations, seems to be 4.5 (Coal–Health–Environment 1983) as is shown in Fig. 1. It may be pointed out that cadmium behaves in a parallel way to zinc which is shown in the figure.

LEVELS OF TRACE ELEMENTS IN NATURAL WATERS

With "eyeglasses" sharp enough it is possible to find more or less the whole periodic system of elements in water. Today we have analytical methods that easily reach the ng/l level. However, this requires sampling, transport and storage of samples performed with the utmost care. An evidence of this is that the so-called "background levels" of trace elements in water has continuously gone down throughout the years.

Among the elements we will look at a few. *Cadmium* is a heavy metal of real concern as the human body burden has increased considerably during this century. In acid ground, waters with pH 5–6 a maximum of 1 μg/l has been detected in Sweden (Monitor 1981) (Fig. 2). The hygienic limit is set at

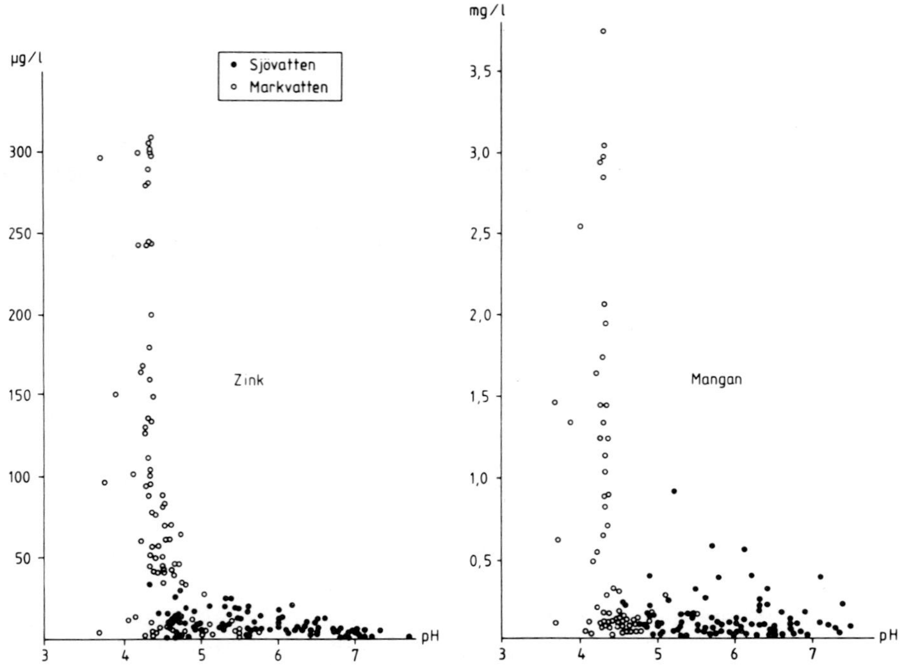

Fig. 1 Contents of zinc and manganese in soil waters (open circles) and lake waters (filled circles) as function of pH
(Coal–Health–Environment 1983; data from Bergqvist, Dickson & Rosén)

5 μg/l. At this level the cadmium intake by water is about 10% of the total intake. However, any increase is of concern for cadmium, and further analysis of cadmium in acid waters is highly desirable.

Lead has increased in the environment during the last century. However, lead is not easily mobilized from soils as is shown by Odén at the Swedish Agric. Univ. (Environment 82) (Fig. 3). In the same set of samples as mentioned above in connection with cadmium, lead showed a median content of about 0.5 μg/l which should be compared with the 50 μg/l which is the present standard in most countries.

Zinc and *copper* are, in natural waters, low in comparison with human daily intake and do not appreciably contribute to it.

Arsenic may sometimes be high in natural waters. Reducing conditions with a fairly low pH favour the dissolution of arsenic from soils and rocks. Arsenic occurs in natural waters in the form of arsenite and arsenate and is likely to be adsorbed on ferric hydroxide surfaces (Matisoff et al. 1982). Removal of iron in water works usually scavenges off the arsenic effectively. In the Netherlands, iron-rich ground waters are common and the iron precipitates that are filtered off are so high in arsenic that they have to be

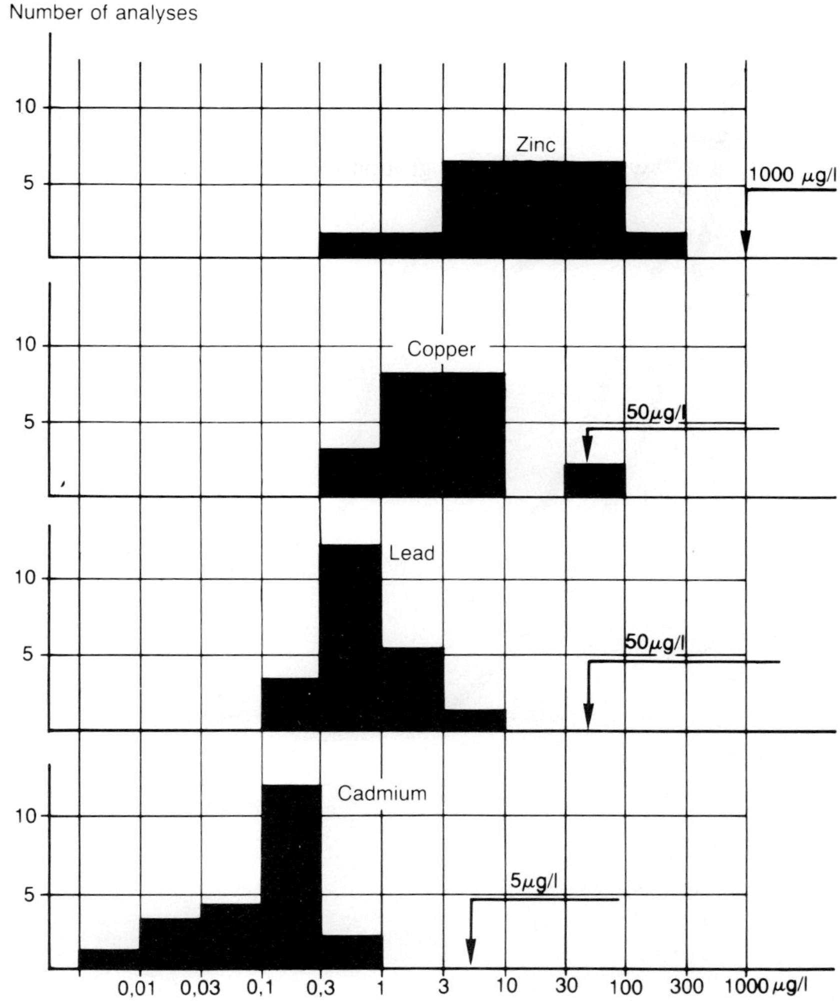

Fig. 2 Heavy metals in acid well and spring waters from two areas in Sweden
pH varied between 5.5 and 6.5
(Monitor 1981)

treated as hazardous wastes (Brinkman, Nat. Inst. for Water Supply, Leidschendam, pers. comm.).

Selenium in natural waters may range from values of a few mg/l to below 1 μg/l. In the Midwest of the USA, toxic amounts of selenium are not uncommon in connection with shales. In Sweden, the content of selenium in natural waters is recorded at levels below 0.2 μg/l in general (Boström & Wester 1967, Lindberg 1968). Again, selenium in drinking water is a small fraction of the human daily intake, which in Sweden is about 30 μg/day. However, selenium content in water is an indication of the generally low

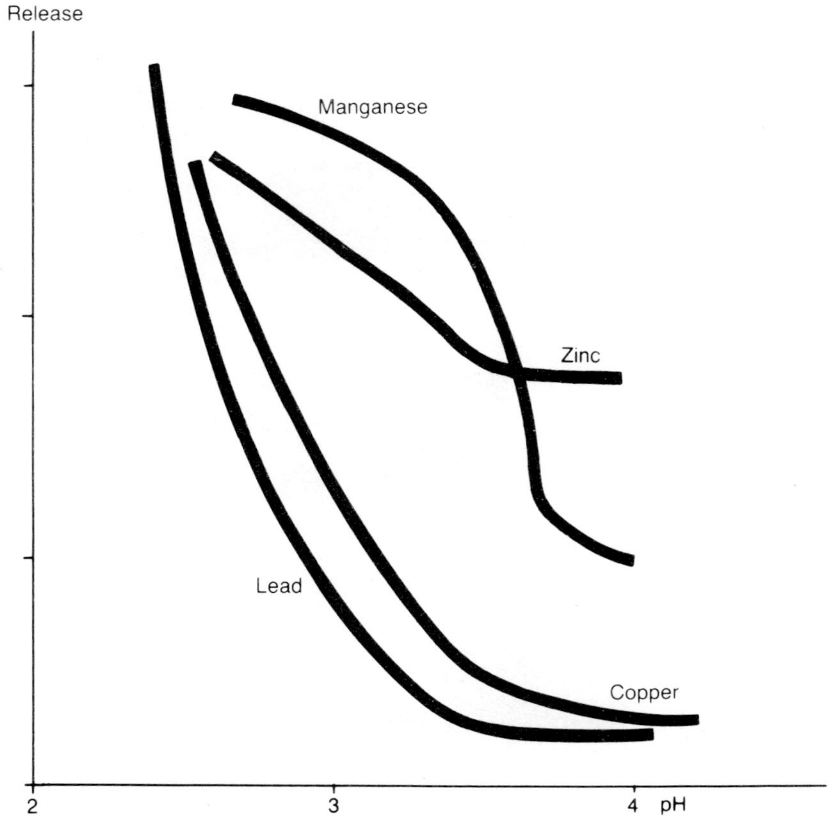

Fig. 3 Leaching of heavy metals from the enrichment layer of the soil

With low pH value in the ground there is an increasing risk that heavy metals will be released from the soil particles. This figure shows how zinc, manganese, copper and lead can be released from the enrichment layer in forestland at various pH levels

(Environment 82; data from Odén)

availability of selenium in Sweden. With acidification the selenium in water seems to decrease (Kjell Johansson, Swed. Nat. Environ. Board, pers. comm.). Acidification of the B-horizons of podsolic soils will tend to increase adsorbtion of anions like selenite and selenate. Selenium acts as an antagonist against mercury uptake in many organisms. Possibly, the increased content in pike in Swedish lakes with lowered pH of the water may be an effect of selenium deficiency.

In near neutral waters, *aluminium* is found only in trace quantities. However, aluminium is mobilized as OH-complexes in the alkaline range and as Al^{3+} in water below pH of 5.5. At pH 5 a few 100 μg/l would be in solution. It is possible that aluminium in acid waters may be harmful to individuals having impaired kidney function (WHO European Office 1984).

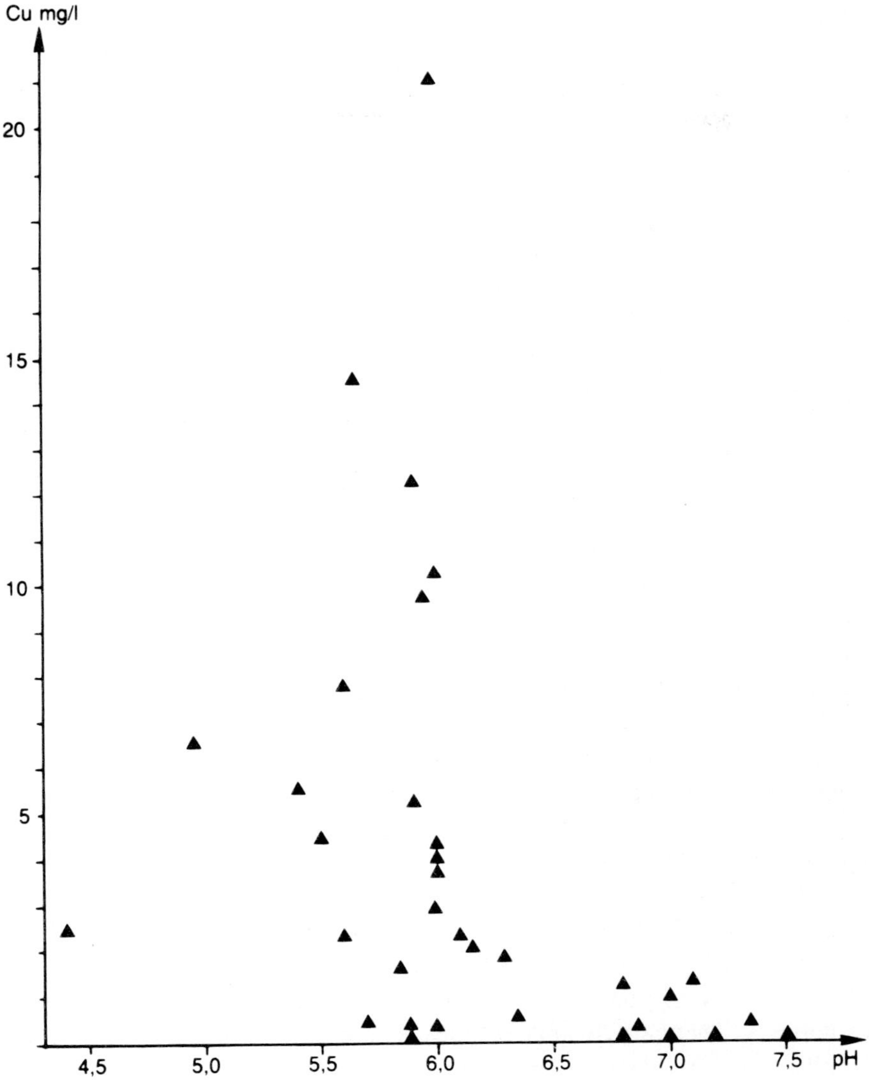

Fig. 4 Copper contents in tap water in western Sweden

High copper contents are liable to be found in tap water that has remained overnight in copper pipes. This is particularly noticeable in the hot water. The concentration of dissolved copper salts increases with declining pH in the water below a certain critical pH value

Source: Public Health Committee of Lilla Edet (Environment 82)

TRACE METALS FROM DISTRIBUTION SYSTEMS

With an adequately treated water, there should be little or no interaction with the pipes during the distribution. Large water works may achieve this as is seen in investigations by Boström and Wester (1967). They investigat-

Table 1 Effects of water treatment on metal contents in tap water

In case A a new effective alkalizing filter was in operation. In case B the filter was largely consumed. T means water standard set for technical reasons (corrosion) and H means a water standard set from strictly hygienic reasons

(Monitor 1981)

			pH	Concentration in μg/l			
				Zinc	Copper	Lead	Cadmium
(A)	Fresh alkalizing filter	raw water	6.0	9.5	1.2	0.4	0.03
		tap water	9.1	0.2	2.3	0.1	0.01
(B)	Used-up alkalizing filter	raw water	5.8	1.7	5.4	0.7	0.03
		tap water	6.3	4,900	83	3.3	3.4
Standards				1,000 (T)	50 (T)	50 (H)	5 (H)

ed a large number of elements in raw water, treated water and tap water from three major towns in Sweden without finding any remarkable changes along the distribution route. However, in small water works the treatment may be less optimal and in private wells there is, in general, no treatment at all.

Lead is a common material in pipes in the UK, USA and Canada. No new installations are done but the ones existing will be used for a few more decades. Any water having less than 100 mg/l alkalinity may give a tap water exceeding 50 μg/l of lead if conveyed through lead pipes (Wong & Berrang 1976). Lead in smaller amounts may come from taps, which contain a few percent of lead. Even plastic pipes may release minor amounts of lead, probably from lead in stearate (Hensgem & DeGraeve 1972).

Copper is a very common material for in-house installations of water in Scandinavia. There are two major types of copper corrosion, cuprosolvency and pit corrosion (Mattson 1980). Sometimes corrosion may be caused by erosion if too narrow sections of tubing are formed (Knutsson 1972). Cuprosolvency may occur in cold water having a low pH and alkalinity. "First flush" waters having concentrations up to 20 mg/l of copper have been found in southwestern Sweden (Environment 82) (Fig. 4). During daytime 2–4 mg/l may appear in acid waters. With such a water the intake of copper from drinking water may be a major portion of the daily intake. Pitting corrosion is common in hot-water systems and is troublesome because it may rapidly lead to water leaks.

Cadmium can sometimes be found in soldering materials. Accidentally, copper–cadmium alloys have been used when manufacturing taps, which has resulted in above standard concentrations of cadmium in tap water (Hareide, Nat. Inst. of Public Health, Oslo, pers. comm). In Sweden up to 3 μg/l have been detected in connection with high zinc concentrations (Monitor 1981). In this case the cadmium is probably occuring as an impurity in galvanization.

Zinc from galvanization may reach a few mg/l in soft acid waters (Monitor 1981). In such cases drinking water may supply a considerable portion of the daily zinc intake.

In this connection, the relation between incidence of cardiovascular diseases and hardness in drinking water that was recognized already in the sixties may be mentioned (Biörck et al. 1965, Masironi 1969). Hard-water areas show a lower incidence than soft-water areas. One possible explanation for this effect could be the presumably more corrosive nature of soft waters leading to higher contents of heavy metals like cadmium. Cadmium is known to raise blood pressure. However, this hypothesis has been challenged by several investigations (Haring & Zoeteman 1980). Selenium which is considered to have a positive effect on cardiac health, is generally positively correlated with hardness (i.e. Boström & Wester 1967). However, so far no unequivocal evidence for any explanation exists.

SUMMARY

When no direct pollution is present, natural waters in general show low contents of most trace metals, both compared to water standards and to human intake from other sources. Under certain conditions arsenic from natural sources may exceed the limits set. Acidification of surface waters especially has brought about increases in heavy metals and aluminium. Aluminium in acid waters may be harmful to individuals having impaired kidney function.

An adequately treated water should have little or no interaction with materials in the distribution system. Small water works and private wells do not in general have any treatment and may be corrosive. This may result in dissolution of lead, copper, cadmium and zinc. The hygienic limits for lead and cadmium may be exceeded. Copper and zinc may appear in amounts of a few mg/l, making drinking water a considerable or even major human source for these metals.

Trace element concentrations in natural waters are generally low as stated above, and their detection may represent some analytical trouble. However, the levels of trace elements in natural waters may indicate the general availability of the respective element to organisms in the given environment. Water is the start of all food chains whether in soils or in lakes.

REFERENCES

ANDERSSON, A. (1977), Heavy metals in Swedish soils, on their origin, distribution and amounts. *Swed. Agric. Res.* 7, 7–20.

BIÖRCK, G., BOSTRÖM, H. & WIDSTRÖM, A. (1965). On the relationship between water hardness and death rate in cardiovascular diseases. *Acta med. scand.* 178, fasc. 2, 239–251.

BOSTRÖM, H. & WESTER, P. O. (1967). Trace elements in drinking water and death rate in cardiovascular disease. *Acta med. scand.* 181, fasc. 4, 465–473.

Coal–Health–Environment Project (KHM) (1983). *Health and Environmental Effects of Coal.* Swedish State Power Board (Statens Vattenfallsverk), Vällingby (in Swedish).

Environment 82 committee (1982). *Acidification Today and Tomorrow.* Swedish Ministry of Agriculture, 231 pp.

HARING, J. A. & ZOETEMAN, B. C. J. (1980). Corrosiveness of drinking water and cardiovascular mortality. *Bull. of Environ. Contamination and Toxicol.* 25, 658–662.

HENSGEM, C. & DEGRAEVE, D. (1972). Importance de l'apport alimentaire en plomb dans l'est de la Belgique. In *Proc. Int. Symp. of Environ. Health Aspects of Lead, Amsterdam, 2–6 Oct. 1972,* Commission of the European Communities, 85 pp.

KNUTSSON, L. (1972). Erosion corrosion in copper tubing. *Brit. Corrosion J.* 7, 208.

LINDBERG, P. (1968). Selenium determination in plant and animal material and in water. *Acta vet. scand.* Suppl. 23.

MASIRONI, R. (1969). Trace elements and cardiovascular diseases. *Bull. WHO* 40, 305–312.

MATISOFF, G., KHOUREY, C. J., HALL, J. F., VARNES, A. W. & STRAIN, W. H. (1982). The nature and source of arsenic in northeastern Ohio ground water. *Ground Water* 20, 446–456.

MATTSSON, E. (1980). Corrosion of copper in fresh waters. *Proc. of Australian Corrosion Ass. Silver Jubilee Conf.,* Adelaide.

MILLOT, G. (1970). *Geology of Clays.* Springer Verlag, N. Y., 429 pp.

Monitor 1981. Acidification of soil and water. Swed. Nat. Environ. Board (in Swedish), 173 pp.

STEELINK, C. (1963). What is a humic acid? *J. Chem. Educ.* 40, 379–384.

WHO European Office 1984, Workshop on health effects of acid rain, Berlin, July 3–6th.

WONG, C. S. & BERRANG, P. (1976). Contamination of tap water by lead pipe and solder. *Bull. Environ. Contamination and Toxicol.* 15, 530.

Health Effects and Environmental Aspects of Trace Elements

By Peter J. Aggett

Although the title of this presentation could imply that this contribution will consider the toxic effects of trace elements on human health this is not the intention. The toxic effects following excessive acute or chronic exposure to metals have been well reviewed and documented elsewhere. The aim of this presentation is to consider the means whereby customary or non-industrial exposure to trace elements in the environment or diet may influence human health, and to indicate the possibility that even this exposure may have an impact on our well-being. Clearly this cannot be a comprehensive review, and some of the examples cited may be conjectural. However, this latter point and some of the polarised and emotive attitudes which develop, as is so often the case, in the absence of factual evidence reflects the difficulties encountered in trying to investigate the possibly more subtle effect of trace elements on human health.

The major features of trace element deficiency in man and some other animals are shown in Table 1. Many of these only develop with gross deficiency of the respective elements. However, it is being increasingly appreciated that other metabolic abnormalities and sub-optimal functions may precede the grosser features of deficiency. For example, studies in animals show that the anaemia and neutropenia of copper deficiency are preceded by impaired oxidative phosphorylation and defective cardiac function (Prohaska 1982). Similarly defective activities of iron-containing enzymes can adversely affect human health, intellectual function and stamina before impairing haematopoiesis (Galan et al. 1984). Since many metabolic mechanisms depend on more than one essential element, they can be disrupted by impaired nutriture with respect to anyone of these. For example, antioxidative mechanisms rely upon copper, zinc, iron, manganese and selenium; optimal carbohydrate metabolism is dependent on zinc, manga-

Table 1 *Features and defects associated with trace element deficiencies in man*

Features in parentheses have only been observed in animal models

Copper	Cardiomegaly and failure, hypercholesterolaemia, defective cross-linkages in elastin and collagen causing skeletal and vascular defects, anaemia, impaired oxidative phosphorylation (impaired immune function).
Zinc	Mood alterations, anorexia, growth retardation, hypogonadism, impaired immune function, dermatitis, reduced dark adaptation, intestinal malabsorption of nutrients and water, altered lipid metabolism.
Selenium	Cardiomyopathy (skeletal myopathy and hepatic necrosis in animals), increased antioxidant damage, (? impaired metabolism of xenobiotics), (impaired leucocyte candicidal activity).
Iodine	Hypothyroidism and its metabolic sequelae.
Manganese	Single case: hypocholesterolaemia, weight loss, prolonged prothrombin time.
Chromium	Growth retardation, altered carbohydrate metabolism, weight loss, neuropathy, encephalopathy.
Molybdenum	Intolerance of sulphur amino acids, encephalopathy, retardation, hypouricaemia, hypouricuria, hypermethioninaemia.
Iron	Apathy, impaired energy and lipid metabolism, defective immune function, anaemia.

nese and chromium whilst deficiencies of anyone of these elements and also of copper, iodine or iron disturb lipid and energy metabolism. Similarly, many aspects of immune competence are susceptible to inadequate nutrition with copper, zinc, selenium or iron. Other pathways and physiological functions have a similar multiple dependence on these trace elements and it is conceivable that absolute deficiencies or relative imbalances amongst these inorganic nutrients themselves or between them and other organic nutrients can seriously derange normal metabolism. This is illustrated by the synergistic interactions between selenium, as a component of glutathione peroxidase, and vitamin E whereby each as an antioxidant can partially compensate for the absence of the other unless factors which cause increased oxidative stress such as cold or exercise; increased oxidisable substrate caused by an increased dietary intake of polyunsaturated fatty acids; and reduced or excessive supply of copper or iron supervene (Editorial 1983). Interactions such as these are being investigated increasingly in animal models but have not yet been examined extensively in man, but the possibility has arisen that the example cited may affect the management of parenteral nutrition.

Another interaction has been invoked to generate the hypothesis that a metabolic imbalance between copper and zinc may predispose to hypercholesterolaemia and thence to ischaemic heart disease (Klevay 1975). However, as is discussed elsewhere in this symposium (Salonen—this volume), other dietary factors, including selenium deficiency, may predispose to cardiovascular disease in man. In examining any of these or similar hypotheses, therefore, all these factors should, ideally, be considered. Our ability to do this, however, is hampered, firstly by an incomplete knowledge of the nature and extent of metabolic interactions described above, and secondly, in the context of environmental exposure (or lack of exposure) to an element, by an inadequate understanding of the environmental factors which affect the directness of the relationship between the health effect and the element. This limitation occurs irrespective of the level at which that element enters the food chain (Table 2). The earlier an element enters the food chain it can be anticipated that it will be correspondingly more difficult to establish any relationship between it and any health effects than it will be to establish an association between a health effect and an element entering as a late dietary contaminant. Both of these aspects will now be considered.

Techniques and approaches to examining human health and environmental geochemistry have been reviewed recently (Tourtelot 1979, Thornton & Webb 1979) but in many cases sufficiently randomised data are not available from either the health bases or the geochemistry to unravel complicated interrelationships. Those associations which have been established are those involving either gross or very small elemental concentrations in the environment and equally extreme pathology. Examples include endemic fluorosis and tooth mottling or, more distressingly, genu valgum (Krishnamachari & Krishnaswamy 1974), and endemic goitre and hypothyroidism in

Table 2 Outline of food chain and some of the geochemical and biological variables which influence body burdens of trace elements

Contamination from industrial and mining sources is not shown

Pathway	Comments
ANIMAL TISSUES growth, maintenance, reproduction	Variable demands with clinical and physiological states
↑	Existence or absence of stores
INTESTINE	Homeostasis mechanisms, adaptive uptake mechnisms, interactions limiting absorption (Table 4)
↑	
DIETARY INTAKE	Losses and contamination Fortification Synthetic foods, novel protein (unknown availability of elements)
↑ FOOD ↑ WATER	
↑ PLANT (→ FOOD)	Strain & species differences in uptake and storage, competitive interactions amongst elements (Table 4)
↑ SOIL SOLUTIONS (→ WATER)	Exchange affected by redox potential of soil, pH, cations and organic ligands
↑ SOIL MATRIX (→ WATER)	
PRIMARY SOURCE (→ WATER)	

iodine deficient regions. More recent examples are the recognition in the Peoples Republic of China of a selenium responsive cardiomyopathy, known as Keshan disease (Chen et al. 1980), and an endemic selenium toxicosis (Yang et al. 1983). The epidemiology of Keshan disease leaves open the possibility that other nutritional, geochemical, climatic, and, possibly, infective factors may compound the disease but the dramatic efficacy of sodium selenite in its prophylaxis and treatment indicates the pathogenic role of a selenium deficiency which can be traced from the soil, through herbage and livestock to man (Chen et al. 1980). Another disabling condition has also been noted to occur in regions where the soil selenium content is low. Its eponomous name (Kaschin–Beck Disease) is derived from its early describers Kaschin, and Beck and Beck who recognised the condition independently in 1859 and 1906, respectively. It is characterised by disturbed endochondrial ossification, especially of epiphyseal cartilage, leading to bilateral and usually symmetrical osteoarthropathies. Many joints are involved leading to dwarfism and deformities. Since these effects are permanent the effect of prophylactic selenium supplements on the incidence of the condition is as yet unknown, but its contrast with Keshan disease although occuring in similar areas would indicate a complex aetiology (Lombeck—personal communication).

The direct relationship encountered in China between soil selenium and health contrasts with experience in some areas where the development of selenium responsive myopathies in cattle bore no demonstrable relationship to the soil selenium content (Arthur et al. 1979). A similar anomaly occurs in pastures where cattle develop symptomatic copper deficiency. This was noted to be due to the prevention of intestinal absorption of copper by molybdenum which was readily available from the soil and the herbage growing on it (Mills 1979). This interaction is further complicated by the direct relationship between the availability of soil molybdenum to plants and the alkalinity and water retention of the soil. Thus, for any given soil copper content, soil pH, drainage and molybdenum content must be considered in assessing the risk of copper deficiency for livestock. The mechanism whereby molybdenum limits the intestinal absorption of copper is attributed to the formation of copper thiomolybolate or sulphide compounds in the reducing environment of the rumen. Consequently, the effects of molybdenum on the metabolism of copper by monogastric species including man was considered to be negligible. This may not be true, however. A study conducted in "molybdenum-rich" provinces in Armenia (Kovalsky et al. 1961) compared both healthy individuals and individuals with arthralgia from a high molybdenum area, with healthy individuals from a relatively low soil molybdenum area. In the high areas the soil and plant molybdenum contents were up to 50 and 260 times higher than those of the reference area. It was presumed that the known increased incidence of gout-like arthralgia in the high molybdenum area was due to increased xanthine oxidase activity

Table 3 *Interaction between molybdenum-rich geochemical environment and human health*

(Abstracted from Kovalsky et al. 1961)

	Dietary intakes (mg/24h) of		Blood content (µg/dl)		Urinary excretion (µg/24h) of		Serum xanthine oxidase activity (minutes)	Blood uric acid (mg/dl)
	Cu	Mo	Cu	Mo	Cu	Mo		
Molybdenum-rich zone								
Patients			113 (25)	3 (8)	304 (14)	29 (2)	4.8 (0.5)	8.1 (1.8)
	5–10	10–15 (both groups)						
Healthy			138 (26)	17 (8)	184 (30)	28 (4)	7.9 (1.0)	5.3 (2.1)
Control zone								
Healthy	10–15	1–2	183 (20)	6 (2)	120 (24)	16 (3)	10.2 (1.4)	3.8 (1.0)

Notes:

The number of observations for each investigation varied.
Figures in parenthesis indicate standard deviations.
Xanthine oxidase activity is time taken to oxidase a standard aliquot of substrate.

secondary to an increased dietary intake of molybdenum. Some results of this study are shown in Table 3. The authors describe, as well as the apparent effect of high dietary intake of environmental molybdenum on purine metabolism, a systemic effect on copper metabolism. This intriguing study bears repitition—it contrasts with observations of elevated plasma caeruloplasmin and copper levels, increased urinary excretion of copper, and raised serum uric acid concentrations in workers exposed to molybdenum dust (Walravens et al. 1979). Nonetheless, both studies suggest that molybdenum can modify systemic metabolism of copper in man as well as ruminants.

Other associations between human disease and geochemistry or soil composition have concentrated extensively on possible causes of human cancer. Regional variations of cancer mortality and incidence have been related to soil composition in England (Smith 1960) but with no particular element being aetiologically incriminated. More recently in Finland increasing manganese content of soils was associated with a diminished incidence of cancer (Marjanen & Soini 1972) and, in the Transkei, corn plants from areas with a high risk of oesophageal cancer were shown to have a lower manganese content than those from low risk areas (Laker et al. 1980). This observation and the possible association of molybdenum deficient soils with oesophageal cancer (Yang 1980) were investigated further in the Transkei. Contour maps of the incidence of oesophageal cancer were compared with soil composition (Kibblewhite et al. 1984). On this occasion the trace element content of soils from areas with a high risk of oesophageal cancer were found to have much lower contents of boron, copper and nickel than those from low risk areas but the contents of manganese, molybdenum and zinc were not so extensively reduced.

The preceding examples show that, although one to one associations may be established, it is invariably necessary to consider other environmental factors, as well as other elements, to avoid detecting spurious relationships between geochemistry and human health. It is also apparent that interactions which affect the passage of elements from the soil to plants and from plants to animals need to be considered as well. Examples of these are listed in Table 4. In the face of such factors it is impressive that geochemical anomalies can extend so far along the food chain. The fact that this is seen in the examples chosen also reflects the relative immobility of the study populations and their dependence on locally grown foodstuffs. With more mobile populations and in those consuming imported foods any local environmental effects of inorganic nutrients on health become more obscure. It is interesting, however, that in some instances where routine supplementation of foodstuffs or of susceptible populations does not occur, abnormalities of thyroid function and dentition still develop. Similarly geographic variation of selenium status in humans is still evident in western cultures (Salonen—this volume).

Table 4 Some interactions reducing passage of essential trace elements from:

Element	Soil to plants	Diet to animals
Cobalt	Mn, Fe, increased pH, good drainage	Fe, Mn, Zn
Copper	High pH	Mo (in ruminants), S, Fe, Zn, Cd, P, phytate
Iodine	—	Co, SCN, F, As
Iron	High pH, P	Mg, Ca, P, Zn, Cd, phytate, Co_3^-
Zinc	High pH	Cu, Ca, Mg, phytates, Fe, Cd
Molybdenum	Low pH, good drainage	W
Selenium	S, Fe	S analogues of Se amino acids, Cu
Manganese	High pH	P, Fe

The use of metal utensils for the preparation or storage of food or both can have either a beneficial or disadvantageous effect. The use of iron utensils can provide a useful source of iron (Baumslag & Petering 1976) but the availability of contaminating iron for intestinal absorption may be quite low and variable, according to the presence, in the diet, of enhancers (e.g. ascorbate, meat, fish) or inhibitors (e.g. phytate, other phosphates, tannins) of iron absorption (Halberg et al. 1983). An example of a possible adverse effect of storage contamination of food comes from Pune, India where Tanner et al. (1983) have been seeking the source of the copper which accumulates in the livers of children with Indian Childhood Cirrhosis (ICC). It has been noted that children with this condition are breast-fed for a shorter duration than non-affected children. Furthermore, the age of presentation of ICC is correlated with the age at which feeding with an alternative animal milk had been commenced. It was also noted that households with a child with ICC were more likely to have exposed the milk to copper contamination by storing and/or heating it in brass utensils. This contamination was less marked from utensils which had been adequately coated with a thin coating, containing tin, called Kallai.

Another effect of extraneous contamination of food has been raised by Johnson et al. (1981) who have proposed that prolonged storage of foods in tinned cans may produce sufficient contamination of the food to interfere with the intestinal absorption of zinc. This interaction and those indicated in Table 4 may all limit the availability of the minerals for absorption. Currently, the most serious consideration in this respect is the widespread use of iron fortification and prophylactic supplementation which may impair human intestinal absorption and metabolism of zinc (Solomons & Jacob 1981). A possible sequel of this has been described by Hambidge et al. (1983) who showed a trend for an inverse correlation between plasma zinc concentrations in pregnant women and the amount of their iron supplementation which in some cases was as high as 260 mg/day. Since zinc may in turn limit the availability of iron for absorption, as well as that of copper, the logical response to this situation is to reassess the need for iron supplements rather than to give additional zinc.

The impact of mineral interactions may also be accentuated by the loss and inadequate replacement of elements during food processing and refining. For example, the chromium content (± SD) of molasses is 266 (± 58) μg/g, whereas in unrefined sugar it is 162 (± 36) μg/g and is only 20 (± 3) μg/g in refined white sugar. Thus, ironically, sugar is deprived of an element needed for its effective metabolism (Masironi et al. 1973). The loss of trace elements during the milling of flour is illustrated in Table 5. Fortification or replacement of only some of the lost elements will clearly exacerbate interelement imbalances. Thus, food processing and fortification can considerably attenuate and obscure any other relationship with environmental trace elements as well as imposing other potential risks.

Throughout this contribution I have tried to avoid any implication of causative associations between these environmental aspects of trace elements and human health effects. All such putative relationships need to be examined by the standard epidemiological criteria of strength, consistency and reproducibility, specificity, temporality, biological dose effect, plausibility, coherence, analogy and experiment (Hill 1965). At least the first five criteria are vulnerable to obfuscation of any casual relationships by other environmental factors which should be examined. These aspects include the relative abundance of other elements, especially since one to one relationships are exceptional. Furthermore other nutritional and environmental influences, such as climate in Keshan disease, need to be assessed. This account has, however, been unable to consider the important effects which physiological demands during growth and pregnancy, genetic variation, intestinal adaptation and the presence or absence of whole body homeostasis may have on the acquired body burden of trace elements and the health effects.

Table 5 The effect of milling on the trace element content (mg/kg) of wheat flour
(Schroeder 1971)

	Wheat	White flour
Percent of wheat	100	72
Chromium	0.05	0.03
Manganese	46	6.5
Iron	43	10.5
Cobalt	5.3	1.7
Zinc	35	7.8
Selenium	0.63	0.53
Molybdenum	0.48	0.25

REFERENCES

ARTHUR, J. R., PRICE, J. & MILLS, C. F. (1979). Observations on the selenium status of cattle in the northeast of Scotland. *Vet. Rec.* 104, 340–341.

BAUMSLAG, N. & PETERING, H. G. (1976). Trace metal studies in Bushman Hair. *Arch. environm. Hlth* 31, 254–257.

CHEN, X., YANG, G., CHEN, J., CHEN, X., WEN, Z. & GE, K. (1980). Studies on the relations of selenium and Keshan Disease. *Biol. Trace Elem. Res.* 2, 91–107.

Editorial (1983). Selenium perspective. *Lancet* i, 685.

GALAN, P., HEREBERG, S. & TOVITOU, Y. (1984). The activity of tissue enzymes in iron-deficient rat and man: an overview. *Comp. Biochem. Physiol.* 773, 647–653.

HALBERG, L., BJORN-RASMUSSEN, E., ROSSANDER, L., SUWANIK, R., PLEEHACHINDA, R. & TUNTAWIROON, M. (1983). Iron absorption from some Asian meals containing contamination iron. *Amer. J. clin. Nutr.* 37, 272–277.

HAMBIDGE, K. M., KREBS, N. F., JACOBS, M. A., FAVIER, A., GUYETTE, L. & IKLE, D. N. (1983). Zinc nutritional status during pregnancy: a longitudinal study. *Amer. J. clin. Nutr.* 37, 429–442.

HILL, A. B. (1965). The environment and disease: association or causation. *Proc. Roy. Soc. Med.* 58, 295–301.

JOHNSON, M. A., BAIER, M. J. & GREGOR, J. L. (1981). Effect of dietary tin on zinc, copper, iron, manganese and magnesium metabolism of adult males. *Amer. J. clin. Nutr.* 35, 1332–1338.

KIBBLEWHITE, M. E., VAN RENSBURG, S. J., LAKER, M. C. & ROSE, E. F. (1984). Evidence for an intimate geochemical factor in the etiology of esophageal cancer. *Environ. Res.* 33, 370–378.

KLEVAY, L. M. (1975). Coronary heart disease: The zinc/copper hypothesis. *Amer. J. clin. Nutr.* 28, 764–774.

KOVALSKY, V. V., JAROVAJA, G. A. & SMAVONJAN, D. M. (1961). Changes in purine metabolism in man and animals in various molybdenum-rich biogeochemical provinces. *Z. Obsc. Biol.* 22, 179 (in Russian).

KRISHNAMACHARI, K. A. V. R. & KRISHNASWAMY, K. (1974). An epidemiological study of the syndrome of Genu valgum among residents of endemic areas for fluorosis in Andhra Pradesh. *Ind. J. med. Res.* 62, 1415–1421.

LAKER, M. C., HENSLEY, M., BEYERS, C. P. DE L. & VAN LENSBURG, S. J. (1980). Environmental association with oesophageal cancer: an integrated model. *S. Afr. Cancer Bull.* 24, 69–70.

MARJANEN, H. & SOINI, S. (1972). Possible causal relationship between nutritional imbalances, especially manganese deficiency, and susceptibility to cancer in Finland. *Ann. Agricultura Fennae* 11, 391–406.

MASIRONI, R., WOLF, W. & MERTZ, W. (1973). Chromium in refined and unrefined sugars from various countries. *Bull. Wld Hlth Org.* 49, 322–329.

MILLS, C. F. (1979). Trace elements in animals. *Phil. Trans. Roy. Soc. (London)* B288, 51–63.

PROHASKA, J. R. & HELLER, L. J. (1982). Mechanical properties of the copper-deficient rat heart. *J. Nutr.* 112, 2142–2150.

SCHROEDER, H. A. (1971). Losses of vitamins and trace minerals resulting from processing and preservation of foods. *Amer. J. clin. Nutr.* 24, 562–573.

SMITH, G. W. (1960). *Soil and Cancer.* Medical Press, London.

SOLOMONS, N. W. & JACOB, R. A. (1981). Studies on the bioavailability of zinc in humans: effect of heme and non heme iron on the absorption of zinc. *Amer. J. clin. Nutr.* 34, 475–482.

TANNER, M. S., KANTARJIAN, A. H., BHAVE, S. A. & PANDIT, A. N. (1983). Early introduction of copper contaminated animal milk feeds as a possible cause of indian childhood cirrhosis. *Lancet* ii, 992–994.

THORNTON, I. & WEBB, J. S. (1979). Geochemistry and health in the United Kingdom. *Phil. Trans. Roy. Soc. (London)* B288, 151–168.

TOURTELOT, H. A. (1979). Geochemical surveys in the United States in relation to health. *Phil. Trans. Roy. Soc. (London)* B288, 113–125.

WALRAVENS, P. A., MOUREERASO, R., SOLOMONS, C. C., CHAPPELL, W. R. & BENTLEY, F. (1979). Biochemical abnormalities in workers exposed to molybdenum dust. *Arch. environm. Hlth* 34, 302–307.

YANG, C. S. (1980). Research on oesophageal cancer in China: a review. *Cancer Res.* 40, 2633–2644.

YANG, G., WANG, S., ZHOU, R. & SUN, S. (1983). Endemic selenium intoxication of humans in China. *Amer. J. clin. Nutr.* 37, 872–881.

Discussion (the papers by Jacks and Aggett)

Chairman: BOSTRÖM

ANDERSON: I have more of a comment than a question. I'm totally amazed by some of these levels of iron that you're talking about, especially in pregnant women where they are talking in excess of 60, 80, 100 or even 200 mg of iron. I can't imagine why a lady would be taking those levels under normal conditions. What are the effects on other trace elements such as zinc, iron and chromium? Hemachromatosis, an iron storage disease, also has a big effect on chromium metabolism and that's only one example. My real point is that I don't think, unless there is an extremely good reason, anyone should be subjected to these high levels of iron.

AGGETT: I'm inclined to agree with you and that's really one of the main theses I was hoping to put over. I think everyone is well aware of the toxic effects of so-called toxic metals. I think we realize, of course, that all metals are potentially toxic as is appreciated with drugs. One should perhaps have far more respect for these metals, regard them as drugs, and realize they're not necessarily benign. I think large levels or chronic exposure to iron certainly can impair the metabolism of zinc and copper. The impairment of copper metabolism by zinc has been used therapeutically in the treatment of Wilson's disease; it has been tried also in primary biliary cirrhosis and in Indian childhood cirrhosis. I think, really, as clinicians we should be far more contemplative about launching in with such large doses of iron. If someone is iron-deficient, we should treat it and if we treat it, perhaps we should use physiological doses. Certainly, I don't think we should use it in such large doses on an empirical basis. I understand in some parts of the U.S.A., people are actually providing zinc supplements on very much the same sort of basis. In fact, I think, in some instances, athletes are being encouraged to take up to 150 mg of zinc a day because it may have some advantageous effect on their performance. I think this approach remains to be justified and I'm rather pleased to hear from Dr Bruce's presentation this morning that, in Sweden, it is intended to establish a ceiling as to the amount which normal individuals should consume.

ANDERSON: Along that same line of 150 mg of zinc for athletes, there have been studies in the U.S. where they've given approximately that amount of zinc and shown that HDL, the protective form of cholesterol, actually has decreased (Hooper et al. *JAMA* 1980: 244, 1960). So rather than an advantageous effect, I think the effects you're going to see will be the opposite.

CHRISTOPHERSEN: I would just like to give a comment to the previous lecture, but I would perhaps like Dr Aggett to comment on it also. It concerns drinking water and cardiovascular disease in Great Britain, because I try to compare the epidemiological patterns in the United States and in Great Britain from the National Academy of Science report on cardiovascular disease and drinking water from some years ago and the patterns are quite different. Not only is there a stronger association but, for instance, you have in Great Britain a negative correlation between calcium in drinking water and mortality but not for magnesium. In the United States, however, the coefficients are similar. In Great Britain you see the association when you compare cities; in the United States you see it better when you compare states. And it can be explained if you assume there is a toxic factor in Great Britain which is not present in the United States, or which is present at much higher levels in Great Britain. And if you ask what is different, I think the most obvious answer would be lead. But I would like to hear your comment on this.

AGGETT: I don't think I'm really well enough informed to make an open comment on that. I don't have enough experience in the field. I don't know if Dr Perry has any comment to make at the moment before his own talk tomorrow? But I'd rather leave it at that and not answer.

ABDULLA: I have two questions, one to Dr Aggett and one to Dr Jacks. Dr Aggett, I wonder if you have considered the interaction between calcium and the other inorganic chemical elements. I think it is important to consider this interaction in view of the fact that the calcium intake in affluent countries is high due to the relatively high consumption of milk and milkproducts. At the same time, the intake of trace elements, such as zinc, copper and selenium, is much lower than the recommended levels. So on a long-term basis, the high calcium intake may influence the bioavialablity of other elements. I wonder if you could comment on this aspect.

The question I want to ask Dr Jacks is about the chemical forms of the trace elements present in water. When we talk about the absorption of inorganic chemical elements from the gut, the chemical form of the element influences a great deal. Now, I wonder how important this aspect is when we are talking about the uptake of these elements by plants from the soil.

AGGETT: Would you like me to answer first? In fact I think I'd like to take your question to me even further and ask me also the relevance of magnesium intake and also perhaps of phosphorus intake, whether it be in the form of inorganic phosphorus or of a phosphorus protein such as casein or of say phosphorus as phytate, because I think all these three factors interact quite considerably in modifying zinc absorption and also the absorption of manganese, iron and copper from the gut. Systematic study of this has been done in this area in animals. Then on top of that there's the work, of course, done by Britt-Marie Sandström and her colleagues in Gothenburg where, as you know, there is obviously some effect of calcium, shown on the bioavailability of some of these metals.

Over and above this, one has to also consider the effect of calcium metabolism on bone turnover and on those elements which get sequestered in bone. If one prevents bone turnover, especially in children by putting them on high-calcium diets, you can, in fact, modify their susceptibility to zinc deficiency and possibly to other toxicities. It's a very complex area and it would take a far longer contribution than this to cover it.

JACKS: If I have understood correctly, you've asked in what form elements are taken up by plants. That should be in free ionic form or in the form of simple inorganic complexes. The organic complexes, for instance, tend to set off toxicity of aluminium in soils, so these complexes are far too big to be taken up as such.

WEISMANN: I want to comment on the question about calcium and zinc. You know, after the war, in America there was a disease among pigs called porcine parakeratosis and it was produced by a high calcium content in the fodder. When it was discovered, all the pigs became normal and their skin diseases disappeared. Of course, no human beings live on a diet similar to that of the pigs, but I think we still need research on this subject especially among pregnant women, because they're also very often taking calcium tablets.

AGGETT: Yes, the pigs, of course, with porcine keratosis were also on a soy-based diet and as was shown subsequently by Boyd O'Dell and others this was related also to the phytate content. There's no doubt that calcium and phytate do interact but there seems to be evidence that calcium, phytate and also magnesium interact synergistically to compromise zinc metabolism and probably that of other elements as well. In terms of direct human experience with calcium, this was actually exploited by two physicians in Manchester, U.K. in one case of acrodermatitis enteropathica where it was wanted to confirm the diagnosis. Their patient, an adolescent, was slow to respond symptomaticaly to a low-zinc diet and they eventually managed to show her susceptibility to zinc deficiency by giving her a high-calcium diet.

WEISMANN: I think the cause of the porcine parakeratosis was due to a diet made of bone. I don't think it was phytate, I think it was calcium from organic material.

ANDERSON: We've heard a number of comments concerning how calcium affects absorption of other trace elements, almost as if calcium is a bad actor, but I really think that we should also point out that low calcium intake, especially in older women, is one of the most serious nutritional problems that we have. For example, more women die from breaking their hips each year, which can certainly be prevented by calcium and exercise, than actually die of breast cancer. So, when saying for example, that calcium adversely affects zinc metabolism, we need to keep it in perspective and, especially in women, the calcium intake, if anything, shouldn't be reduced but it definitely should be increased.

HURLEY: I think this is just another example, a very good example, showing the problems of interactions and that it's hard to do only one thing. Everything that we do affects something else and so we have to have enough calcium, but we also have to have enough zinc so that the additional calcium doesn't produce zinc deficiency.

CHRISTOPHERSEN: I would just like to ask somebody about possible causes of geographical differences in calcium metabolism, because it is known from studies in Britain, at least, that one can achieve a neutral calcium balance in post-menopausal women by giving them about 1.5 g of calcium per day. So, apparently, calcium deficiency is very common in some of the industrial countries of Western Europe. But, if we compare this with other parts of the world, for instance, Norway (Oslo) is on the top of the list on the prevalence of osteoporosis and, at the same time, Norway is one of the countries in the world with perhaps the highest milk consumption, only Finland is still higher. On the other hand Singapore, with a population many of whom are ethnic Chinese who don't drink milk, has much less osteoporosis as indicated, say, by the frequency of hip fracture. So I think one may conclude that the calcium requirement for women in Singapore is probably much lower than it is in Norwegian or British women, but why?

AGGETT: I have a basic comment. I think, first, that the only constructive thing I can say is that it sounds like a topic which could well, in terms of the high incidence of mortality associated with it, benefit from a further Skandia symposium. But I think, as you imply, it's more than just calcium intake. It is a matter, as I understand, of exercise. It's also a matter of knowing how that calcium is metabolized in general terms, in terms of vitamin D and protein and osteoid metabolism as well. I just don't know enough about calcium metabolism to actually comment on that area.

BOSTRÖM: Perhaps I could add a little to this discussion. As far as I know, it's well known by Professor Nikolaussen's studies in Norway some decades ago that you can have an adaptation on various levels of calcium. You can have a normal calcium balance on various levels due to adaptation, not necessarily genetic. I think this was shown in people who were kept on an extremely low calcium diet for a very long time and finally they showed up with a normal calcium balance on a very, very low level.

HURLEY: Another problem is that calcium balance is a very poor index of calcium needs and requirements because of the release of calcium from bone, so that you can have calcium balance but still be releasing calcium from the bone in order to maintain plasma calcium levels. It's not a very good way of measuring calcium status.

KIILERICH: In Denmark, we have made a study where we have treated patients with chronic renal failure with calcium and different vitamin D metabolites and we saw, of course, that the concentration of calcium in serum and in urine was increased. But there was no difference in the values of zinc in serum or urine even if you corrected it for albumin. So we don't think that zinc and calcium are absorbed in the same way from the gastrointestinal tract.

FRANK: I would like to leave this very interesting discussion about calcium, and comment on Dr Aggett's presentation of Kovalsky's results from 1961. In Scandinavia, we have a disease in sheep, the chronic copper toxicosis. This is a problem in both Sweden and Norway. A research group in Norway has been working with this problem and they have found very interesting results. They found that sheep sometimes get copper toxicosis but also copper deficiency in places located very close to each other. Their investigation showed that it is not the absolute value of copper and molybdenum which is important, but the relationship between the molybdenum and the copper in this case.

AGGETT: Yes, that's quite right. I was hoping perhaps Dr Jacks could comment and I think I'll still leave an open end for him if he can but, for example, it certainly is a question of the alkalinity of the soil and the redox potential as well. Molybdenum is far less available from an acid soil than it is from an alkaline soil. I think one of the fascinating things that occurred in Norway was, in fact, that in some areas where the condition occurred, nitrate fertilizers were actually being used. I think this would increase the acidity of the soil and at the same time reduce the bioavailability of molybdenum. It just goes again to show how all of these sort of technological innovations, and implementation of them at no matter what level of the food chain, have the most unexpected results.

AHLROT-WESTERLUND: I would like to try to answer or at least comment on Dr Christophersen's question about possible causes of the differencies in calcium metabolism between post-menopausal women in Singapore and, for instance, those in Norway. Apart from what has been said about influences from hormones, vitamins and other substances interfering with calcium metabolism, the diet in Singapore is mainly of a vegetable kind and this makes calcium more available. In

Norway, the food is mainly based on animal proteins which might influence the metabolism in an acidic direction and as a consequence decrease the calcium uptake.

SALONEN: Coming back to the osteoporosis, I think Finland is a good example of a case where there is an extremely high intake of calcium from the diet. There is a low intake of fluoride from the diet and there are several studies that point out that the low intake of fluoride is also increasing the risk of osteoporosis in post-menopausal women.

JACKS: I would first like to direct a question to Dr Salonen. Do you have less osteoporosis in Karelia, then, because you have lots of fluoride there?

SALONEN: Well, we know that the fluoride intake is low in the eastern parts of Finland using a method based on urine determinations. There are differences in the soil. I don't know details, but I do know that the incidence and the prevalence of osteoporosis is generally high in Finland and the fluoride intake, estimated, based on urinary excretions of fluoride is low.

JACKS: You should have high contents of fluoride in southeastern Finland because you have such rocks there.

SALONEN: Let me point out that there is a big geographical difference between southern eastern parts and eastern parts of Finland so that the soil content and drinking water content of fluoride is high in the southern parts only but not in the middle parts of eastern Finland.

JACKS: I could comment on the alkalinity of soils. As far as I know there are examples from Great Britain where you had cattle grazing on coal ashes covered by a very thin soil cover. Coal ashes are alkaline and I think you had copper deficiency in those cases.

ANDERSON: We've heard a number of things about high calcium intake, for example, in the Scandinavian countries where you have high calcium intake and you also have high incidences of osteoporosis. But I think another thing that hasn't been mentioned here is phosphate intake itself. In the United States, especially in young women who try to watch their weight by drinking diet colas, they have found that the bone strength, the bone mineral content, is greatly decreased in these people, lower than one would expect just from their calcium intake and they think this may be related to their high phosphate intake from the colas.

HALL: I would like to ask if it is recommendable to give iron supplementation to blood donors or shouldn't I do it at all?

AGGETT: Are they anaemic? Do they need iron?

HALL: I don't think most of them need it. Very few are anaemic. We can find low serum ferritin but, mostly, no sign of anaemia at all.

AGGETT: If they have a low serum ferritin and you have reason to suspect the iron stores are reduced, do you think that it's right that they should actually be giving blood?

Sample Collection, Treatment, Preservation and Storage of Biomedical Specimens for Trace Element Analysis

Quality Assurance Considerations

By Venkatesh Iyengar

Among trace element researchers dealing with biological systems, there is mounting concern that the elemental composition data, especially for trace elements at lower concentration levels, are inaccurate (Iyengar et al. 1978, Parr 1980, Versieck & Cornelis 1980, Iyengar 1982a & b, Talanta 1982, Heydorn 1984, Versieck 1984). Major efforts are therefore necessary to generate reproducible and reliable results to build up a reference data base for human tissues and body fluids. Unless this is achieved, true variations in elemental concentrations arising from physiological changes, pathological influences and occupational and environmental exposures remain submerged in the wide ranges of the largely uncontrolled analytical data. This being the case, very little progress can be achieved in applying the knowledge gained from trace element studies to practical problems in human health.

The purpose of this report is to identify the special difficulties associated with biomedical systems which are aimed at elemental composition studies as opposed to inorganic systems. The main emphasis will be placed on the *quality* of the sample by elaborating the influence of various presampling factors and other problems related to sampling, preservation, storage and specimen preparation for assay, as illustrated in Fig. 1.

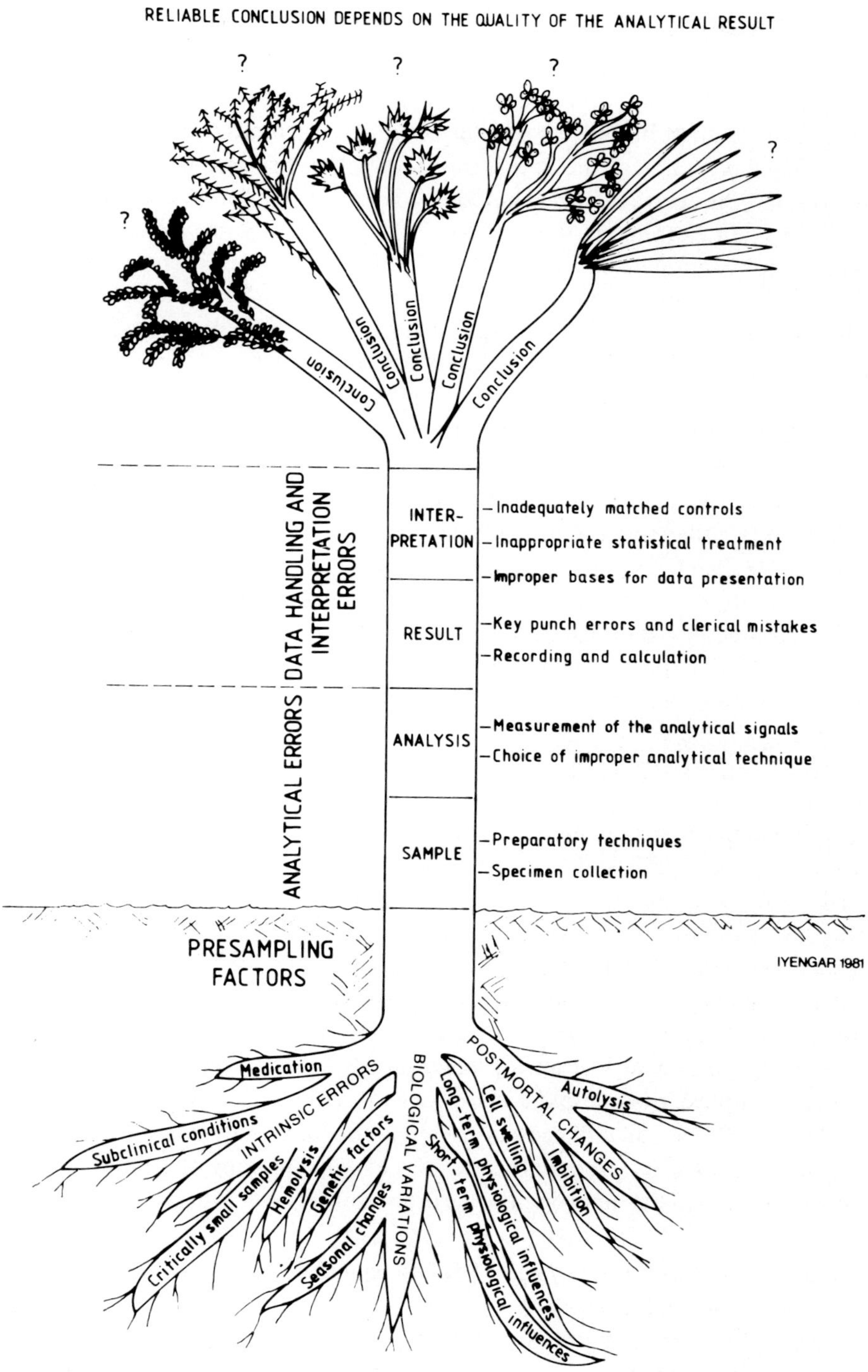

Fig. 1 Elemental analysis of biological systems

QUALITY, QUALITY ASSURANCE AND QUALITY CONTROL

A major consideration in any analytical measurement is the *quality* of the sample, where quality refers to the degree to which a sampled portion retains its original properties after it is removed from its original environment. However, not all the properties in the parent source may be retained always and the consequenses should be viewed in relation to the problem at hand. A good example is that of blood plasma and serum. Plasma is more suitable for a number of clinical investigations but when it comes to trace element determinations serum is to be preferred because of the problems of contamination from anticoagulants. This is very well illustrated with an element such as Cr. Considering that one needs about 4 mg of ethylene diamine teatraacetic acid (EDTA) per ml of blood, and assuming that the entire EDTA remains with plasma, it can be seen that the absolute content of 1.2 ng of Zn introduced as contamination does not affect the analysis of Zn, whereas, for Cr, the quantity introduced (0.2 ng) is entirely unacceptable, and the analysis is invalid (Table 1).

It should also be recognised that the analysis of trace elements in biological materials is more meaningful when the elemental data are related to other parameters such as certain cells, cellular components, enzymes or proteins. Under these circumstances, the specimen collection and preparatory techniques must be capable of preserving the biological integrity of the sample.

Quality assurance involves a set of measures that should be looked upon as mandatory. These involve among others, development of an adequate sampling approach well ahead of the start of an investigation, steps to avoid contamination and loss of the analyte as well as retaining the integrity of the analytical signal. Several aspects of a good protocol have been discussed by Heydorn (1984). For example, every sample should have an individual record revealing details of the health status of the subject, habits, etc. It must be emphasized that there is no match for a thorough documentation of the history of the sample. This may save much of the frustration while interpreting the results of an investigation. It is apt to quote Thiers in this context: "unless the complete history of the sample is known with certainty, the analyst is well advised not to spend his time analyzing it."

Quality control is essentially the process of ensuring the factors mentioned under quality and quality assurance. However, in practice several

Table 1 Elemental impurities in EDTA (ng/g dry substance)[1]
Data from Behne 1983

Element	Ag	Co	Cr	Cs	Fe	Rb	Sb	Se	Zn
Impurity	1	3.2	50	0.2	1100	10	1.5	15	300

[1] Merck, p.a. quality

difficulties are encountered, especially in testing the various stages of sampling and handling. The best way is to carry out replicate analysis of both known (e.g., standard reference materials) (SRM) and unknown compositions. Use of simulated samples of high purity components (e.g., high purity water) and matrices of low levels of concentration for trace elements (e.g., potato powder or animal muscle in some cases) is helpful to detect the pick up of contamination, if any.

PRESAMPLING FACTORS

Essentially, presampling factors may be defined as events associated with a biological specimen *in situ* and before the arrival of the sample at the laboratory for analysis. Thus, a host of factors such as biological variations, post-mortem changes, intrinsic and inadvertent errors, preferential accumulation in selected organs or within an organ, etc. fall in this group.

Several examples may be offered to illustrate the effect of these factors (Iyengar 1982a). "Status at sampling" (physiological and others, Table 2) is a good example that is relevant to routine sampling situations and reflects the numerous sources of variability. Concerning normal human tissues, barring a few specimens such as blood, excretory products and occasional

Table 2 Influence of "status at sampling" on the concentration of selected elements in human subjects: Some examples.

Sample	Element	Condition	Influence	Remarks
Serum	Zn	Fasting	Elevated	Elevated also during overnight fasting
		After food	Lowered	Lowered during the first few hours
		Stress	Elevated	Standing posture
		Sea food	Elevated	E.g., oyster
		Low Zn intake	Lowered	Effect rather sudden
		Pregnancy	Lowered	Progressive decline
Serum	F	Fasting	Normal	Overnight fasting
		After food	Variable	Sampled immediately
		Intake of tea	High	Sampled immediately
		Low F intake	Lowered	Over a few days
Serum	I	High I intake, e.g., sea food, excess intake of iodinated salts, etc.	Elevated	Uptake is rapid but decline is slow because of 2.5 weeks biological half life
Serum	As	Consumption of shrimps	Normal	Negligible absorption
		Consumption of fish	Elevated	Well absorbed and slowly excreted
Blood	Cd	Smoking	Elevated	Remains chronically high in smokers
	Pb	Alcohol	Elevated	E.g., wine drinkers

biopsy samples which are obtainable from living subjects, most other samples must be sought during an autopsy. Under these circumstances, presampling factors play a large role and sample characterization is not easy.

Biological variations. These may be divided into genetic factors, long- and short-term physiological influences and seasonal changes.

Genetic predisposition of human subjects belonging to different racial groups is an example in this context.

Long-term physiological influences include age, sex, geographical and environmental factors, diet, habit, pregnancy and lactation, to mention a few. These involve many *in-vivo* factors that may influence the analytical result. *Short-term influences* can be regarded as those which affect the system over short periods. Thus, circadian rhythm, recent food, posture and stress can be grouped under this. However, the definition of long- and short-term influences is somewhat arbitrary since such factors as diet and habit (e.g., smoking) often overlap. Thus, habitual diet may be regarded as a long-term effect, while a single meal may be looked upon as a short-term effect.

Seasonal changes can be grouped as either physiological or climatic. The combined influence of these two factors has been previously illustrated through various examples by Iyengar (1981a). In humans, changes brought about by summer may be explained through recreational activities, differences in diets due to the availability of fresh fruits and vegetables, and changes in the excretory patterns because of excessive sweating.

Post-mortem changes. These changes mainly involve three stages: cell-swelling, imbibition and autolysis. These changes can introduce great variations in elemental concentration and content. For example, it has been shown that retaining the liver inside intact carcasses for prolonged periods of time under different conditions induces fluctuation in tissue weight and elemental composition. Both concentration and content of electrolytes and trace elements, such as Co, Cs, Cu, Fe, Mn, Rb, Se and Zn, varied up to 50 per cent with respect to control values. The levels of Ca were shown to increase to very high levels extending to a factor of 6 due to mobilization from residual food in the stomach (Iyengar 1981b).

Intrinsic errors. These errors reflect the factors inherently present in the sample that may falsify the results. These errors, as the definition itself suggests, are difficult to detect and the analyst has little or no control over them. Good examples in this context are medication, haemolysis, subclinical conditions and certain inescapable medical restrictions.

Besides intrinsic errors, sometimes errors may be introduced *inadvertently*. These may happen while dealing with critically small samples (e.g., needle biopsies) due to changes in humidity in the sample environment thereby presenting formidable difficulties in assessing the correct weight of the sample material. Retaining viability of the cells in some cases (e.g., platelets) until the samples are safely contained is yet another example of this situation.

Differences between organ segments. Significant differences in trace element concentrations among specific segments of an organ such as kidney, brain and bone are well known. Careful sectioning is necessary in order to appreciate these differences.

SAMPLING

It should be mentioned at the outset that there is no single best method of sampling. Further, sampling errors are rather special in that they cannot be controlled by the use of blanks, standards or reference materials and require to be treated separately. No amount of care during the analysis can compensate and guarantee reliable information if an error has been introduced during the collection of specimens and subsequent handling. Thus, the problem of an "invalid" sample is something inherent in nature, and considerable thought should therefore be devoted to procure "valid" samples by introducing stringent precautions already at the planning stage of the investigation so that the specimen analysed truly represents the object under study. Also, as analytical methodologies have improved, the need for smaller analytical portions or aliquots has also been growing. This has increased the risks of errors from sampling operations since sample heterogeneity can pose a major problem.

As a general rule, the analyst himself should be directly involved in the sampling procedure in order to ensure that the samples are representative, and that no significant changes in composition occur during sampling, transport and storage. When medical restrictions prevent the analyst from applying special sampling procedures, the medical staff should be familiar with the requirements of valid sampling.

Basic hazards. There are a few basic hazards faced in all the steps of sampling, storage, pretreatment and analysis. These are contamination by elements, loss of elements and changes in mean composition with respect to the elements to be determined (Sansoni & Iyengar 1980). Contamination is by far the most serious threat, especially at ultra trace level analysis. A striking, but by no means atypical, illustration of this problem is provided by observations of inadequately collected and processed serum samples for the determination of Mn (Versieck 1983). In nine samples transferred with an automatic dispenser (inadequate procedure), the following results were obtained: 4.83 ± 5.17 micro g per L with a range of 0.61 to 16.81 micro g per L. On the other hand, with inadequately handled samples from the same serum pool, using exactly the same analytical procedure, the following values were measured: 0.72 ± 0.1 micro g per L with a range of 0.56 to 0.89 micro g per L, i.e., a factor of almost 7 lower.

Sampling procedures for solids. Sampling of solids is often more complex than that of pure liquids. As a general rule, the homogeneity of the total sample and of subsamples should never be assumed to be satisfactory until this has been proved. Because of the lower reactivity of solids, the dangers of contamination from container walls, etc., losses of trace elements due to absorption and other effects and changes in mean composition are generally smaller than with liquids. Autopsy sampling from human cases needs to be carried out under standard conditions, e.g., time of sampling after death. These aspects have been dealt with by Iyengar previously (1980).

Sampling procedures for liquids. For liquids the problems of heterogeneity and sampling statistics are generally less difficult than for solids because of the relatively high degree of homogeneity. In the case of suspensions or emulsions it has to be decided whether these should be sampled whole or whether the phases should be sampled separately. If necessary, the phases of suspensions or emulsions can be separated and weighed before analysis, in order to determine their elemental contents separately and to arrive at the values of the whole sample by calculation.

Timed collection is necessary for several body fluids, for example a 24-hour collection period for urine samples.

Transporting liquid samples to the laboratory presents more difficulties than dealing with solid samples. Stringent precautions are necessary as discussed elsewhere (Sansoni & Iyengar 1980).

PRESERVATION AND STORAGE

Preservation essentially relates to the process of retaining morphological and cellular integrity of an organ or tissue. Therefore, under ideal preservation conditions, specimens so protected may be expected to retain the natural chemical forms of the elements. *Storage*, on the other hand, especially from the trace element studies point of view, basically implies an overall safe, clean, uncontaminated and non-degraded containment.

Preservation of a sampled specimen is largely dependent upon the matrix properties, the time span available between collection and transport to the laboratory and subsequent handling for analysis. For example, preserving bone, hair or nail is relatively simple when compared to brain, liver, lung or kidney. The conventional method of treating the latter group of samples with formaldehyde is generally unacceptable due to contamination and leaching problems. Therefore, the alternate method of preservation by freezing should be preferred. For short-term preservation temperatures of 2–4°C (normal refrigeration) are low enough. Long-term preservation should generally be done by deep-freezing below −15°C. Where possible, e.g., autopsy cases, animal experiments, whole organ or big chunks of tissues, such as muscle, should be preserved with original capsules. Samples can be sealed in clean polyethylene (PE) bags and packed in plastic

Table 3 Some examples of established storage conditions for blood and urine

Lead in blood Human and cow blood	Conditions: EDTA used as anticoagulant, haemolysed by ulstrasonication, stored for 4 weeks in polypropylene tubes and recovery investigated at				
Vahter (1982)	−20°C	+4°C	+20°C	+37°C	
	(recovery 100 per cent)		Unpredictable, clotting at 6 h		
Cadmium in blood	Conditions same as for lead, 12 weeks				
Vahter (1982)	Recovery 87–100 per cent Temperatures tested: +4 and +22°C				
Mercury in urine	Days	0	3	7	14
Trujillo et al. (1974)	Polyethylene	100[1]	101	87	6
	Pyrex glass	100	94	85	93
	+ $K_2S_2O_8$ (preservative) 100% for both				

[1] per cent recovery

containers with tight caps and enclosing the whole thing in an additional PE bag, if necessary.

Storage of specimens either directly afte sampling or from primary preserved material may become necessary for several reasons. In such cases, freeze-drying is well suited. Even oven-drying at relatively low temperatures, e.g., at 80°C, may be employed. In all cases, certain basic precautions are necessary and exceptions have to be made with respect to some elements. Storage containers should be made of non-porous, smooth and non-wettable, e.g., teflon, walls. The total surface area of the container and the free space in it should be kept to a minimum. Prevention of humidity and a dust-free storage compartment is mandatory. If suitably packed, dry samples can be stored for long periods of time under cold storage.

Container material, humidity, pH, temperature and duration of storage are firmly linked to contamination and originality of the sample because of adsorption, leaching and biochemical interactions. Extensive trials were needed to optimize conditions for storing blood for Pb and Cd (Vahter 1982) and lyophilized serum proteins for Se and other elements (Thomassen 1982). In freeze-dried form serum protein can be stored for up to three years at −20°C. After reconstruction, the duration of storage is reduced drastically: one month at −20°C, four days at 2–8°C and only eight hours at room temperature. Use of polycarbonate tubes is adequate for storage of serum and plasma for up to two weeks under refrigeration temperature. Table 3 elucidates a few conditions that are very useful.

SAMPLE PREPARATION

The sample obtained by a sampling operation generally has to be reduced in amount by subsampling in the laboratory to provide the much smaller size of sample that is actually analysed. Such operations with solid samples involve washing, drying, ashing, powdering, homogenization and homogeneity tests, if required. Body fluids are generally heterogeneous suspensions or emulsions. For these, a separation into pure liquid and solid phases or stabilization and homogenization of the suspension or the emulsion, followed by homogeneity tests, have to be considered. The reader may refer to the generalised sample preparation scheme which may be used as a check list for outlining the working steps (Iyengar & Sansoni 1980).

All the above mentioned sample manipulations are prone to contamination, loss of elements and change in mean composition of the sampled material and call for careful selection of methods of sample treatments, clean handling environment and tools that are compatible with the analytical requirement. Therefore, it is a good practice on the part of the analyst, firstly, to assess all the potential sources of error within his working environment under realistic conditions; secondly, to take measures to minimise the impact of such errors, and thirdly, to maintain appropriate monitoring of surface and other contaminations at regular intervals. For example, contamination introduced (leaching) or analyte lost (adsorption) can be studied by preparing a particular type of sample in containers of different materials as illustrated by Damsgaard et al. (1973) for Mn in serum.

The analytical laboratory. The danger of contamination by elements is a relative concept, and as a rule, the hazards of potential contamination should be kept small in relation to the concentration level sought in the sample. For example, Cr, Mn and Pb are more easily susceptible to airborne contamination than a few other elements. An example is given in Table 4 which shows a comparison of particulates in the air of an ordinary laboratory, a clean room and a class 100 hood (Murphy 1976). Both the clean room and the class 100 hood air showed a dramatic reduction in contamination. The concentrations of Pb were reduced by a factor of 200, and other elements which were already low to start with were further reduced by a factor of 10.

The impact of operating personnel in the laboratory through sweat, cosmetics, tobacco ash and smoke poses a real threat. Strict adherence to good laboratory practices such as use of separate sets of plastic and glassware for handling of standards; separate cleaning of these wares; and not preparing the standards in the same room as the sample, keeping the working table

Table 4 Particulate concentration in laboratory air (micro g/cubic m)

Element	Iron	Copper	Lead	Cadmium
Ordinary lab	0.2	0.02	0.4	0.002
Clean room	0.001	0.002	0.0002	nd
Clean hood	0.0009	0.007	0.0003	0.0002

nd=not detected

free of loose surface contamination and factors that contribute to it, e.g., marking pens, used hand gloves and tissue paper, etc., are all helpful aspects.

Materials. The primary concern from sample handling point of view is to obtain tools and containers made of materials of very low concentration of trace elements of interest. At the moment there seem to be no good alternatives to plastic, quartz and some high purity metals of which Ti has been slowly gaining popularity. If technical problems in obtaining a durable sharp edge for the sample handling tools made of Ti can be overcome, this should help solve an important problem of manufacturing a standardized kit of instruments for tissue handling. Efforts on these lines are required rather urgently.

Use of stainless steel knives continues to be controversial (Versieck & Speecke 1972, Heit & Klusek 1982). Heit and Klusek (1982) compared the effects of dissecting tools made of stainless steel, Lexan plastic, titanium and teflon-coated stainless steel and concluded that for Al, Cd, Cr, Cu, Hg, Ni, Pb, Se, Sn, Te and V there were no significant differences in fish or muscle samples. However, the purpose of the analysis, i.e. the elements determined and the levels of concentration involved, is the deciding factor for the handling of the samples and many practical solutions are possible. For example, use of a Ti knife or a Ni needle should not present any problems as long as these elements are not sought in the respective samples. Therefore, depending upon the analytical purpose, e.g., Se, Hg and Pb, even stainless steel knives may be acceptable for use. In all cases, disposable plastic gloves, teflon tweezers, PE and teflon foils and wax paper are very useful aids.

Cleaning procedures. Since the sample container represents one of the principal sources of sample contamination, much of the analytical accuracy will not only depend on the choice of the container materials but also on the procedures used to clean them. For example, the need for etching the inner surface of quartz tubes to a depth of about 20 micro metres using HF in order to remove surface contamination from Cr, La, Co, Zn, Fe and Au has been demonstrated by Maziere et al. (1976). This is crucial if samples are irradiated in quartz tube for neutron activation analysis (NAA). Several laboratories have established standard washing procedures to clean laboratory wares. For example, the methods used to clean glassware (Levi & Purdy 1980), plastic containers (Moody & Lindstrom 1975), quartz (Cornelis et al. 1978) and metal knives (Harrison 1981) are adequate and may be followed.

Practical handling steps for fluids. Biological fluids are more susceptible to bacterial growth in an unfrozen state and sample preparation should be finished preferably within 24 hours. Since most biological fluids are suspensions or emulsions, care should be taken to select the phase of interest, or in the case of the whole sample, to ensure that the phases are properly mixed.

Handling of blood to obtain serum or plasma is a common requirement in many laboratories. In this case, it is important to minimize haemolysis by gentle handling, use of dry syringe, slow transfer to dry test tube and sufficient time for clotting. The clotting of blood takes about 15 minutes at room temperature, but is delayed if siliconized glassware, teflon or PE-containers are used. Fractionation of blood by centrifugation is done at about 300 revolutions per minute for 5 to 10 minutes. The contents of the tube should be kept closed to avoid contamination and evaporation. For plasma, blood containing an anticoagulant is handled in the same way as obtaining serum. Depending upon the degree of *haemolysis*, serum values of elements such as K, Zn and Fe may be affected. Kasperek et al. (1981) investigated the influence of haemolysis on serum elemental concentrations of Cs, Co, Fe, Hg, Rb, Se and Zn. Of these elements, Fe, Rb and Zn showed significantly higher concentrations in serum than in plasma; the average differences were 320, 12 and 20 ng per ml for Fe, Rb and Zn, respectively.

Individual working steps for handling various other body fluids such as urine, milk, cerebro-spinal fluid and sweat are discussed in earlier reports (Iyengar & Sansoni 1980, Iyengar 1983).

Practical handling steps for solids. The rationale of washing some type of samples such as autopsy specimens, hair and nail prior to analysis is to minimize the influence of residual blood or its components for the former and to remove non-intrinsic elemental contamination for the latter two tissues. In the case of hair, this prewashing step is also helpful in eliminating most of Na, an advantageous factor for gamma ray measurements. Because of the diversity of this problem, consensus on the type and extent of washing to be undertaken in the case of hair and nail, and whether the excised tissue from autopsy should be washed or merely just rinsed with water, is a very difficult proposition. Depletion extending up to 30 per cent has been reported for the electrolyte elements whereas protein-bound elements such as Cu and Zn are affected to a much lesser extent by washing samples of liver with water (Iyengar 1981).

Concerning hair there appears to be controversial findings as a result of various washing procedures, some adopted as standard methods. For example, a mild and highly reproducible preirradiation washing procedure using succesively acetone, water, water, water and acetone (Ryabukin 1980), has been found to be unsuitable for Cr analysis (Kumpulainen et al. 1982), because the Cr concentration continued to decline with lengthy washing. According to the latter investigator, sodium lauryl sulphate and hexane ethanol are the most reliable washing agents for hair intended for Cr analysis. Similarly, doubts are also expressed concerning Cd (Salmela et al. 1981). Further evidence of the unsuitability of the acetone wash has been reported by Das et al. (1981) who found that levels of As, Co, Cr, Fe and Hg dropped sharply after the first wash and remained approximately constant thereafter.

On the whole, the effects of washing treatments on the elemental composition profiles of biological specimens is still an open question and a few selected combinations of treatments may be necessary to answer different analytical situations. More investigations are needed to draw firm conclusions.

Drying. It is important to control temperature while oven-drying biological specimens. Temperatures exceeding 100°C are not recommended since this leads to matrix decomposition depending upon the type of the tissue. Elements such as Hg, I and Sn are lost from urine, muscle and liver even at 80°C. These and other aspects concerning a few more elements such as Cd and Cr are discussed elsewhere (Iyengar & Sansoni 1980, Iyengar 1983).

Freeze-drying is also known as lyophilization or vacuum freeze-drying and is basically well suited for drying biological samples. It involves three stages: namely prefreezing, primary and secondary drying. Ensuring an adequate vacuum and prefreezing the samples before lyophilization are important to achieve good retention yields and for preventing contamination. Failure of the vacuum may lead to thawing of the frozen sample promoting sample container interactions thereby losing the advantage of the frozen state. For this reason, it is better to control the sample-cooling separately by an additional pump which is not part of the freeze drier system. Also, care should be taken to prevent metallic contamination from the housing of the freeze drier, using non-metallic components, e.g., perspex for sample housing. One disadvantage of freeze-drying is that fluids such as urine are hygroscopic (Cornelis et al. 1975) and care is necessary to avoid errors from this source. For these reasons, if the analytical technique permits, analysis of whole urine is recommended. Freeze-drying has been used satisfactorily and for several elements in a variety of samples with occasional exceptions for Hg (Iyengar 1983).

Ashing. Ashing is the process of removal of the organic matrix by converting to gaseous components, then eliminating them to obtain a solid inorganic residue. Among the various ashing methods, dry-ashing with air in an open muffle furnace, or by oxygen plasma at temperatures below 150°C and wet-ashing with various acid mixtures are of importance. Dry-ashing around 500°C is effective even for big samples but has the disadvantage of voltilization of a number of elements. On the positive side, dry-ashing does not require the addition of chemicals. In low-temperature ashing, the decomposition which is brought about by nascent oxygen is essentially a surface phenomenon and, therefore, some sort of a sample agitation will be required to accelerate the rate of ashing. It is effective for small-size samples only and the method is not totally safe for volatile elements. Wet-washing, where applicable, is recommended since it is faster, efficient and results in lower losses of trace elements. A survey of the loss of elements from different biomatrices under different ashing conditions has been presented by Iyengar and Sansoni in their earlier report (1980).

Homogenization. Where possible, liquid biological samples should be aliquoted in fluid state since it is relatively simple to retain homogeneity in this form and to dispense efficiently. With adequate care, even fluids such as whole blood can be dealt with satisfactorily, provided that care is taken to recover the entire sample aliquot during the analysis. Frozen fluids should be allowed to thaw completely and be stirred well to overcome concentration gradients before dispensing.

With the exception of a few solid tissue samples such as hair and nail, most biological tissue samples are intricately mixed with other body components such as connective tissue, capsule, layers of skin, fat, blood vessels, nerves, hair (during sampling of skin), glandular parts, GI-tract contents, residual blood, decidual tissues, sweat, extracellular fluids, etc. Some of these interfering components are very difficult to remove without severely damaging the integrity of the parent tissue. Since the interfering components have differing elemental composition profiles, and their total exclusion from a given sample is not always possible, for this reason alone, basically, some degree of heterogeneity should always be anticipated among aliquots of a particular sample analysed without prior homogenization. Moreover, at cellular level also, the distribution may be expected to be non-homogeneous because of the structure of the cell itself. Therefore, strictly speaking, there is an inherent lack of homogeneity in biological tissue samples. However, with adequate precautions it is possible to collect a satisfactory sample of a certain tissue for practical use.

In general, the problem of homogenization of biological materials may be viewed as follows:

As the quantity of the sample material increases, the need for homogenization also increases. This, for example, is the case with SRMs.

For samples such as composite meal and faeces, although these are smaller in volume with respect to SRMs, homogenization is inevitable.

On the other hand, for muscle and liver, if the interfering components are carefully sorted out to minimize their presence during the sample handling stage as shown by the example of liver (Iyengar & Kasperek 1976, Lievens et al. 1977), the problem of heterogeneity, e.g., for an element such as Zn, does not appear to be serious. By analysing multiple aliquots from such sample sources, reasonably good results can be obtained without having to place the blame entirely on heterogeneity.

Brain and lung present a mixed situation. By proper segregation of anatomical regions which are more meaningful to analyse, inhomogeneity can be vastly controlled. In the case of lung, special treatment may be necessary if there is visible deposition of particles. However, when the information is needed for whole brain or lung, then one should resort to homogenization.

The case of kidney is somewhat different and provides a good example where even small sections of anatomically segregated parts such as cortex and medulla require homogenization prior to analysis. This is because metal sequestration within the kidney is site-dependent (Livingstone 1971).

Sample homogenization, when necessary, may be achieved for both wet and dry tissues. Cryogenic homogenization techniques (Iyengar & Kasperek 1976) are generally well suited to powder the samples. For samples which are of the order of a few hundred g, the disc mill type (Zeisler et al. 1983) which is in use at the National Bureau of Standards, Washington, is recommendable. The disc mill mode is an improved version of the brittle fracture technique proposed by Iyengar and Kasperek (1976).

CONCLUSIONS

Greater effort is needed on the part of biomedical trace element researchers to obtain "valid" samples for the analysis. Unless sample quality is improved by taking adequate precautions against presampling factors, poor results continue to pile up.

There is a need for standardizing sampling and storage conditions for autopsy samples aimed at elemental composition studies. Presampling factors should be considered carefully in this context. Unless these measures are incorporated into the sampling plans it will not be possible to reveal the true biological variations of the elemental composition of biological systems. Therefore, very little progress may be anticipated in terms of practical applications.

Much has been learned in the past years about quality control factors that play a vital role starting from the presampling stage to data interpretation of trace element studies in biological systems. However, much of the information on quality control has not yet reached the bench workers, who are ultimately behind the large mass of analytical data that enter the literature. The implications of the many intriguing factors and their control or even recognition at the right time involve the competence of several disciplines.

Thorough documentation of the sample history should be practised in every laboratory as a routine.

It is imperative that analysts be associated with trace element investigations in biological systems at the planning stage and not just from the moment a sample arrives at the laboratory.

REFERENCES

BEHNE, D. (1983). Personal communication.

CORNELIS, R., SPEECKE, E. & HOSTE, J. (1975). NAA for bulk and trace elements in urine. *Anal. Chim. Acta* 78, 317–27.

CORNELIS, R., MEES, L., HOSTE, J., RYCKENBUSCH, J., VERSIECK, J. & BARBIER, F. (1978). *Determination of V in Human Blood Serum and Liver by Radiochemical NAA*, pp. 165–177. Vienna, IAEA-SM-227.

DAMSGAARD, E., HEYDORN, K., LARSEN, N. A. & NIELSEN, B. (1973). *Simultaneous Determination of As, Mn and Se in Human Serum by NAA*. RISO Report-271, Roskilde.

DAS, H. A., DEJKUMHANG, M., HERBER, R. F. M., HOEDE, D. & VAN DER SLOOT, H. A. (1981). *Instrumental NAA of Human Hair and Related Radiotracer Experiments on Washing and Leaching*. ECN Report-107, Petten.

HARRISON, S. H. (1981). Personal communication.

HEIT, M. & KLUSEK, C. S. (1982). The effect of dissecting tools on the trace element concentrations of fish and mussel tissues. *Sci. total Environ.* 24, 129–134.

HEYDORN, K. (1984). *Neutron Activiation Analysis for Clinical Trace Element Research,* Vol. I, pp. 36–50. CRC Press, Boca Raton, Fl.

IYENGAR, G. V. (1980). Post-mortem changes of the elemental composition of autopsy specimens: Variations of K, Na, Mg, Ca, Cl, Fe, Zn, Cu, Mn & Rb in rat liver. *Sci. total Environ.* 15, 217–36.

— (1981a). Problems in trace element analysis of biological systems. In *Trace Element Metabolism in Man and Animals—4,* pp. 697–701. Ed by J. Howell. Australian Academy of Sciences, Canberra.

— (1981b). Autopsy sampling and elemental analysis: Errors arising from post mortem changes. *J. Path.* 134, 173–80.

— (1982a). Presampling factors in the elemental composition of biological systems. *Anal. Chem.* 54, 554A–558A.

— (1982b). *Elemental Composition of Human and Animal Milk: A Review*. IAEA TECDOC-269, Vienna.

— (1984). Preservation and preparation of biological materials for trace element analysis: Quality assurance considerations. In *Quality Assurance in Biomedical Neutron Activiation Analysis*, pp. 83–105. IAEA TECDOC, Vienna.

IYENGAR, G. V. & KASPEREK, K. (1976). Application of brittle fracture technique (BFT) to homogenize biological samples and some observations regarding the distribution behaviour of the trace elements at different concentration levels in a biological matrix. *J. Radio. Anal. Chem.* 39, 301–316.

IYENGAR, G. V. & SANSONI, B. (1980). Sample preparation of biological materials for trace element analysis. In *Elemental Analysis of Biological Materials,* pp. 73–101. IAEA Technical Report 197, Vienna.

IYENGAR, G. V., KOLLMER, W. E. & BOWEN, H. J. M. (1978). *The Elemental Composition of Human Tissues and Body Fluids*. Verlag Chemie Publishers, Weinheim.

KASPEREK, K., KIEM, J., IYENGAR, G. V. & FEINENDEGEN, L. E. (1981). Concentration differences between serum and plasma of the elements Co, Fe, Hg, Rb, Se and Zn determined by NAA. *Sci. total Environ.* 17, 133–143.

KUMPULAINEN, J., SALMELA, S., VUORI E. & LEHTO J. (1982). Effects of various washing procedures on the Cr content of human scalp hair. *Anal. Chim. Acta.* 138, 361–64.

LEVI, S. & PURDY, C. (1980). Continuous sampling of dialysate for the atomic absorption spectrometric determination of Cu and Zn from haemodialysis patients. *Anal. Chim. Acta* 116, 375–381.

LIEVENS, P., VERSIECK, J., CORNELIS, R. & HOSTE, J. (1977). The distribution of trace elements in normal human liver determined by semiautomated radiochemical NAA. *J. radioanal. Chem.* 37, 483–496.

LIVINGSTONE, H. D. (1971). Distribution of Zn, Cd and Hg in human kidneys. In *Trace Substances in Environmental Health–V,* pp. 399–411. Ed by D. D. Hemphill. University of Missouri, Columbia, Mo.

MAZIERE, B., GAUDRY, A., GROS, J. & COMAR, D. (1976). Biological sample contamination due to quartz container in NAA. In *Accuracy in Trace Analysis—Sampling, Sample Handling, Analysis,* pp. 593–604. Ed by P. D. LaFleur. National Bureau of Standards, Washington, D. C.

MOODY, J. R. & LINDSTROM, R. (1975). Selection and cleaning of plastic containers for storage of trace element samples. *Anal. Chem.* 47, 2264–67.

MURPHY, T. J. (1976). The role of the analytical blank in accurate trace analysis. In *Accuracy in Trace Analysis— Sampling, Sample Handling, Analysis,* pp. 509–539. Ed. by P. D. LaFleur. National Bureau of Standards, Washington, D. C.

PARR, R. M. (1980). The reliability of trace element analysis as revealed by analytical reference materials. In *Trace Element Analytical Chemistry in Biology and Medicine,* pp. 631–55. Ed. by P. Braetter and P. Schramel. De Gruyter & Co, Berlin.

RYABUKIN, S. (1980). Nuclear based methods for the analysis of trace element pollutants in human hair. *J. Radio Anal. Chem.* 60, 7–30.

SALMELA, S., VUORI, E. & KILPIO, J. O. (1981). The effect of washing procedures on the trace element content of human hair. *Anal. Chim. Acta* 125, 131–37.

SANSONI, B. & IYENGAR, G. V. (1980). Sampling of biological materials for trace element analysis. In *Trace Element Analysis of Biological Materials,* pp. 57–71. IAEA Technical Report 197, Vienna.

Talanta Special Issue (1982) 29, 963–1056.

THOMASSEN, Y. (1982). Personal communication.

TRUJILLO, P., STEIN, P. & CAMPBELL, E. (1974). The preservation and storage of urine samples for the determination of Hg. *Amer. Ind. Hyg. Ass. J.* 35, 257–261.

VAHTER, M. (1982). *Assessment of Human Exposure to Cd and Pb through Biological Monitoring,* Institute of Environmental Health, Stockholm, WHO/UNEP Report.

VERSIECK, J. (1984). Collection and manipulation of samples for trace element analysis: Quality assurance considerations. In *Quality Asurance in Biomedical Neutron Activation Analysis.* IAEA TECDOC, Vienna.

— (1984). Trace element analysis: A plea for accuracy. *Trace Elem. Med.* 1, 2–12.

VERSIECK, J. & CORNELIS, R. (1980). Normal levels of trace elements in human blood plasma or serum. *Anal. Chim. Acta,* 217–54.

VERSIECK, J. & SPEECKE, A. B. H. (1972). Contaminations induced by collection of liver biopsies and human blood. *Proc. IAEA Symp. on Nuclear Activiation Techniques in the Life Sciences,* Vienna, 39–49.

ZEISLER, R., LANGLAND, J. K. & HARRISION, S. H. (1983). Cryogenic homogenization of biological tissues. *Anal. Chem.* 55, 2431–34.

Discussion (the paper by Iyengar)

Chairman: WALDENSTRÖM

PERRY: One thing that has bothered me for some time and continues to bother me has to do with what one really means by normal, when one talks about autopsy tissue. One of the problems that I have run across, and I don't see an easy solution to, is what one uses as the normal data bank. I had an interesting experience a few years ago which left me bothered and which, I think, illustrates the problem. We were asked to look at a series of trace metals in individuals who had died in the Miami area in driving accidents, the thesis being that these were people who had smoked, had gotten too much carbon monoxide, had had some problems with cerebration, and had died in automobile accidents. We said this was fine, but what we really needed was a group of controls who were non-smokers and who otherwise were similar. We were very promptly told by the coroner that there was no such group, that the individuals who had died in automobile accidents of any kind by and large matched a particular type, that there was a life style involved, that these were smokers, drinkers, people who drove too fast, people who had a very different life style from the majority of the population. And when one stops to think of it, with relatively young age groups, any group that has died is different from the majority of the population. One can speculate that this is going to make some real difference and that the normal liver trace metal, not blood but liver or some other organ, is really going to be very difficult to obtain under these circumstances. Now, obviously, certain things are not going to change as a result of this life style, but it's very difficult to be sure what, and certain things are going to change. Do you have any suggestions as to how to get around this problem?

IYENGAR: Yes. It's something very similar to what you think: I have stopped referring to human values as "normal" values. I call them "reference values" or "reference range of values". Gross abnormalities, if any, I guess will still show up if you are using a range of values. It would be extremely impossible to pin up a single normal value, at least for human populations, and in my new report which will come out in a couple of months, I have got rid of the words "normal values". We should simply take some regional ranges. If we are lucky, we may be able to identify such ranges, even if I am not very sure of this because not all of us, unless some new experiments are undertaken with meticulous care, are ever too sure, as we showed in the case of the milk sample.

PERRY: This still leaves you somewhat uncertain, though, as to what kinds of effects the values that you find are associated with. In other words, you have a group now who you quite directly say is not normal, but it leaves you uncertain as to whether there are significant biologic effects associated with these abnormalities.

IYENGAR: I would say there's one partial way of overcoming it. Suppose we are able to pick up some truly rural populations who have not moved out much. I'm quite sure their habits would not have changed drastically. The unfortunate thing about trace element research, as I see it, is that in most of these population studies about 80% are from urban populations. Nobody has gone to the remote parts. Of the few results recorded, low values are from interior regions. We must produce more data from unexposed and geochemically different populations.

HURLEY: I was just wondering, Dr Perry, what about the victims of these drivers? There are often innocent victims who do not follow the life style that you describe; why can't they serve as controls? And, just as a comment on Dr Iyengar's response, it seems to me that you've gone around the problem by not using the word "normal" but you haven't really changed the problem at all. If you go into rural areas, you may have normal baseline levels for lead, but how do you know that would be true for zinc or some of the other essential trace elements? People in remote areas often have unusual diets and they may be either excessive or deficient.

IYENGAR: I guess I partially answered this question by saying that we should adopt a certain "range" and not a fixed value. For example (if you are really looking into two distinctly different populations, but not within the same population), in the so-called zinc deficiency areas, I could see hair values being reported as 140, 130 μg/g, while from normal areas 250, 300 μg/g. Like that you are able to pick up some gross differences. I still agree with you that this is something very difficult to reveal. For example, what sort of serum zinc value should be taken as the lower minimum for comparisons?

PERRY: Dr Hurley, we actually thought of the idea of looking at victims. There were two problems. One is that there weren't as many of them and it was hard to get them. But, in addition to that, the comment was made to me by the Dade County coroner that, really, these people weren't typical either. Most of the accidents occurred late at night and the people who were out being hit late at night were not typical of the population. There's no real way of going any further than that, but it does raise the question that the people being killed, by whatever mechanism, are really different from the rest of the population.

IYENGAR: This is a new difficulty. I am willing to keep it in mind.

ANDERSON: I'm not sure I agree that everyone who is killed is abnormal but my comment has nothing to do with that. I have a couple of comments. As far as your in-house standard for your milk samples, you concluded that the samples from Nigeria were much higher than those from Sweden and you thought that was a real difference. But with the in-house standards used by the Sweden group, you had the number one and the one used by Nigeria, you had an in-house standard of eleven. Did anyone check the in-house standard from Nigeria to see if they got the same values the Nigerians did?

IYENGAR: No. The in-house standard was not different in all of the different places. It was also developed by the central laboratory and distributed among the groups.

ANDERSON: If that's the case, why was the Nigerian group getting eleven for that value and the Swedish group getting one?

IYENGAR: What you can see in Table 1 is not Mn value but figures indicating the number of aliquots of Hm-1 analysed. HM-1 means Human Milk Standard 1.

Table 1 Total number of samples analysed
Reference samples/Actual samples = 15%

	Actual samples	HM-1	A-11
Guatemala	84	5	2
Philippines	65	11	4
Zaire	69	2	5
Sweden	32	4	3
Nigeria	18	1	2
Hungary	71	8	3
Total	339	31	19

CHRISTOPHERSEN: I would just like to ask about the manganese values. Are you planning to follow these, studying other tissue samples and enzyme values, for instance, manganese superoxide dismutase, to see if the differences you found in milk may reflect real geographical differences in the manganese status of the populations, implying that people living in many of the industrial countries have a certain optimal manganese status?

IYENGAR: We are not planning any additional biochemical studies. I agree that it would be interesting to see where these differences are, where this extra manganese is sitting.

Analytical Methods for Trace Elements in Biological Material

By Lars-Olof Plantin

Elements present in tissues or any material in lower concentrations than 100 parts per million (PPM) or 0.01% are commonly defined as trace elements. Those trace elements that are necessary for maintenance of a normal life and normal body functions are called essential trace elements. They are thus present and effective in human tissues and body fluids at extremely low concentration levels. Table 1 shows the gross elemental composition of the human body according to ICRP (1). These elements are of course not uniformly distributed in all tissues. The iron concentration in the erythrocytes is, for example, around 1,000 PPM but only a few PPM in serum. Calcium constitutes around 30% of the bone but only 40 PPM in cerebrospinal fluid. Thus, calcium is a trace element in CSF but a major constituent of bone. Trace elements are classified as essential or accidental. Table 2 shows the normal concentration of the essential trace elements in human blood

Table 1 Elemental composition of the human body
(Adapted from ref. 1)

Element	Per cent
Oxygen	63
Carbon	20
Hydrogen	10
Nitrogen	3
Calcium	1.5
Phosphorus	1.0
Potassium	0.25
Sulphur	0.2
Chlorine	0.1
Sodium	0.1
Magnesium	0.04
Iron	0.008
Trace elements	0.045

Table 2 Normal concentrations of essential trace elements in serum

Element	mg/L (PPM)
Arsenic	0.02
Cobalt	0.0003
Copper	1.0
Chromium	0.0025
Fluorine	0.02
Iodine	0.066
Iron	1.1
Manganese	0.0006
Molybdenum	0.01
Nickel	0.003
Selenium	0.08
Silicon	6.9
Tin	0.03
Vanadium	0.00003
Zinc	1.15
Possibly essential elements	
Cadmium	0.002
Lead	0.05
Mercury	0.012

serum. The table is compiled from the work by Iyengar et al. (2) with the exception of the value for Se which is the concentration found in the Swedish population (3). As we can see, many of these elements function in extremely low concentrations. Their analysis is very difficult. Several of them can be determined only with great effort and the use of the most sophisticated (and expensive) analytical equipment. Our knowledge about the concentrations of these elements in other tissues and body fluids is far from complete. It is much more fragmentary than the serum values in Table 2. Much work remains to be done in order to establish the normal concentration ranges of all elements in all body tissues and fluids. Unless we have that information we can never decide with certainty if the concentration of a specific element in a tissue sample is at a toxic, a normal or a subnormal level.

Many methods have been used for trace element analysis. In this short review, emphasis will be placed on those methods that are more general and are most used. They are listed in Table 3. Before any analytical procedure can be applied it is necessary to obtain a sample. It is no exaggeration to say that the most important steps in all analytical procedures are the sampling and the sample treatment. There is always a method or several methods available for the analysis but if the sampling is not done correctly or if the sample is treated in a wrong way it is meaningless to make the analysis. A thorough treatment of the considerations that are necessary has been given by Sansoni and Iyengar (4). See also Iyengar's contribution in this book.

Table 3 Useful methods for analysis of trace elements in biological material

---

A. *Chemical methods*
   1. Catalytic reactions
   2. Complexometric titration

B. *Electrochemical methods*
   1. Ion-selective electrodes
   2. Polarography
      a. Pulse polarography (DDP)
      b. Anodic stripping voltammetry (ASV)

C. *Optical spectrometry*
   1. Emission spectrometry
      a. Flame excitation
      b. Arc excitation
      c. Plasma excitation
      d. Laser excitation
   2. Absorption spectrometry
      a. Colorimetry
      b. Atomic absorption
   3. Fluorimetry

D. *X-ray spectrometry*
   1. Selectivity
      a. Energy dispersive
      b. Wave-length dispersive
   2. Excitation method
      a. X-ray beam (XRF)
      b. Electron beam (EMP)
      c. Proton beam (PIXE)

E. *Nuclear methods*
   1. Isotope dilution (RIA)
   2. Activation analysis
      a. Activation by thermal neutrons (NAA)
      b. Activation by photons
      c. Activation by charged particles

F. *Mass spectrometry*

CHEMICAL METHODS

There are numerous chemical analytical procedures for every element in the periodic table but very few of them possess the sensitivity and specificity necessary for trace element determination. These are procedures like catalytic reactions and complexometric procedures that are used for specific purposes (5). The expenditure for equipment and chemicals is low but these methods demand a lot of skill and time.

ELECTROCHEMICAL METHODS

A very large number of electroanalytical methods have been published. Some of them have potentially very high sensitivities such as the ion-selective electrodes. The most common of these, the pH electrode, has been around for some time for measuring the acidity of solutions. Electrodes for other ions have been available for a little more than 20 years. Some practical difficulties have limited their use. They are not as specific as the name implies and the conditions for the analysis must be rigidly controlled. Cu, F and I are the main trace elements that are measured by this technique.

Polarographic methods are based on the electrochemical reactions that occur at the surface of a newly formed mercury electrode when a potential is applied between this electrode and a reference electrode in a solution. A very large number of techniques have been developed to measure and characterise the variable current that passes between the electrodes when the potential is applied in various ways. This technique is theoretically very sensitive but the sensitivity is difficult to realise because of all sorts of parasitic reactions of a chemical and electrical nature. It has mainly been used to measure the metals Cu, Ni, Cd and Pb, for which it is very suitable and with high realistic sensitivity (of the order of nanomoles/litre). (See ref. 6 and 7.)

OPTICAL SPECTROMETRY

Optical spectrometric methods cover a great number of techniques and it could be said that the sensitivity of spectrometric methods has enabled the original detection, identification and quantitation of the trace elements. It is impossible to go into details about the different applications of these techniques. Fundamentally they work by supplying so much energy to the atoms in the sample that electrons in the outermost orbits around the nucleus are moved from one orbit to an orbit further out. The atom is said to be excited. Then the electron falls back to its original orbit and a package of energy is emitted. It is specific for the atom and the orbit and if a sufficient number of atoms are excited the emitted energy can be quantitatively measured. That is called emission spectrometry. In absorption spectrometry the cloud of excited atoms is irradiated with a beam of light formed in a special lamp by exciting the metal one wishes to determine. When this light strikes atoms of the same kind it is absorbed according to the principle just described above. The amount of absorption of the incident energy is thus a measure of the amount of that element. The higher the temperature is, the higher the sensitivity that can be obtained. The sensitivity of the emission spectrographic methods has therefore increased with the different excitation techniques that have evolved. Excitation by an electrical arc or spark was used in the original emission spectrographic methods. Flame excitation is used in flame photometers and flame atomic absorption. Plasma and laser excitation techniques are recent developments. Emission spectrometric methods have the great advantage of being multi-element methods. Absorption spectrometry can only handle one element at a time. In atomic absorption spectrometry one excitation lamp is needed for every element to be determined. This is an excellent method and it is probably the one most used for trace element analysis today. Almost all elements in the periodic system can be analysed and the sensitivity is very high. The method is also fast and it can be run completely automatically with samplers. It is necessary to realise, however, that with this method the risk for contamination is not over until the result has been read or printed. For multi-element analysis the new so-called ICP (Inductively Coupled Plasma) spectrometers as well as DCP (Direct Coupled Plasma) instruments show great promise for the future. In this method the sample is introduced in an argon plasma with very high temperature (up to 8,000°K). The light from the plasma can be analysed by several element-specific detectors or by an adjustable spectrometer. These types of instruments are being rapidly developed to an increasing technical sophistication and versatility.

X-RAY SPECTROMETRY

Methods utilising X-ray spectrometry are gaining in popularity. This technique depends on the possibilities of exciting electrons in the inner shells of atoms with different energy sources so that they move to shells further out. From there they fall back to their original shell emitting X-rays that are characteristic of the atom and the electron shell. Other more energetic X-rays can be used as energy sources, in which case we talk about X-ray fluorescence methods or XRF (9). An energetic electron beam can also be used as is the case with electron microprobe instruments or EMP (10). Finally, proton beams from some accelerators are used for the excitation, in which case we talk about proton-induced X-ray emission or PIXE spectrometers (11). These techniques are multi-element methods capable of analysing almost all elements in the periodic system above sodium. The absolute sensitivities are about the same for all elements and 10^{-12} g or better. In practice, it is difficult to realise relative sensitivities better than around 1 PPM. The sample must be presented to the beam, preferably as a thin layer. The precision can be good with very thin samples but not so good for thick layers. The necessary investment in such a machine is very high. X-ray fluorescence machines are not quite so expensive. Such a machine, although it is a very complicated instrument, is rather easy to use and it has high productivity which leads to comparatively low analytical costs per sample.

RADIOISOTOPE METHODS

Detectors for nuclear radiation have extreme sensitivity. In fact they can detect one single atom or rather the radiation it emits. This makes very sensitive analytical techniques possible—the most sensitive that exist. Trace elements can be determined by isotope dilution techniques. This is not practised very much, however. A refinement of isotope dilution techniques is radioimmuno assays (RIA) which as we all know are extremely sensitive methods for determinations of all sorts of molecules. Much more practised for trace element determination are the activation analysis methods. In this context we mean by activation that some sort of energetic particle or radiation interacts with the atomic nucleus in such a way that it changes to an unstable state—it becomes radioactive. The activating radiation used can be either thermal or fast neutrons, photons (usually intense gamma rays), or charged particles such as electrons, protons, deuterons or alfa particles. Thermal neutrons are the particles that are most often used. A neutron can easily enter the atomic nucleus because it is electrically neutral. If it has low energy it will stay in the nucleus. In many cases, but not all, this leads to instability in the nucleus and we have obtained a radioactive isotope of the same atomic species as we irradiated. Irradiation by thermal neutrons of copper leads to the formation of ^{64}Cu, a radioactive copper isotope with a half-life of 12.8 hours. In the same way irradiation of selenium leads to several selenium isotopes. ^{75}Se with a half-life of 120 days is most used for neutron activation analysis of selenium. All elements in the periodic system react in this way but not all neutron additions lead to a radioactive isotope. The resulting nucleus may also be stable. Not all radioactive isotopes can be measured either because the half-life can be extremely short (10^{-15} sec) or extremely long, meaning thousands of millions of years. These facts limit the number of elements that can be profitably analysed with this technique to little more than 70.

The sensitivity obtainable with this technique is different for every element and varies from about 10^{-6} PPM to 100 PPM (see ref. 12). One great advantage of this method is that it is a multi-element technique. All elements in a sample that can be activated are activated and can, in principle, be determined together with all the others. The result can depend on the mixture of elements, the matrix in other words, and the counting equipment. The radiation from the activated elements can be of any sort: gamma rays, negatrons, positrons, X-rays and more. Most laboratories prefer to measure the characteristic gamma rays that the majority of radioisotopes emit, because this can be made even on rather complex mixtures without too much interference from one isotope with another. Nowadays a gamma spectrum is usually registered with the aid of a Ge(Li)-semiconductor detector and a multichannel analyser which may be a computer or coupled to a computer for the rather complex data reduction necessary. It is not necessary to have a nuclear reactor as irradiation services are available in most countries. It is, however, necessary to have a laboratory for work with radioactive isotopes and a gamma spectrometer and detector. In addition a microcomputer or an advanced programmable calculator is necessary.

REFERENCES

1. SNYDER, W. S., COOK, M. J., NASSET, E.S., KARHAUSEN, L. R., PARRY HOWELLS, G. & TIPTON, I. H. (1975). *Report of the Task Group on Reference Man*. ICRP publication no. 23.
2. IYENGAR, G. V., KOLLMER, W. E. & BOWEN, H. J. M. (1978). *The Elemental Composition of Human Tissues and Body Fluids*. Verlag Chemie, Weinheim, New York.
3. PLANTIN, L.-O., MEURLING, S., NYQUIST, O., STRANDVIK, B. & TUNELL, R. (1981). Selenium in blood in health and in certain diseases. In *Trace Element Metabolism in Man and Animals*, pp. 510–513. Ed. by Howell et al. Australian Academy of Science, Canberra.
4. SANSONI, B. & IYENGAR, V. (1978).*Sampling and Sample Preparation Methods for the Analysis of Trace Elements in Biological Material*. Spezielle Berichte der Kernforschungsanlage Jülich, Nr 13.
5. BINNERTS, W. T. (1980). Search for sensistive catalytic methods in analysis of trace elements in biological material: iodine, cobalt and selenium. In *Trace Element Analytical Chemistry in Medicine and Biology*, pp. 553–558. Ed. by Brätter and Schramel. Walter de Gruyter, Berlin, New York.
6. FLEET, B. & JOE, R. D. (1976). Advances in voltammetric techniques. In *Annual Reviews of the Analytical Sciences*, pp. 1–35. Ed. by L. S. Bark. Chemical Society, 1976: 4, London.
7. NURNBERG, H. W. (1977). *Electrochimica Acta* 22, 935–949.
8. VEILLON, C. (1976). Optical atomic spectroscopic methods. In *Monographs on Analytical Chemistry and Its Application*, Chapter 6. Wiley-Interscience, New York.
9. BERTIN, E. P. (1975). *Principles and Practice of X-ray Spectrometric Analysis*. Plenum Press, New York.
10. BIRKS, L. S. (1971). *Electron Probe Microanalysis*. Vol. 17 in the series Analytical Chemistry and Its Application. Wiley-Interscience, New York.
11. JOHANSSON, S. A. E. & JOHANSSON, T. B. (1976). *Nuclear Inst. Methods* 137, 473–516.
12. DE SOETE, D., GIJBELS, R. & HOSTE, J. (1972).*Neutron Activation Analysis*. Vol. 34 in the series Analytical Chemistry and Its Application. Wiley-Interscience, New York.

Discussion (the paper by Plantin)

Chairman: WALDENSTRÖM

ANDERSON: I have a comment. Among the numbers shown in your Table 2, the value for chromium is 10–20-fold too high. There you have .0025 which is 2.5 ppb and the correct value *has* to be less than .2.

PLANTIN: Yes, that's right, these tables grow old with time.

ANDERSON: But your publication is new and I think you should correct those values.

PLANTIN: Yes, you're quite correct. That was the value I had available at the time. We have seen now that the chromium values are still lower. This has been the tendency. If you plot the normal level considered at the time you will find a sloping line and if you miss some publications you will be in error.

CHRISTOPHERSEN: I would just like to make one comment regarding the multi-element method. I think today we know quite a little about the biochemical functions of many of the trace elements. But, for example, we know nothing about arsenic and as for selenium, we know of only one function quite well in mammals, so it undoubtedly has several unknown functions. There are several trace elements that are even not known to be essential at all, maybe possible candidates, like titanium for instance. I think it is very important to use these multi-element methods in a very systematic way, to study what we may call especially important enzymes and transport systems, etc. themselves in order to find out which elements they contain. I think they would find out there would be many surprises. If we should find, for instance, that titanium might be present in an insulin receptor, then perhaps we should start making a clinical study. Maybe some of the diabetics are deficient in titanium. I think this is another strategy which should now be very important if one wants to make more rapid progress towards an understanding of the pathogenesis of trace element-related diseases.

PLANTIN: I agree completely with you. I have always been for multi-element methods. I have no opinion about how it should be, I am very interested in finding how it is. There is certainly a lot of interaction between trace elements. Elements which we do not know are essential and may not be essential, can still interact with essential trace elements. That's why we should always strive to get multi-element analyses.

SHAMBERGER: I would like to agree that multi-element analysis is certainly quite desirable. Fortunately I had saved the samples from looking at individual elements of selenium, cadmium and zinc because I found later that the selenium/cadmium ratio, the selenium/zinc ratio, the zinc/cadmium ratio, or the zinc/copper ratio was far more important than what I had wanted to look at in the beginning.

I would like to ask a question about ICP and how you feel about this emerging technique. Do you think ICP will replace neutron activation analysis in analysis of biological samples?

PLANTIN: I'm not sure it will replace it altogether, but it certainly will be a strong candidate for that. There may still be specific elements that may be better analysed by neutron activation and the instruments are not yet precise enough, I should say, for multi-element analysis. But, with the development of this technique, that is foreseeable, I think it will compete very heavily with neutron activation analysis. It will have a very strong factor speaking for it and that is that it will be much faster. If you want to do neutron activation analysis, you may radiate for a week and cool the samples for a week and take another few days to analyse the samples. You usually cannot get fast results if you do not have the reactor in the house, which very few people have, so you have to send it to some centre. In Sweden we have to send samples abroad for radiation. That will speak very strongly for the ICP method.

FRANK: I just want to agree with Dr Plantin about the usefulness of multi-element measurements. So far we have talked about the ICP. At the National Veterinary Institute we have experience of another plasma technique, the DCP (direct current plasma), which we have used in simultaneous measurements of as much as 17 elements in animal tissues. That means, when analysing for only 14 elements in the routine procedure, we are doing 700 metal determinations per day with not more than two co-workers. The method has an enormous capacity and good reliability. The detection limit is, however, something we always have to consider.

Although plasma techniques are excellent to use in the simultaneous multi-element determinations they are not applicable to all elements in general. Unfortunately the important and essential element selenium cannot be included in the simultaneous routine determination of metals, but has to be determined with special techniques separately.

ABDULLA: I have a question to Dr Plantin. We have recently made a decision to buy an ICP instrument. I was in Frankfurt to look at the instrument and according to the experts, the instrument is good for multi-element analysis, but may not be the ideal one to measure the concentration of trace elements such as chromium and selenium. For these elements, atomic absorption spectrophotometry with Zeeman background correction and graphite furnace is the ideal choice. I wonder if you have any comments on the ICP instrument?

PLANTIN: I couldn't say. I haven't used it. Referring to what I said, the ICP instrumentation is developing at the moment very fast and it is not at its optimum yet. There will certainly be improvements in the next few years.

AGGETT: Could I just take the discussion slightly further away from straight analysis and in fact put forth a challenge to the rest of the members of the conference as well as to the two speakers. I think we have partially answered why we are measuring trace elements in tissues but I think we have to ask that all the time. So, what I would specifically like to ask you is what do you really measure? What tissue do you measure? What facilities are available to tell us what chemical form these elements are in, what the tissue compartmentalisation of that element is or the subcellular distribution, and whether, in fact, there is any metabolic compartmentalisation? How do we take this all into consideration because, if we're going to answer these things effectively and make use of the data which you are providing from these analytical instruments, I think we, as the people who provide the samples, need to know how you can answer these kind of questions, so that we are achieving more than giving you something to exercise your analytical abilities with.

PLANTIN: Yes, you've put your finger on a very sore point. These implications complicate still further the analytical programs for trace elements. Dr Iyengar talked about a lot of things you have to think of when you want to take a sample but, of course, as you say, it is also interesting to know the subsample. If you go down into the matter further and further, you will see that it is, of course, not a continuous concentration of the trace element in a tissue. It is concentrated to some carrier of this trace element and the biological effect it carries—enzymes, vitamins, hormones and so on. They are not evenly distributed within the cells and in the cells themselves you still have substructures of microsomes, mitochondria, everything. You have to analyse them too and see where in the cell this trace element is doing its thing, in which form. This is another difficult question. It depends on what method you use. If you use neutron activation analysis you cannot say anything about the form, in which molecule this element is contained, because it's just an elemental method and that's that. But with the other techniques, combined with the analytical, you may separate cell organelles, cells of different kinds and tissues of different kinds and get much more information about this.

AGGETT: Could things like electron spin resonance or NMR help at all in some of these respects?

PLANTIN: I don't think it can be used at this time. It has been used with some specific tracers, but I don't see it as a technique that could now give you very much. NMR gives you, of course, some idea in which type of molecule a certain element may be situated and that might help in the most refined aspects of it.

JOHANSSON: I would like to ask you about your Table 2. You mentioned possible essential elements and you mentioned mercury. Can you comment about that?

PLANTIN: This is nothing that I have studied myself. It's just that Klaus Schwarz during his last years was rather convinced that both mercury and cadmium were essential trace elements. That was based on a technique using isolators and giving rats diets deficient in one element at a time. He had observed effects that suggested to him that even these elements might be essential, but he had no time to finish his investigations so that this is an open question. But there are indications and if he thought it was worthwhile to pursue, I believe these indications were rather strong.

WALDENSTRÖM: Perhaps I might ask a question myself. Being a hematologist, of course I think that cobalt is a very important substance as far as vitamin B_{12} is concerned. Would anybody like to talk a little bit more about cobalt or has that been treated so well in the morning that nobody has anything to add? Dr Frank, for instance?

FRANK: Cobalt is very important for human and animal health. At this symposium we are discussing trace elements in human health, our experiences at the National Veterinary Institute are from the field of veterinary medicine. The geographical areas of Sweden are differently mineralised, some even show very low levels in metals important to life. Such an area is Gotland, an island in the Baltic Sea, which is very poor in, i.a., cobalt and copper.

Last year we investigated 82 lambs, which were growing poorly and generally in bad condition. Our analyses displayed serious cobalt deficiency in 66 percent of the investigated animals.

In this connection I would like to mention another project at our Institute. We have collected and are analysing samples of organ tissue from 4,300 moose from all over Sweden. Thanks to the DCP-technique it is possible to perform such a huge investigation. Our aim is to determine the availablity of cadmium via plants to the moose in the different geographic areas of Sweden. The simultaneous multi-element determination will give us renal contents of 14 elements in total and ideas about the metals in Swedish nature available to the moose via plants, e.g., in addition to cadmium also cobalt.

IYENGAR: Just a short comment since we were speaking about nickel. I don't know which samples you were referring to, but if the sample is whole blood or serum, there doesn't seem to be any more doubt about nickel levels. There are very many new reports which are in the reference value report I am planning to bring out.

If I may take this opportunity, also, just to answer part of your question as to how we go about selecting samples. For example, we were quite successful in showing that if your problem is selenium, it's quite useful to look at selenium in platelets. We found quite a rich sample for selenium. We are also in a position now to answer questions. If, for example, your problem is cadmium, routine monitoring of faeces can give you very useful information. Similarly, it's very well known that hair can be a useful indicator for methyl mercury.

AGGETT: May I come back to Dr Iyengar's presentation and ask: Are you implying that even though multi-element analysis may be useful, in terms of, say, optimising information, for looking at marginal status, whatever that may be, we have to choose the tissue to go with the element and the particular situation? For example, there may be many practical problems, say for children, in choosing platelets, but there may well be other good reasons for not choosing platelets for other elements. One can run through the whole gamut for other tissues. If one is worried about cadmium or mercury status, perhaps we could go for the liver or the kidneys. Are there situations where multi-element analysis would not be of much use for the clinician?

IYENGAR: I would say that if you can afford to do multi-element analysis, it's a good thing to do. You get some basic information. Also, on many elements, you probably end up with many unexpected situations if your analysis is correct. Otherwise, probably you have missed some of the very useful side information. But, as I said in the beginning, there are always going to be some conflicting situations. For instance, you take blood serum from fasting subjects and it may not be useful for the zinc level, whereas the fluoride will be perfectly all right. The same thing would also apply to arsenic. Depending on the food you have eaten it may take your body a week before its level normalises. There are many reports on that. Therefore, I personally feel we simply have to know the problem as intimately as possible.

AGGETT: May I ask Dr Iyengar another question going even further? How should we ask or actually express results? We're talking here of ppb in terms of dry weight or wet weight. I know you've thought about this. What about expressing it in terms of protein or nuclelic acids as markers or, for example, even the intracellular content of another element such as magnesium which has been used to express the zinc content of cirrhotic livers?

IYENGAR: I certainly agree with you that we need different methods. For example, we have done this already for the milk project where we have used the wet, dry and also the protein has been taken into account. The fat content has been provided so that you were able to compare results. As far as the general situation is concerned, I'm afraid there is something that cannot ultimately be imposed. There are various arguments on this. In fact, I am trying to get this into an editorial right now. Irrespective of what base one uses to express one's results, I think the relations between wet and dry or dry and protein etc. should be provided, so that at least others who use the data are able to interpret it. This seems to be the only compromise I can think of, because there is also the question of the practical aspects. Suppose the sample is collected in the field, it is unrealistic to ask for the result on the wet basis. Under such circumstances it should be on the dry basis. However, the authors should provide information on water content of the tissue.

SALONEN: I was going to follow the line that Dr Aggett started and point out that at least in human studies, and especially in epidemiologic studies, determinations of trace elements and minerals are often made to have an indicator of dietary intake of those elements. And, in that kind of situation, some additional requirements are there, like the fact that one needs to know what is the best tissue sample for an indicator of tighter intake. Where large numbers of persons are concerned, the accuracy and sensitivity of those analyses do not have to be as high as in smaller clinical studies. In epidemiology, we also often use dietary recordings to measure dietary intake of trace elements. I wonder, if you are aware of comparisons between dietary recordings and determinations of various trace elements, for example, from blood? Could dietary recordings be used to determine whether the chemical determinations are, for instance, uncontaminated and so on?

IYENGAR: May I answer this question please? I guess this is very well known, at least for elements such as mercury. There are several sets of publications that have come out connecting high mercury with fish eaters. But these are isolated cases. I agree with you that there is no systematic study carried out in several countries to show such pattern of dietary conditions.

We are actually embarking on a study of this problem on a global level. We are going to involve about 15 different countries on a trace element dietary-intake study-project which is just in the beginning stages.

FRANK: There are two subjects I would like to comment on. One concerns the choice of organs for investigations, which Dr Aggett was discussing. At the National Veterinary Institute we do not have any problems with the choice of suitable tissues for our purposes. Since we work with slaughterhouse and cadaverous materials, we have access to satisfactory amounts. The most frequently analysed tissues are liver and kidneys in determination of poisonings, deficiency of elements and in investigation of the metal status in domestic and wild animals.

The other subject concerns the interesting question from Dr Waldenström about our work on cobalt. In addition to our cadmium project on the Swedish moose we also get the renal values of cobalt. As we have collected also liver samples from the moose, the cobalt content in the liver should be of great interest to get analysed. It would elucidate the geographical distribution of cobalt availability in Sweden. Such studies would have great importance due to the interesting research of Dr Engel into the prevalence of pernicious anaemia in Sweden. It is fascinating to look forward to the ability of correlating the cobalt content in the liver of this wild ruminant to the frequency of this disease in different regions of Sweden.

ENGEL: I have been studying pernicious anaemia all my life and in different parts of Sweden and observed an unequal distribution of this disease. In later days I started using our modern hospital morbidity and drug consumption statistics to clear out the geographical distribution. These studies are facilitated by the fact that B_{12} is delivered free of cost for pernicious anaemia patients. I was happy to get in touch with Dr Frank's cobalt studies and we will together look for any correlation of distribution figures.

NORRMAN: Dr Iyengar, you have shown us some very interesting figures about the selenium content in human milk. As we saw, the values for Sweden, Hungary and some other countries were quite low. Are you aware of some earlier measurements to see if there have been any changes in time? As a comparison, I can tell you that I made some analyses of the selenium content in Swedish crops and found it to be about 40% lower today than it was only 20 years ago. I have also measured the selenium content in cow's milk and today it is about 40 to 50% lower than it was 20 years ago.

IYENGAR: I don't have those levels of selenium.

PERRY: I would like to comment on the question about the tissue one should use. I'd like to second very strongly the idea that this has to be highly individualised. It *really* does depend on the tissue in question. To make a comment about cadmium with which I spend a great deal of my time, I think that probably blood is not a very good tissue, because this is an element that stays for a very long time in the body and what's in the blood probably represents much more recent exposure. But I think, in addition to this, that liver and kidney, where I have been wont to look for a long while, may not be the right tissues either. Recently, we have found much bigger chemical differences when we looked at the heart which has very low concentrations but, because it has no metallothionine, it's possible that the effect in the heart is really much larger than what we are looking at. What we should be looking at is unbound metallothionine. At least what we seem to be seeing in the heart are marked changes in high-energy phosphate in particular. When we use NMR to give us a pattern of the phosphate metabolites, there is much less high-energy phosphate in the heart than with cadmium-exposed animals, animals with very small exposures. Even though the amount of cadmium is very much less than in the kidney and the liver, we can find the same sort of change in kidney and liver but it's much less than the change in heart. So I think that sometimes our tendency to look at the tissue in which the highest concentration occurs really may not be the right case, and, again, one has to individualise.

SALONEN: If I may continue from that, from living humans we sometimes are not able to obtain samples of liver or kidney. Sometimes we have to use serum, blood, even urine or adipose tissue. For epidemiological studies, urine is very frequently used, for instance for cadmium, even for fluorine and several others. I think for cadmium and fluorine, urine concentrations respond much better to dietary exposure than serum concentrations.

The Role of Zinc in Diabetes Mellitus

By Søren Kiilerich

ZINC AND THE INSULIN MOLECULE

In 1921, Banting and Best discovered insulin, but the content of insulin in the pancreas from patients with diabetes mellitus was not examined before 1938, when Scott and Fischer quoted that the total content of insulin present in the pancreas of diabetics amounted to only one quarter of that found in the pancreas of normal individuals. At the same time they stated that the amount of zinc contained in the pancreas of diabetics is only one-half that normally present. Scott (1934) also stated that crystalline insulin contains relatively large quantities of zinc. More recent crystallographic studies (Harding et al. 1966) have clearly demonstrated the presence of zinc in crystals of insulin, confirming the close relationship between zinc and insulin.

INFLUENCE OF ZINC ON THE INSULIN ACTION

It has been reported that the removal of zinc can reduce immunological insulin activity due to changes in antigenic determinants of insulin (Arquilla et al. 1978b). In the same year the same authors demonstrated (Arquilla et al. 1978a) that pretreatment of normal mice with zinc caused an accelerated and enhanced binding accompanied by an attenuation of degradation of (^{125}I) iodoinsulin by the liver compared to pretreatment with Na. *In vitro* experiments employing isolated liver plasma membranes demonstrated that added zinc increased the binding and inhibited the degradation of insulin.

Coulston and Dandona (1980) showed that zinc had a stimulatory effect upon lipogenesis by rat epididymal adipocytes, even in the absence of insulin. They also showed that zinc has an additive effect with insulin upon lipogenesis by adipocytes. At the clinical level these observations raise the possibility that relative or absolute zinc deficiency may have a role to play in the pathogenesis of maturity-onset diabetes in which insensivity to insulin is considered to be an important contributory factor (Reaven et al. 1976,

Olefsky & Reaven 1977). May and Contoreggi (1982) showed that the insulin-like effect of zinc in adipocytes is caused not only by direct effects of the ion on the intracellular metabolism, but, also by direct effects related to H_2O_2 generation.

In order to see if zinc has any influence on the organism's capability to receive glucose, the glucose tolerance levels of different animals were determined. Hendricks and Mahoney (1972) have shown that zinc-deficient rats slowly develop a decreased tolerance for glucose which is administered directly into the peritoneal cavity and that this impairment is rapidly corrected by zinc supplementation. This was not the case when glucose was given orally, perhaps because the insulin response is greater to this form of administration (McIntyre et al. 1965). Other investigators have confirmed these observations (Bouquist & Lernmark 1969, Roth & Kirchgessner 1981) (Fig. 1).

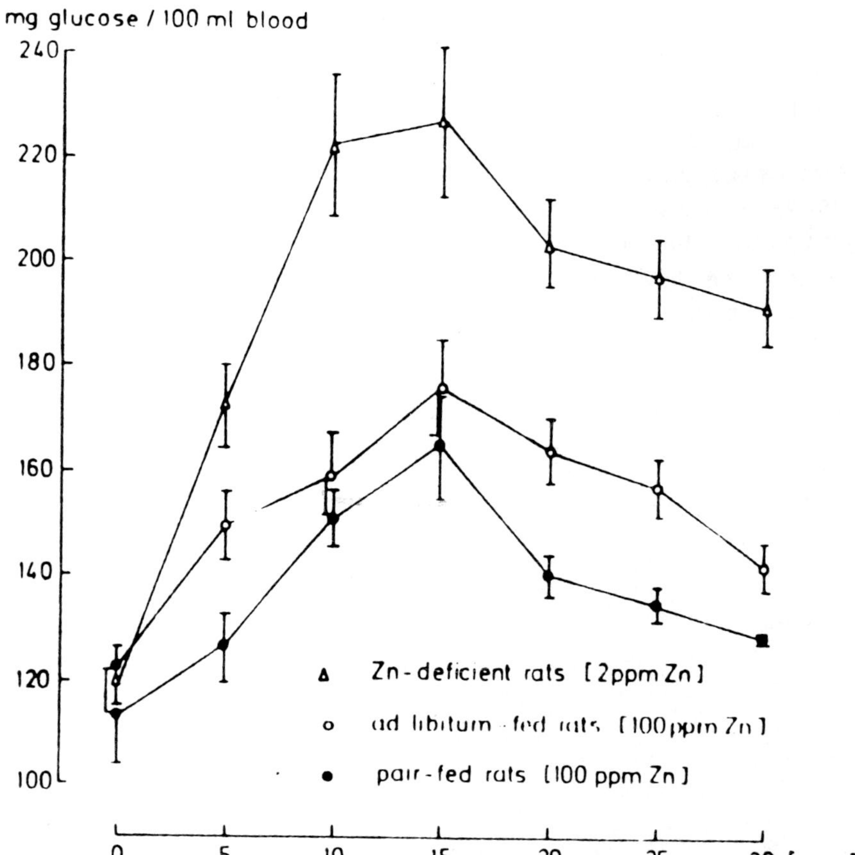

Fig. 1 Glucose tolerance curves of zinc-deficient rats in comparison to ad libitum and pair-fed rats
(Roth et al. 1981)

Table I Clinical data in 60 insulin-treated diabetic out-patients

	Mean	Range
Age (years)	40.4	23 – 64
Age at diabetes onset (years)	34.5	16 – 58
Duration of diabetes (years)	5.9	1 – 11
Body height (cm)	172	153 –191
Body weight (kg)	65.7	46 – 88
Insulin dose (U/kg/24 h)	0.47	0.05– 1.01
Creatinine clearance (ml/min)	94.7	52 –170

ZINC AND DIABETES MELLITUS IN HUMANS

The afore-mentioned observations have caused many speculations about the role of zinc in diabetes mellitus in humans.

Patients and control

In order to elucidate the zinc metabolism in patients with diabetes mellitus, we studied 60 adult insulin-dependent diabetic out-patients (40 males and 20 females) (McNair et al. 1981b). All patients selected had normal serum creatinine (<115 μmol/1) and none had other diseases or received drugs known to interfere with mineral metabolism. Pertinent clinical data for these patients are given in Table I. The body weight of each patient had been constant during the year previous to the study. One hundred and four normal subjects (aged 21–70 years, mean 41 years) gave reference values for serum zinc, protein, albumin and α_2-macroglobulin; 28 of these persons served as a control group for the urine data. The control group has been described in detail elsewhere (Kiilerich et al. 1980).

Methods

Fasting blood samples were collected between 8 and 10 a.m. before the administration of morning insulin. A 24-hour urine collection was completed on the morning of the study day. The concentration of zinc in serum was measured by atomic absorption spectrophotometry taking great care to avoid zinc contamination in all steps of the analysis. The method has been described in detail elsewhere (Kiilerich et al. 1980, Kiilerich et al. 1981). Blood and urine glucose were determined routinely in the laboratory by enzymatic analysis. Serum and urine creatinine were determined by the Jaffé reaction, modified for the SMA 6/60 autoanalyzer. Serum albumin was measured by the bromcresol green method, using a reaction time of 10 sec. (Gustafsson 1976). Serum α_2 -macroglobulin was determined by Laurell's electroimmunoassay (Laurell 1972).

Table II *Serum zinc, serum albumin, serum α_2-macroglobulin and urinary excretion rates of zinc and glucose per mmol creatinine excreted by diabetic patients compared with normal subjects*
(Mean ± S.E.M.)

	Diabetic		Normal	
	40 males	20 females	37 males	67 females
Serum zinc (μmol/l)	14.7 ±0.21	14.8 ± 0.35	15.3 ± 0.35[b]	14.1 ±0.24
Serum albumin (μmol/l)	684 ±7	664 ±12	663 ±10	652 ±7
Serum α_2-macroglobulin (μmol/l)	2.97±0.13[c]	3.91± 0.18[d]	2.78± 0.13[c]	3.33±0.10
Urinary zinc excretion rate (μmol/mmol creatinine)	1.14±0.06[a,d]	1.37± 0.10[d]	0.55± 0.06 (n = 14)	0.48±0.08 (n = 14)
Urinary glucose excretion rate (mmol/mmol creatinine)	23.2 ±3.1	35.8 ± 7.5		

Significance of difference between male and female: [a]$p<0.05$; [b]$p<0.01$; [c]$p<0.001$
Significance of difference between diabetic and correspondent control value: [d]$p<0.01$

Results

The diabetic patients had a normal serum concentration of zinc and albumin, but showed increased concentrations of α_2-macroglobulin (Table II). The urinary excretion rates of zinc relative to the creatinine excretion was almost doubled in the diabetic patients compared with normal subjects.

The diabetic hyperzincuria was associated with the degree of glucosuria (Fig. 2) ($r = 0.36$, $p < 0.01$). The zincuria also correlated with the creatinine corrected water diureses ($r = 0.27$, $p < 0.05$). The correlation between glucosuria and water diuresis was $r = 0.47$, $p < 0.001$. Serum zinc and albumin decreased with increasing duration of the disease ($r = -0.33$, $p < 0.01$; $r = -0.31$, $p < 0.02$, respectively). Serum α_2-macroglobulin was not related to the duration of the disease, nor was the urinary zinc excretion rate. There was no association between the dosage of insulin and the urinary excretion rate of zinc, nor between the amount of zinc contained in the insulin administered and the excretion rate of the ion. The amount of zinc injected per 24 hours averaged 0.6 μmol/l (range 0–1.5) which is about 5% of the amount excreted in the urine of the diabetic patients.

Discussion

In the present cross-sectional study of 60 insulin-dependent diabetic out-patients, no difference in serum zinc was observed between normals and diabetics. This is in conflict with some reports (Constam et al. 1964, Kumar et al. 1974, Mateo 1978) but agrees with other studies (Khattab et al. 1976, Davies et al. 1968, Pidduck et al. 1970a, Chooi et al. 1976). The discrepan-

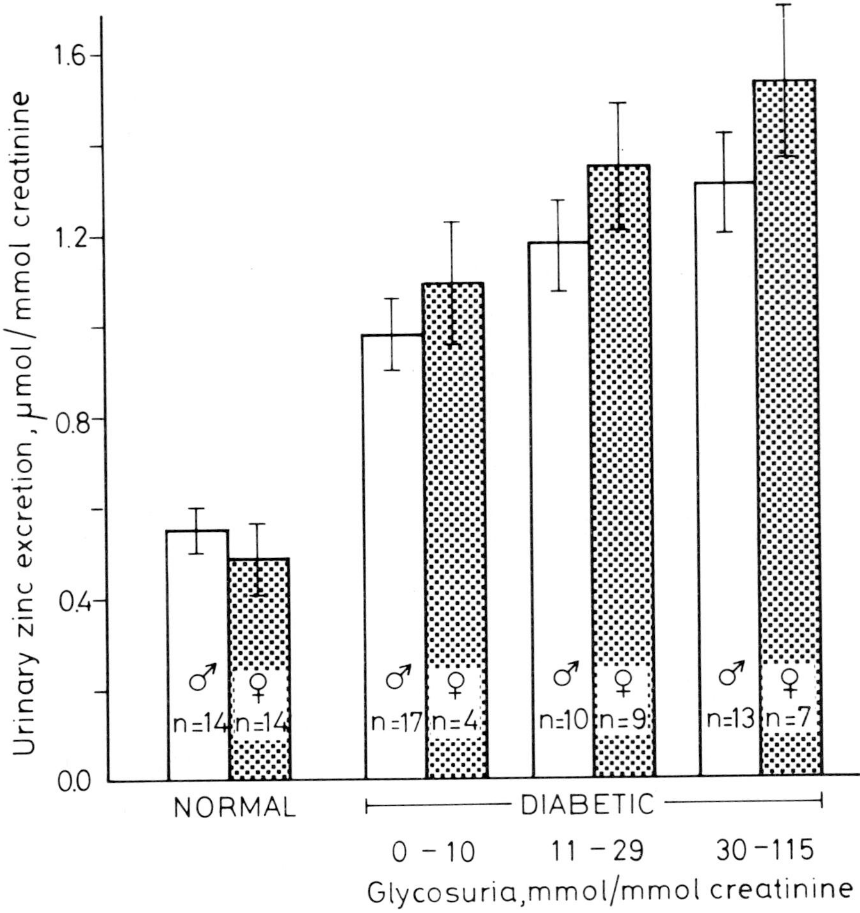

Fig. 2 Urinary excretion rate of zinc in 28 normal and in 60 diabetic subjects, grouped according to sex and degree of glucosuria

cies might be explained by the great possibilities of contamination of the assay and the biological conditions such as non-fasting, diural variation (Kiilerich et al. 1980) and proteinbinding of serum zinc (Kiillerich et al. 1984). Evidence of a progressing zinc depletion was, however, not present. The slight decrease in serum zinc with increasing duration of diabetes could easily be explained by the simultaneous decrease in serum albumin. The state of hyperzincuria in diabetes is normally accepted (Meltzer et al. 1962, Pidduck et al. 1970b, Kumar et al. 1974, Hägglöf et al. 1983), but the reason is obscure. In our study patients with high urinary glucose excreted more zinc than patients with moderate to lower glucosuria and almost three times more than normal individuals. The phenomenon was to some extent explained by the concomitant increase in water diuresis. The loss of bone which has been described in these insulin-dependent diabetics (McNair et

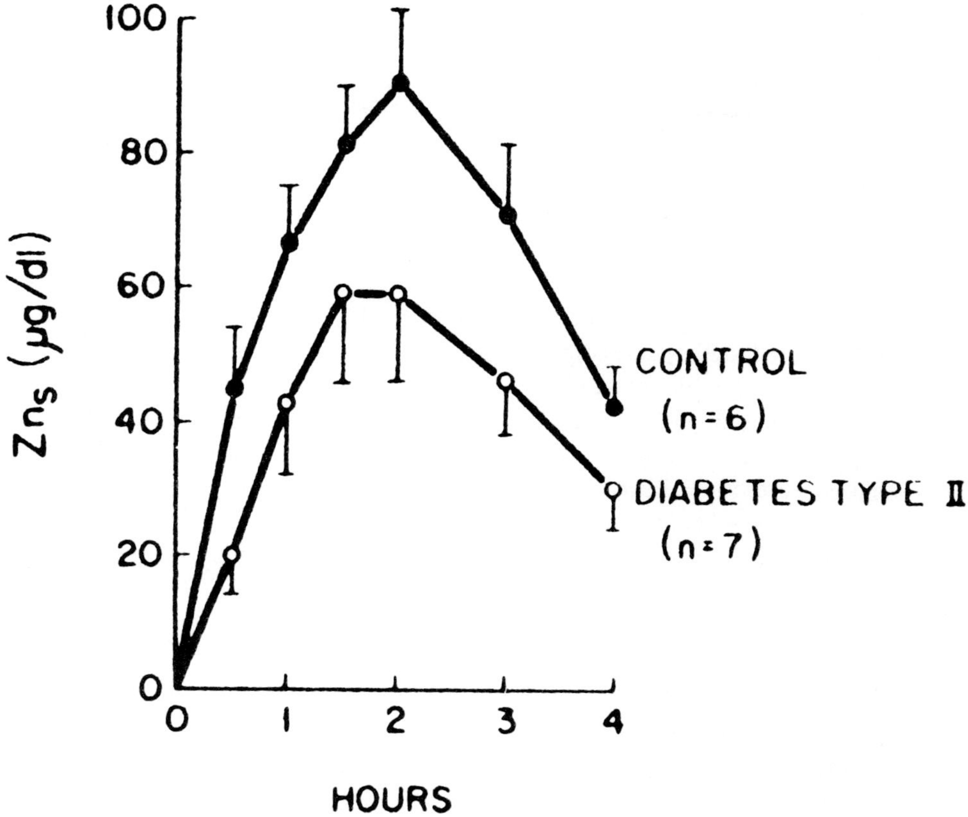

Fig. 3 Oral zinc tolerance test in control subjects and diabetic patients
Means ± standard deviations are indicated
(Kinlaw et al. 1983)

al. 1981) and the amount of zinc administered through the insulin injection is only an insignificant amount of the observed hyperzincuria.

The cause of the hyperzincuria could be a renal abnormality or enhanced production of endogenous chelating agents (Tarui 1960).

It has been proposed that the ability of the human organism to keep the concentration of zinc in serum within the normal range is the effect of a hyperabsorptive gastrointestinal mechanism. However, Kinlaw et al. (1983) has recently demonstrated a reduced absorption of zinc in patients with insulin-dependent diabetes (Fig. 3). It is therefore possible that diabetic patients develop a state of intracellular zinc depletion.

CONCLUSION

The mutual connection between insulin and zinc has been clearly demonstrated. That zinc has a certain influence on the function of insulin has been rendered probable. Earlier, the hypothesis has been stated that relative zinc deficiency may play a role in the pathogenesis of maturity-onset diabetes. The possibility that the addition of zinc to insulin preparations may significantly enhance the biologic potency of insulin *in vivo* had also been stated. The condition of decreased glucose tolerance seen in animals fed a zinc-deficient diet has not been studied in humans. Whether patients with zinc deficiency in general have concomitant glucose intolerance has not been elucidated.

It has been described that patients in the initial stage of insulin-dependent diabetes have a decreased concentration of zinc in serum. As zinc is essential for the body's defence against infections, these authors advance the possibility that a decrease in the zinc concentration in insulin, e.g., evoked by some diabetogenic agent, can lead to an increased sensitivity for isletotropic viruses in patients with heriditary disposition for insulin-dependent diabetes mellitus. Finally it can be concluded that the true role of zinc in the metabolism of insulin and in the development and medical treatment of the different types of diabetes mellitus needs further investigation.

REFERENCES

ARQUILLA, E. R., PACKER, S., TARMAS, W. & MIYAMOTO, S. (1978a). The effect of zinc on insulin metabolism. *Endocrinology* 100 (108), 1440–1499.

ARQUILLA, E. R., THIENE, P., BRUGMAN, T., RUES, W. & SEGIYAMA, R. (1978b). Effects of zinc ion on the conformation of antigenic determinants on insulin. *Biochem. J.* 175, 289–297.

BANTING, F. G. & BEST, C. H. (1921). The internal secretions of the pancreas. *J. Lab. clin. Med.* 7, 251–266.

BOUQUIST, L. & LERNMARK, Å. (1969). Effects of the endocrine pancreas in chinese hamsters fed zinc deficient diets. *Acta path. microbiol. scand.* 76, 215–228.

CHOOI, M. K., TODD, J. K. & BOYD, N. D. (1976). Influence of age and sex on plasma zinc levels in normal and diabetic individuals. *Nutr. Metabol.* 20, 135–142.

CONSTAM, G. R., LEEMANN, W., ALIMASY, F. & CONSTAM, A. G. (1964). Weitere Beobachtungen über den Zinc Stoffwechsel bei Diabetes Mellitus. *Schweiz. med. Wschr.* 32 (94), 1104–1109.

COULSTON, L. & DANDONA, P. (1980). Insulin-like effects of zinc on adipocytes. *Diabetes* 29, 665–667.

DAVIES, I. J. F., MUSA, M. & DORMANDY, T. R. (1968). Measurements of plasma zinc. *J. clin. Path.* 21, 359–363.

GUSTAFSSON, J. E. C. (1976). Improved specificity of serum albumin determination and estimation of "acute phase reactants" by use of brom cresol green reaction. *Clin. Chem.* 22, 616–622.

HARDING, M. M., HODGKIN, D. C., KENNEDY, A. F., O' LONNOR, A. & WEITZMANN, P. D. J. (1966). The crystal structure of insulin. *J. molec. Biol.* 16, 212–226.

HENDRICKS, D. G. & MAHONEY, A. W. (1972). Glucose tolerance in zinc-deficient rats. *J. Nutr.* 102, 1079–1084.

HÄGGLÖF, B., HALLMANS, G., HOLMGREN, G., LUDVIGSSON, J. & FALKMER, S. (1983). Prospective and retrospective studies of zinc concentrations in serum, blood clots, hair and urine in young patients with insulin-dependent diabetes mellitus. *Acta endocrin.* 102, 88–95.

KHATTAB, M., DANASOURY, M., SHARAF, M. & SHERBENY, A. (1976). Zinc in serum and urine of diabetics. *J. Egypt. Med. Assoc.* 59, 597–601.

KIILERICH, S. & CHRISTIANSEN, C. (1984). Distribution of serum zinc between albumin and α_2-macroglobulin estimated by ultracentrifugation. *Clin. chim. Acta* 142, 273–280.

KIIERICH, S., CHRISTENSEN, M. S., NAESTOFT, J. & CHRISTIANSEN, C. (1980). Determination of zinc in serum and urine by atomic absorption spectrophotometry; relationship between serum levels of zinc and proteins in 104 normal subjects. *Clin. chim. Acta.* 105, 231–239.

— (1981). Serum and plasma zinc concentrations with special reference to standardized sampling procedure and protein status. *Clin. chim. Acta* 114, 117–121.

KINLAW,W. B., LEVINE, A. S., MORLEY, J. E., SILVIS, S. E. & MCCLAIN, C. J. (1983). Abnormal zinc metabolism in type II diabetes mellitus. *Amer. J. Med.,* 75, 273–277.

KUMAR, S. & JAYA RAO, K. S. (1974). Blood and urinary zinc levels in diabetes mellitus. *Nutr. Metabol.* 17, 231–235.

LAURELL, C. B. (1972). Electroimmuno assay. *Scand. J. clin. Lab. Invest.* 29, Suppl. 124, 21–37.

MATEO, M. C. M., BUSTAMTE, J. B. & CONTALAPIEDRA, M. A. G. (1978). Serum zinc, copper and insulin in diabetes mellitus. *Biomed. (Express)* 29, 56–58.

MAY, J. M. & CONTOREGGI, C. S. (1982). The mechanism of the insulin-like effects of ionic zinc. *J. biol. Chem.* 257 (8), 4362–4368.

MCITYRE, N., HOLDSWORTH, C. D. & TURNER, D. S. (1965). Intestinal factors in the control of insulin secretion. *J. clin. Endocr.* 25, 1317–1321.

MCNAIR, P., CHRISTIANSEN, C., CHRISTENSEN, M. S, MADSBAD, S., FABER, O. K., BINDER, C. & TRANSBØL, I. (1981a). Development of bone mineral loss in insulin treated diabetes mellitus. A 1 1/2 years follow up study in 60 patients. *Eur. J. Clin. Invest.* 11, 55–59.

MCNAIR, P., KIILERICH, S., CHRISTIANSEN, C., CHRISTENSEN, M. S., MADSBAD, S. & TRANSBØL, I. (1981b). Hyperzincuria in insulin treated diabetes mellitus—its relation to glucose homeostasis and insulin administration. *Clin. chim. Acta* 112, 343–348.

MELTZER, L. E., RUTMAN, J., GEORG, P., RUTMAN, R. & KITCHELL, Y. R. (1962). The urinary excretion pattern of trace metals in diabetes mellitus. *Amer. J. med. Sci.* 44, 282–289.

OLEFSKY, Y. M. & REAVEN, G. M. (1977). Insulin binding in diabetes. Relationship with plasma insulin and insulin sensitivity. *Diabetes* 26, 680–688.

PIDDUCK, H. G., WREN, P. J. J. & PRICE EVANS, D. A. (1970 a). Plasma zinc and copper in diabetes mellitus. *Diabetes* 19, 234–239.

PIDDUCK, H. G., WREN, P. J. J. & PRICE EVANS, D. A. (1970 b). Hyperzincuria of diabetes mellitus and possible genetical implications of this observation. *Diabetes* 19, 240–247.

REAVEN, G. M., BERNSTEIN, R., DAVIS, B. & OLEFSKY, J. M. (1976). Nonketotic diabetes mellitus: insulin deficiency or insulin resistance. *Amer J. Med.* 60, 80–88.

ROTH, H.-P. & KIRCHGESSNER, M. (1981). Zinc and insulin metabolism. *Biol. Tr. El. Res.* 3, 13–32.

SCOTT, D. A. (1934). Crytalline insulin. *Biochem. J.* 28, 1592–1598.

SCOTT, D. A. & FISCHER, A. M. (1938). The insulin and the zinc content of normal and diabetic pancreas. *J. clin. Invest.* 17, 725–728.

TARUI, S. (1960). Studies on zinc metabolism. *J. Osaka Univ.* 10, 499–505.

Discussion (the paper by Kiilerich)

Chairman: WRETLIND

JAMESON: I want to add some information to the paper you gave. Table 1 shows our data on zinc in a cross-sectional study of diabetics. Study group I had in the uncomplicated cases the same mean value as you had, but the difference between our material and yours is that our patients had a longer duration of diabetic state. We had a group of 30 uncomplicated cases and 20 complicated cases. The group with complications had significantly lower mean serum zinc level. This is also true for study group II which is a group of 61 male diabetics with polyneuropathy and impotence. This group also had significantly lower mean serum zinc level than the uncomplicated diabetic patients.

Figure 1 shows quite a difference between the uncomplicated and complicated group I patients. The lowest level of zinc in the uncomplicated group is in an alcoholic and the two lowest in the complicated group are in fact diabetic patients with concomitant coeliac disease. Coeliac disease is more frequently found in diabetics. That could be one of the reasons why zinc uptake is decreased when testing the uptake from a pharmacological dose and when measuring the area under the curve. So it's very important to investigate these diabetic patients with low zinc levels with gastric endoscopy and duodenal biopsy because it's important for them to have their coeliac disease revealed and treated. They do better with their diabetes also. Anyway, to us, it seems that if the diabetes is of a long duration there is a steady loss of zinc as you have shown and we also find a negative correlation between the glucosylated hemoglobin values and the serum zinc levels. The higher the glucosylated hemoglobin values, the lower are the zinc levels. It fits well with your data and to me it's more a matter of time before the low circulating zinc levels develop.

ABDULLA: Zinc is not the only element that is related to diabetes and insulin-resistance. Recently some workers have shown that magnesium may play even a bigger

Table 1 (From S. Jameson, A. Brattberg, J. Fagius, K. Hellsing & C. Berne. In *Trace Element Metabolism in Man and Animals—5*. Ed. by C. F. Mills. Commonwealth Agricultural Bureaux, Slough, U.K. In press)

	S-Zn μmol/l		Age years		HbA1c %		n
	mean	SD	mean	SD	mean	SD	
Study group I	13.5	2.5	52.8	15.9	11.2	2.3	50
uncomplicated cases	14.7	1.8	49.1	15.6	10.9	2.1	30
complicated cases	11.7	2.2	58.3	15.0	11.8	1.8	20
Study group II	10.6	1.6	51.2	10.3	11.2	1.8	61

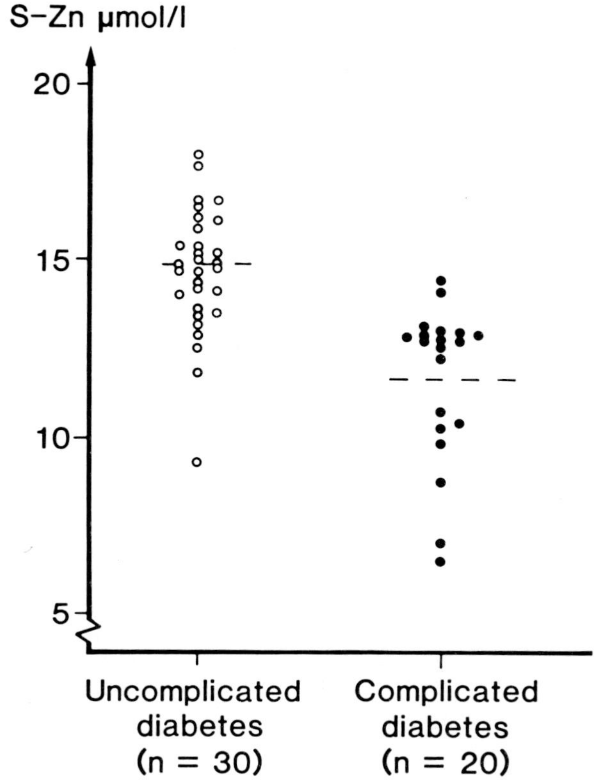

Fig. 1 (Ref. see Table 1)

role than zinc in diabetic patients. I wonder if you have measured any elements other than zinc in your material. We have also done some studies in Lund. In diabetic patients, of course, we found low zinc values, but we also found low magnesium and high copper levels in plasma.

KIILERICH: In this study we have only measured the zinc values just to start somewhere. Of course, it is nice to see that we have got the same values when we are looking at patients with the same duration of the disease and, with time, it has to go wrong when the patients are excreting three times more than normal persons.

CHRISTOPHERSEN: I would like to ask you if you have tried to consider the possible interrelationship between disturbances of zinc metabolism in diabetes and disturbances of protein metabolism. I think it is possible to imagine that many of the disturbances of zinc metabolism in some way may be regarded as secondary to disturbances of protein metabolism, especially as regards the membrane transport of amino acids. It is also known, of course, that insulin is important for the control of the membrane transport of amino acid by sodium-dependent uptake systems.

Then there is also another aspect. I wonder if you have considered that since zinc is needed for protein synthesis, it must also be needed for the synthesis of insulin. One might imagine that if you have an intracellular zinc depletion in the beta cells, this might be one cause for the reduced rate of insulin synthesis.

One final point I'd like to mention. Magnesium was also discussed here and when you have a sodium-dependent transport system for organic solute, the rate of transport may also depend on the electrochemical potential difference for sodium across the membrane. It has been shown in malnourished children that the rate of sodium uptake may be reduced because of zinc deficiency, and magnesium has, of course, the same effect. So it seems possible that these transport systems may be affected in a similar way both by magnesium and by zinc deficiency.

KIILERICH: To the first point, the only proteins we have looked at in these patients are albumin and α_2-macroglobulin and the results were as you saw here. When you study zinc in serum, it's, of course, necessary to look at the proteins albumin and α_2-globulins, because nearly 100% are bound to these proteins. We found that only about 7% of the total serum zinc are bound to α_2-macroglobulin in normals and so it is in diabetic patients.

We haven't been studying intracellular zinc depletion in these patients. We have done that in alcoholics but not in these patients. The third question—I can't give you any qualified answer to that.

WESTER: I should like to ask you if you know if the diabetogenic effect of thiazides relates to the zinc deficiency, because if you treat patients with thiazides, the urinary zinc will increase about 50%. I have shown in patients on thiazides that there is no change in the balance of zinc, no change in absorption, but, there is a depletion of zinc, first in the liver but also in the muscles. But I don't know if the zinc deficiency in thiazide-treated patients is related to diabetes.

KIILERICH: We are talking about diuretics? I can say that none of these patients have got diuretics at all. I know there is a problem with zinc and diuretics but we have not encountered it.

HURLEY: I would like to ask if these patients maintained their body weight during the period you were doing these studies?

KIILERICH: Yes, they were followed over a period of a year and a half and the body weight was constant during that time.

HURLEY: It would be interesting to know something about the body composition as well, to try to get some explanation as to where this zinc was coming from. Also, I believe you said that the α_2-macroglobulin levels were higher in the patients than in the controls although the albumin was the same and the serum zinc was the same on the average. Do you have any explanation for this higher concentration of α_2-macroglobulin?

KIILERICH: No, I haven't, but you see it in other disease groups. You see it in alcoholics, in cirrhosis of the liver, in many other diseases. It is a common clinical finding that α_2-macroglobulins are increased in these disease states, but I don't know why.

AGGETT: My first point relates to the comments made by Dr Christophersen and Dr Hurley about protein turnover. I think we are thinking too narrowly about insulin in assuming that its primary role is to do something to plasma glucose. I think that this is possibly the wrong way of looking at insulin overall. As far as I know there's no per se first class evidence that that's what insulin really does. It might well have intracellular effects to which glucose uptake is a secondary phenomenon. From that point of view I would really support the interests of people who suggest you take into account amino acid metabolism. For example, do you still have the urines? Could you measure the urine nitrogen in these patients in relation to the zincuria?

KIILERICH: No, we don't have them.

AGGETT: The second question I wanted to ask was, how you are concluding that these patients are zinc-depleted intracellularly?

KIILERICH: In our patients with about six years' duration of the disease, we could find no decrease in serum zinc values and that is what we have been looking at in combination with the urine data. So it's my thought that when you have got a state of hyperzincuria, three times as high as in normal persons, and these patients don't look to have a high absorptive mechanism, it has to go wrong at some point.

AGGETT: You haven't looked at any cells to work out the intracellular zinc content?

KIILERICH: No, not with these patients.

AGGETT: Have you done it with alcoholics?

KIILERICH: Yes, with alcoholics we have done it. We have looked at the concentrations of zinc in the hepatocytes in living, normal persons and in patients with cirrhosis of the liver and the zinc content is decreased with about 30% in the cirrhotic liver tissue.

AGGETT: So this again hinges back to what Dr Hurley was suggesting, that studies of body composition would be very useful.

KIILERICH: Absolutely.

WRETLIND: My question is, if you have noted any clinical symptoms of zinc deficiency in your diabetic patients? There are several reports on overt zinc deficiency symptoms such as dermatitis in patients on parenteral nutrition regimens with no or inadequate amounts of zinc. Do you happen to know if any changes of carbohydrate metabolism have been observed in these patients?

KIILERICH: In answer to your first question, none of these diabetic patients showed any symptoms of zinc deficiency. As for the next question, I have never seen any of these patients, but I know that Dr Weismann has.

JAMESON: I wanted to add some information about zinc and diabetes. In at least two studies of the threshold of taste in diabetics, it is amply shown that there is a decrease in the acuity of taste. There are also at least two studies concerning the dark adaptation in diabetics. With advanced disease, they have a decreased dark adaptation probably due to damage in vitamin A utilisation.

Then I want to add more data about the trace element handling in diabetics with a bad diabetic state. There are data from several groups, for instance Dr Gunnar Johansson in Uppsala, showing that diabetics also have a magnesium deficiency. We also have the same data on selenium in complicated diabetics as we have on zinc. With increased duration of the diabetes, there are lower serum levels of selenium and lower glutathione peroxidase levels in the red blood cells. It's probably also interesting to look into manganese status, but to my knowledge there are no manganese data yet. And, of course, all the other trace elements, as Dr Wester noted, are most interesting. To my knowledge there are no data trying to understand why the treatment with diuretics increases the possibility of getting an impaired glucose tolerance. It would be interesting to look into the trace element balance in these patients.

CHRISTOPHERSEN: I just wanted to comment on the question of zinc balance. I don't think one can necessarily conclude that there will be a zinc deficiency even if you have a combination of increased urinary excretion and reduced intestinal absorption, because the main route of excretion in normal individuals is by way of the intestine. So it is possible, in principle, that a reduction of absorption combined with increased urinary excretion can be compensated by reduced secretion to the intestine. I think it is most probable that you will have deficiencies when you have this combination, but it is not a logical necessity.

KIILERICH: The main route of excretion is through the intestinal canal, but not by secretion. Only a little amount is being absorbed and the rest is going out so you don't absorb all your zinc and then secrete it afterwards.

CHRISTOPHERSEN: I'm talking about endogenous secretion to the intestine which is more important than the urinary excretion.

THEORELL: Will you comment on the possible connections between the elevated α_2-macroglobulin levels and the lowered zinc levels? I assume you have a relatively homogeneous diabetes control and you have eliminated renal function impairment and other complicating diseases. However, since α_2-macroglobulin is first of all an enzyme inhibitor and secondly an inflammatory reactant, could there be a correlation between the α_2-macroglobulin levels and the metabolic control of the diabetic state? Is there an elevated α_2-macroglobulin level and a lowered zinc level?

KIILERICH: All we know is that when you have diabetes, your α_2 is elevated. As far as I'm concerned the explanation for that is unknown. I haven't seen any studies that can answer that question, if it has anything to do with the severity of the disease.

WESTER: I should like to ask if there is anyone who can tell me, which is the best way to make the diagnosis of zinc deficiency in humans?

KIILERICH: We would like to make serum zinc a reliable measurement for it. We do know it is not without difficulties, but we try to optimate it, looking at the different proteins to which zinc has been bound. It would be the easiest way not to have to get tissues from here, there and everywhere to estimate the zinc status. But, I can't give you the final answer to it.

WEISMANN: I have a remark on the question concerning α_2-macroglobulin. We have found that in severely zinc-depleted patients total serum zinc is very low, but there's a relative increase in the α_2-macroglobulin. I don't know why that is so, but we have found it in two patients.

I would like to ask Dr Kiilerich: From your study it is clear that the serum zinc remains normal during the time of study. This is despite an increased urinary zinc excretion. The question then arises, where does the zinc come from? I think the absorption curve you mentioned, made by Kinlaw, is perhaps not the best way to discuss it, because this was an oral-loading test. Are you aware of any more specific absorption studies in diabetes? These oral-loading tests are very intriguing because what you measure actually is the serum department of the whole body and if you have a rapid turnover, which may be the case in diabetes because of a latent zinc deficiency, you will have a rapid transfer of zinc from the serum into the tissues. So what you have is a flat curve which actually represents an increased absorption. To discuss this, I think we have to have more sophisticated methods to study the zinc absorption in diabetes.

KIILERICH: I absolutely do agree, but I don't think that there are any other studies concerning these aspects today.

AGGETT: I, too, wanted to discuss that point. What was the oral-loading dose that Kinlaw was using?

KIILERICH: 25 mg.

AGGETT: So that was a fairly pharmacological dose in any case. Our experience, say with coeliac disease, is that whereas we can get abnormalities using something like 25 mg of zinc it seems to be more physiologically relevant to use a lower dose of zinc of 2 mg. Then we see no difference at all between the zinc absorption as assessed by ^{65}Zn and whole-body monitoring of patients with coeliac disease and normal volunteers. Following on from Dr Weismann's point, it could well be that your patients are maintaining a normal serum zinc, because that zinc is actually coming out of muscle or out of some other rapidly turning-over tissue pools of zinc. In fact, you are seeing your patients in a fairly acute state and if you hang on to them and see them later on, such as Dr Jameson has, perhaps you will then start to see a correlation in the slightly suboptimal diabetic control and a decline in zinc status.

KIILERICH: I can follow that point. We saw that the body weight was constant for one and a half years and we took that as an expression of a relatively constant metabolic level. We don't know the body's composition.

AGGETT: No, that's the net result. I was just wondering if there was increased turnover all the time, synthesis going much faster, breakdown much faster, with the zinc being lost adventitiously even though you're maintaining your body mass.

HURLEY: I agree with what Dr Aggett said but, also, I wonder if you were careful to measure the zinc levels in your patients at certain times of the day, at the same time of the day and also in a non-fasting state?

KIILERICH: Yes, we have done a methodological study before this and studied the importance of the diurnal variation, protein binding, interference of other metals and so on. Of course, we took these samples in a fasting state between 8 and 10 a.m.

HURLEY: You took them in a fasting state? Then I think that in itself could explain the higher levels. If you took them in a fed state you would get lower levels. Fasting increases turnover of gluconeogenesis which is multiplied in a fasting state. Therefore, protein is broken down and cells are broken down and that releases zinc. You can take a rat that is severely zinc-deficient and if you fast it, the plasma zinc level will become normal.

KIILERICH: Yes, but our control persons with the control urines have also been taken in a fasting state. So the normal persons have been fasting as well as the diabetics who were excreting three times as much zinc in the urine.

Chromium Supplementation: Effects on Glucose Tolerance and Lipid Metabolism

By RICHARD A. ANDERSON

GLUCOSE intolerance is usually one of the first measurable signs of chromium (Cr) deficiency and also diabetes. In the early experiments of Schwarz and Mertz (1957, 1959), which led to the discovery of Cr as an essential nutrient in preventing and reversing glucose intolerance, supplementing the apparently low Cr diet of rats with Cr led to rapid improvements in glucose tolerance. Chromium supplementation of patients on total parenteral nutrition also led to significant improvements in several diabetic-like symptoms including glucose intolerance (Jeejeebhoy et al. 1977, Freund et al. 1979). These symptoms were not improved with increased caloric intake, exogenous insulin or any other conventional methods of treatment. However, Cr supplementation of the total parenteral nutrition solutions caused reversal of the diabetic-like symptoms and exogenous insulin was no longer required. Chromium supplementation of children with protein calorie malnutrition (Gurson & Saner 1971), diabetics (Glinsmann & Mertz 1966, Nath et al. 1979, Mossop 1983), elderly (Levine et al. 1968), individuals of varying ages with marginally impaired glucose tolerance (Anderson et al. 1983b) and hypoglycemic patients, have all been shown to respond to supplemental Cr (Anderson et al. 1984).

Chromium also functions in lipid or fat metabolism. Evidence of a role of Cr in lipid metabolism and resulting detrimental effects of insufficient dietary Cr in the development of atherosclerosis is accumulating from animal and human studies. Chromium affects serum cholesterol (Schroeder & Balassa 1965, Abraham et al. 1982), cholesterol : high density lipoprotein cholesterol ratio (Riales & Albrink 1981), arterial plaque size (Abraham et al. 1980), and serum insulin (Nath et al. 1979, Mossop 1983, Anderson et al. 1984), all of which affect the development of atherosclerosis.

Table 1 Signs and symptoms of chromium deficiency
(Source: Adapted from Anderson 1981)

Functions	Animal
Impaired glucose tolerance	Human, rat, mouse, squirrel monkey
Elevated circulating insulin	Human, rat
Glycosuria	Human, rat
Fasting hyperglycemia	Human, rat, mouse
Impaired growth	Rat, mouse, turkey
Decreased longevity	Rat, mouse
Elevated serum cholesterol and triglycerides	Human, rat, mouse
Increased incidence of aortic plaques	Rabbit, rat, mouse
Neuropathy	Human
Encephalopathy	Human
Reduction in aortic intimal plaque areas	Rabbit
Corneal lesions	Rat, squirrel monkey
Decreased fertility and sperm count	Rat

DIETARY Cr INTAKE

The signs and symptoms of Cr deficiency listed in Table 1 appear to be widespread and are not limited to any particular socioeconomic group or geographical area. In 1980 the suggested safe and adequate intake for chromium was established at 50–200 μg/day for adults and 10–120 μg for infants, children and adolescents (National Research Council 1980). A limited number of people appear to meet the minimum suggested Cr intake and the remaining individuals are often well below this level. Well-balanced diets designed by a nutritionist to meet the requirements for most nutrients often contain less than the minimum suggested intake for Cr.

Reported Cr content of foods and diets varies depending upon methods of collection, homogenization and analysis. For example, stainless steel containers and/or stainless steel blender blades (stainless steel is approximately 18% Cr) are usually used for homogenizing of samples. When using these the apparent Cr content of foods depends more upon duration of blending than on the endogenous Cr content of the foods. Methods of food preparation also affect Cr intake. Chromium tends to leach from stainless steel cookware (Offenbacher & Pi-Sunyer 1983) and Cr that is incorporated into foods during preparation may be utilized. For example, Cr in beer, some of which originates from contamination, was absorbed and therefore presumably utilized similar to Cr found endogenously in foods (Anderson & Bryden 1983). The relative distribution of Cr among food groups is similar for fruits, vegetables, dairy products, beverages and meats with lesser amounts from cereal products and negligible dietary Cr from most seafoods and drinking water. Foods high in Cr are listed in Table 2. In general, most nonprocessed, high fiber foods, which are usually good sources of other trace elements, are also high in Cr.

Table 2 Foods high in chromium

Mushrooms
Brewer's yeast
Prunes
Nuts
Asparagus
Rhubarb
Black pepper
Wine
Beer

We have recently completed a study involving the dietary Cr intake of 10 adult male and 22 female subjects consuming self-selected diets (Kozlovsky et al. 1984). Daily diet samples were collected for seven consecutive days and analyzed for Cr. Chromium daily intake ranged from 8 to 89 μg with a mean (± S. E.) intake of 27 ± 1 μg. Chromium intake per 1,000 calories was approximately 15 μg, therefore to obtain the minimum suggested intake of 50 μg would necessitate consuming more than 3,000 calories per day and to consume the upper range of the suggested safe and adequate intake of 200 μg, more than 13,000 calories would need to be ingested!

An important question is, "Is the suggested safe and adequate intake realistic or is a large segment of the population consuming suboptimal amounts of Cr?" To answer this question the effects of supplemental Cr on subjects consuming normal self-selected diets need to be determined. These are discussed in the following sections.

CHROMIUM SUPPLEMENTATION AND GLUCOSE TOLERANCE

Chromium functions in glucose tolerance primarily through its action of insulin potentiation; much higher amounts of insulin are required at suboptimal Cr levels both *in vivo* and *in vitro*. In Fig. 1 is shown the effect of an organic chromium complex on the insulin dependent breakdown of glucose to carbon dioxide. Overall glucose breakdown can be increased by increasing insulin concentration but also by adding biologically active Cr and keeping the total amount of insulin constant. Similar results are obtained using Cr complexes extracted from natural resources (Anderson et al. 1978). Since some of the secondary complications linked to diabetes, including the increased incidence of cardiovascular disease, have been associated with elevated insulin (Stout 1977), it is advantageous to keep circulating insulin levels well within the normal range. Chromium functions not only in increasing the activity of insulin but also with this increased activity less insulin is required. Therefore, if the dietary intake of Cr is sufficient, lower levels of insulin are usually present.

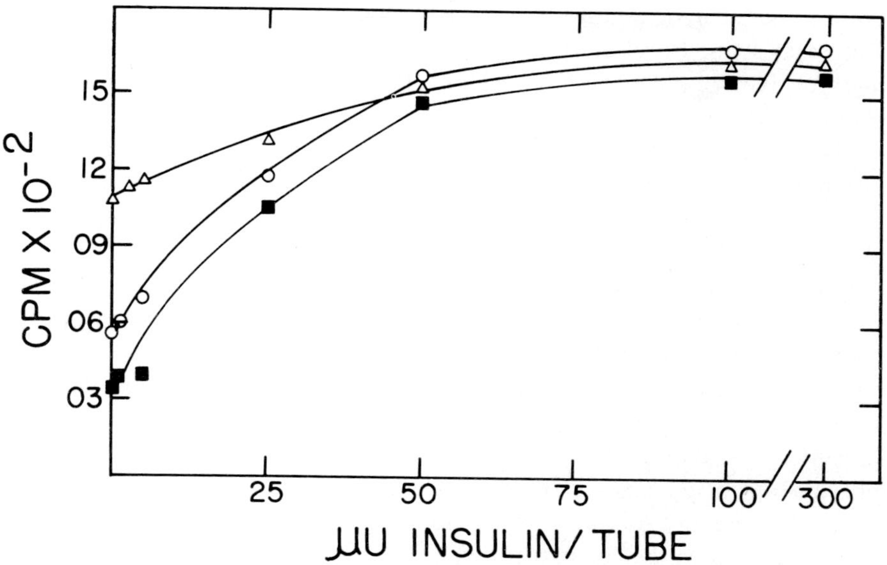

Fig. 1 *Effect of synthetic Cr complex on rat insulin stimulation of glucose oxidation by fat cells*

Epididymal fat cells isolated from two 125 g rats were suspended in Krebs Ringer phosphate-albumin buffer pH 7.4, 37°C. Closed squares (■) represent insulin dose response of glucose oxidation by fat cells; (○) designated levels of insulin +75 μg of Cr-complex containing 1 μg of chromium; (△) insulin +750 μg of Cr-complex containing 10 μg of Cr. All data points are an average of at least four separate determinations

(Source: Anderson et al. 1978)

Exogenous insulin requirement of a female patient receiving total parenteral nutrition (TPN) decreased from 45 units per day to zero following Cr supplementation (Jeejeebhoy et al. 1977). The patient had been on TPN for three years and had severe diabetic-like symptoms including glucose intolerance, inability to utilize glucose for energy, neuropathy, high fatty acid levels, low respiratory quotient and abnormalities of nitrogen metabolism. Addition of 250 μg daily of Cr as chromium chloride restored intravenous glucose tolerance and respiratory quotient to normal. The subject was then placed on a daily maintenance dose of 20 μg and symptoms mentioned above were eliminated. Similar results were reported for a female patient that had been receiving TPN for five months following complete bowel resection (Freund et al. 1979). Symptoms included severe glucose intolerance, weight loss and metabolic encephalopathy-like confusional state that were alleviated following addition of Cr to her TPN solutions.

Since Cr is present in TPN solutions as a contaminant, its concentration varies depending upon the lot, manufacturer, type of solution and other unknown variables. Chromium concentration is usually higher in protein or protein hydrolysates than in synthetic amino acid mixtures, fat, carbohydrate or electrolyte solutions (Seeling et al. 1979, Fell et al. 1979, Hauer & Kaminski 1978, Borel et al. 1984). Therefore, the amount of Cr a patient may receive fluctuates widely and Cr intake of subjects on long-term TPN should be monitored.

The American Medical Association (1979) recommends daily supplementation of TPN solutions with 10–15 μg of Cr for stable adult patients and 20 μg/day for stable adults with intestinal fluid losses. No definite amount is recommended for patients in acute catabolic states.

Improvements in glucose tolerance following Cr supplementation are not limited to patients on TPN. Children with protein-calorie malnutrition, the elderly, insulin and non-insulin dependent diabetics, hypoglycemics and subjects of varying ages with marginally impaired glucose tolerance have all been shown to respond to supplemental Cr (Table 3). Malnourished children in Turkey, Jordan and Nigeria responded to Cr supplementation with improvements in glucose tolerance (Hopkins et al. 1968, Gurson & Saner 1971). The glucose tolerance of malnourished children from Egypt was not improved following Cr supplementation; however, dietary Cr intake of those children was high relative to the Cr intake of the children whose glucose tolerance improved following supplemental Cr. Supplemental Cr has also been shown to improve the glucose tolerance of elderly subjects, maturity-onset diabetics and insulin-requiring diabetics; however, not all studies have reported improvements in glucose tolerance (see review Borel & Anderson 1984). This may be due in part to the habitual Cr intake of the particular groups of subjects (as discussed above for the children that responded to supplemental Cr) or the cause of the glucose intolerance. Obviously, not all glucose intolerance is due to Cr deficiency, therefore

Table 3 Studies reporting improved glucose tolerance following Cr supplementation

Cr supplementation refers to supplementation with inorganic Cr compounds. Several studies have reported significant improvements in glucose tolerance following brewer's yeast supplementation but in those studies, improvements may not be due solely to Cr but to other nutrients present in brewer's yeast (for review see Borel & Anderson 1984)

Subject description	Reference
Maturity-onset diabetics	Glinsmann and Mertz 1966 Nath et al. 1979
Malnourished children	Hopkins et al. 1968 Gurson and Saner 1971
Elderly	Levine et al. 1968
TPN patients	Jeejeebhoy et al. 1977 Freund et al. 1979
Insulin requiring diabetics	Mossop 1983
Marginally glucose intolerant	Anderson et al. 1983b
Hypoglycemics	Anderson et al. 1984

Table 4 *Effect of Cr supplementation on 90-min serum glucose of subjects with varying degrees of glucose tolerance*

Subjects	90-min serum glucose (mg/dl)	
	Placebo	Cr-supplemented
Marginally hyperglycemic (20)[1]	135 ± 9	116 ± 11
Hypoglycemic (35)[2]	70 ± 1	81 ± 4
Normal (21)[3]	86 ± 2	85 ± 3

Number in parentheses denotes number of subjects. Glucose values are an average of 2- and 3-month values during each portion of the study.

[1] Marginally hyperglycemic subjects are defined as those subjects that are not yet classified as diabetic but have 90-min glucose values (average of pretest and 2- and 3-month placebo values following a glucose load, 1 g/kg body wt) greater than 100 mg/dl.

[2] Hypoglycemic subjects are defined as subjects with 90-min glucose values less than fasting.

[3] Normal subjects are the remaining subjects with near-optimal glucose tolerance.

supplemental Cr will only help those subjects whose abnormalities in glucose utilization are due to insufficient dietary Cr. Chromium functions as a nutrient and not as a therapeutic agent.

We have recently reported that response to Cr varies with degree of glucose intolerance (Table 4) (Anderson et al. 1982, 1983b). Our study design was double-blind crossover with each test period lasting three months. Subjects were tested after two and three months during each portion of the study; values after two and three months of the study were similar and therefore combined. There were 76 total subjects in the three groups defined in Table 4, 20 of these comprised the marginally hyperglycemic group (90-min glucose greater than 100 mg/dl following a glucose load of 1 g glucose/kg body wt). The glucose tolerance of 18 of the 20 subjects in this group improved following supplementation of 200 μg of chromium as chromium chloride, glucose tolerance of one subject was unchanged and that of one subject continued to decline during both the placebo and Cr supplementation periods. The glucose tolerance of subjects with 90-min glucose less than 100 mg/dl but greater than fasting denoted as "normals" in Table 4 was not changed following Cr supplementation. These subjects have near-optimal glucose tolerance and presumably adequate Cr stores and therefore would not be expected and in fact do not respond to supplemental Cr. The 90-min glucose of subjects with 90-min glucose values less than fasting increased following Cr supplementation (Table 4). Therefore, supplemental Cr tended to normalize glucose tolerance, namely, Cr supplementation decreased glucose levels of subjects with elevated glucose, increased glucose of subjects with low blood sugar and had no effect on serum glucose of subjects with near-optimal glucose tolerance. We have also determined the effect of Cr supplementation on subjects that are either diabetic or borderline diabetics. The percentage of subjects that responded to supplemental Cr in this group is usually quite low. Similar results were reported in a Finnish study involving subjects with advanced stages of glucose intolerance (Uusitupa et al. 1983). Subjects appear to be less likely to respond to supplemental Cr with increasing degrees of glucose intolerance.

Subjects with low blood sugar responded to supplemental Cr with an increase in blood sugar (Table 4). Many of the subjects in this group, characterized by 90-min glucose values less than fasting, would be normal, but some may be truly hypoglycemic. Minimum hypoglycemic values are usually reached two to three hours following a sugar challenge, therefore 90-min glucose values may not be an accurate measure of the degree of hypoglycemia. To determine if Cr would improve the symptoms of patients diagnosed as hypoglycemics, eight female patients, under treatment for hypoglycemia, were supplemented with Cr (Anderson et al. 1984). Study design was similar to the previous study and was double-blind crossover with each test period lasting three months. Serum samples were obtained at fasting and 30, 60, 90, 120, 180, 240 and 300 min following a glucose load. The area of the glucose tolerance curve (glucose concentration vs. time) less than fasting was compared during the placebo and Cr supplementation periods. There was a significant improvement in hypoglycemic glucose values following Cr supplementation. Immunoreactive serum insulin also improved in five of the eight patients. Therefore, supplemental Cr appears to not only lead to a decrease in the blood sugar of subjects with elevated serum glucose following a glucose load but also leads to an increase in blood sugar of subjects being treated for hypoglycemia.

CHROMIUM AND LIPID METABOLISM

Evidence linking marignal Cr intakes with abnormal lipid metabolism and ultimately atherosclerosis is accumulating from both animal and human studies. Animal studies indicate that with increasing age, rats fed a low Cr diet have increased serum cholesterol, aortic lipids and plaque formations (Schroeder & Balassa 1965). In rabbits fed a high-cholesterol diet to induce atherosclerotic plaques, subsequent intraperitoneal administration of 20 μg potassium chromate per day led to a reducion in the size of aortic plaques and a decrease in aortic cholesterol concentration (Abraham et al. 1980). Chromium supplementation of a high-cholesterol diet resulted in significantly less aortic cholesterol and plaque area (Abraham et al. 1982). Individuals that died of coronary artery disease were also reported to have lower Cr concentration in aortic tissue compared to subjects dying from accidents, although the Cr concentration of other tissues analyzed was similar (Schroeder et al. 1970). Subjects with coronary artery disease have also been reported to have lower serum chromium than subjects without symptoms of disease (Newman et al. 1978). In that study decreased serum Cr correlated highly ($p < 0.01$) with the appearance of coronary artery disease, whereas elevated serum triacylglycerol correlated less significantly ($p < 0.05$) and there was no correlation between other risk factors, such as serum cholesterol, blood pressure or body weight. Chromium supplementation (200 μg daily, 5 days a week for 12 weeks) of 12 adult men resulted in significant decreases in serum triglycerides and increases in high-density lipoprotein cholesterol compared to the placebo subjects (Riales & Albrink 1981). Chromium supplementation (600 μg Cr as chromium chloride daily) of patients being treated for diabetes also resulted in a significant increase in high density lipoprotein cholesterol and a decrease in total cholesterol (Mossop 1983). Numerous studies have also reported beneficial effects on serum lipids following supplementation with brewer's yeast that is high in Cr (see review Borel & Anderson 1984).

SUMMARY

Chromium is an essential trace element required for normal carbohydrate and lipid metabolism. Insufficient dietary Cr leads to signs and symptoms similar to those observed for individuals with diabetes and/or cardiovascular disease. Dietary intake of Cr from self-selected diets appears to be approximately half of the minimum suggested safe and adequate intake. Children with protein calorie malnutrition, diabetics, elderly, individuals of varying ages with marginally impaired glucose tolerance and hypoglycemics have all been shown to respond to supplemental Cr by improvements in glucose tolerance and/or serum lipids.

REFERENCES

ABRAHAM, A. S., SONNENBLICK, M., EINI, M., SHEMASH, O. & BRATT, P. (1980). The effect of chromium on established atherosclerotic plaques in rabbits. *Amer. J. clin. Nutr.* 33, 2294.

ABRAHAM, A. S., SONNENBLICK, M. & EINI, M. (1982). The action of chromium on serum lipids and on atherosclerosis in cholesterol-fed rabbits. *Atherosclerosis* 42, 185.

American Medical Association Department of Foods and Nutrition (1979). Guidelines for essential trace element preparations for parenteral use. A statement by an expert panel. *J. Amer. Med. Ass.* 241, 2051.

ANDERSON, R. A. (1981). Nutritional role of chromium. *Sci. Total Environ.* 17, 13.

ANDERSON, R. A. & BRYDEN, N. A. (1983). Concentration, insulin potentiation and absorption of chromium in beer. *J. agric. Food Chem.* 31, 308.

ANDERSON, R. A., BRANTNER, J. H. & POLANSKY, M. M. (1978). An improved assay for biologically active chromium. *J. agric. Food Chem.* 26, 1219.

ANDERSON, R. A., POLANSKY, M. M., BRYDEN, N. A., ROGINISKI, E. E., PATTERSON, K. Y., VEILLON, C. & GLINSMANN, W. (1982). Urinary chromium excretion of human subjects: Effect of chromium supplementation and glucose loading. *Amer. J. clin. Nutr.* 36, 1184.

ANDERSON, R. A., POLANSKY, M. M., BRYDEN, N. A., PATTERSON, K. Y., VEILLON, C. & GLINSMANN, W. H. (1983a). Effect of chromium supplementation on urinary Cr excretion of human subjects and correlation of Cr excretion with selected clinical parameters. *J. Nutr.* 113, 276.

ANDERSON, R. A., POLANSKY, M. M., BRYDEN, N. A., ROGINSKI, E. E., MERTZ, W. & GLINSMANN, W. H. (1983b). Chromium supplementation of human subjects: Effects on glucose, insulin and lipid parameters. *Metabolism* 32, 894.

ANDERSON, R. A., POLANSKY, M. M., BRYDEN, N. A. & CANARY, J. J. (1984). Chromium supplementation of humans with hypoglycemia. *Fed. Proc.* 41, 471.

BOREL, J. S. & ANDERSON, R. A. (1984). Biochemistry of chromium. In *Biochemistry of the Elements,* pp. 175–199. Ed. by E. Frieden. Plenum Publishing Co., N. Y., N. Y.

BOREL, J. S., MAJERUS, T. C., POLANSKY, M. M., MOSER, P. B. & ANDERSON, R. A. (1984). Chromium intake and urinary chromium excretion of trauma patients. *Biol. Trace Element Res.* 6, 317.

FELL, G. S., HALL, D. & SHENKIN, A. (1979). Chromium requirements during intravenous nutrition. In *Chromium in Nutrition and Metabolism,* pp. 105–112. Ed. by D. Shapcott and J. Hubert. Elsevier/North Holland, Amsterdam.

FREUND, H., ATAMIAN, S. & FISCHER, J. E. (1979). Chromium deficiency during total parenteral nutrition. *J. Amer. Med. Ass.* 214, 496.

GLINSMANN, W. H. & MERTZ, W. (1966). Plasma chromium after glucose administration. *Science* 152, 1243.

GURSON, C. T. & SANER, G. (1971). Effect of chromium on glucose utilizations in marasmic protein-calorie malnutrition. *Amer. J. clin. Nutr.* 24, 1313.

HAUER, E. C. & KAMINSKI, M. V. (1978). Trace metal profile of parenteral nutrition solutions. *Amer. J. clin. Nutr.* 31, 264.

HOPKINS, L. L., Jr., RANSOME-KUTI, O. & MAJAJ, A. S. (1968). Improvement of impaired carbohydrate metabolism by chromium (III) in malnourished infants. *Amer. J. clin. Nutr.* 21, 203.

JEEJEEBHOY, K. N., CHU, R. C., MARLISS, E. B., GREENBERG, G. R. & BRUCE-ROBERTSON, A. (1977). Chromium deficiency, glucose intolerance, and neuropathy reversed by chromium supplementation in a patient receiving long-term total parenteral nutrition. *Amer. J. clin. Nutr.* 30, 531.

KOZLOVSKY, A. S., HALLFRISCH, J. & ANDERSON, R. A. (1984). Chromium intake, excretion and absorption by adult subjects consuming self-selected diets. *Fed. Proc.* 43, 471.

LEVINE, R. A., STREETEN, D. H. P. & DOISY, R. J. (1968). Effects of oral chromium supplementation on the glucose tolerance of elderly subjects. *Metabolism* 17, 114.

MOSSOP, R. T. (1983). Effects of chromium (III) on fasting glucose, cholesterol and cholesterol HDL levels in diabetics. *Cent. Afr. J. Med.* 29, 80.

NATH, R., MINOCHA, J., LYALL, V., SKUNDER, S., KUMAR, V., KAPPOR, S. & DHAR, K. L. (1979). Assessment of chromium metabolism in maturity onset and juvenile diabetes using chromium-51 and therapeutic response of chromium administration on plasma lipids, glucose tolerance and insulin levels. In *Chromium in Nutrition and Metabolism,* pp. 213–222. Ed. by D. Shapcott and J. Hubert. Elsevier/North Holland, Amsterdam.

National Research Council (1980). *Recommended Dietary Allowances.* National Academy of Sciences, Washington, D. C.

NEWMAN, H. A. I., LEIGHTON, R. F., LANESE, R. R. & FREEDLAND, N. A. (1978). Serum chromium and angiographically determined coronary artery disease. *Clin. Chem.* 24, 541.

OFFENBACHER, E. B. & PI-SUNYER, F. X. (1983). Temperature and pH effects on the release of chromium from stainless steel into water and fruit juices. *J. agric. Food Chem.* 31, 89.

RIALES, R. & ALBRINK, M. J. (1981). Effect of chromium chloride supplementation on glucose tolerance and serum lipids including high-density lipoprotein of adult men. *Amer. J. clin. Nutr.* 34, 2670.

SCHWARZ, K. & MERTZ, W. (1957). A glucose tolerance factor and its differentiation from factor 3. *Arch. Biochem.* 72, 515.

— (1959). Chromium (III) and the glucose tolerance factor. *Arch. Biochem.* 85, 292.

SCHROEDER, H. A. & BALASSA, J. J. (1965). Influence of chromium, cadmium and lead on rat aortic lipids and circulating cholesterol. *Amer. J. Physiol.* 209, 433.

SCHROEDER, H. A., NASON, A. P. & TIPTON, I. H. (1970). Chromium deficiency as a factor in atherosclerosis. *J. chron. Dis.* 15, 941.

SEELING, W., AHNEFELD, F. W., GRUNERT, A., KIENLE, K. H. & SWOBODNIK, M. (1979). Chromium in parenteral nutrition. In *Chromium in Nutrition and Metabolism,* pp. 95–104. Ed. by D. Shapcott and J. Hubert. Elsevier/North Holland, Amsterdam.

STOUT, R. W. (1977). The relationship of abnormal circulating insulin levels to atherosclerosis. *Atherosclerosis* 27, 1.

UUSITUPA, M. I. J., KUMPULAINEN, J. T., VOUTILAINEN, E., HERSIO, K., SARLUND, H., PYORALA, K. P., KOIVISTOINEN, P. E. & LEHTO, J. T. (1983). Effect of inorganic chromium supplementation on glucose tolerance, insulin response, and serum lipids in noninsulin-dependent diabetics. *Amer. J. clin. Nutr.* 38, 404.

Discussion (the paper by Anderson)

Chairman: WRETLIND

EKMAN: I would like to ask about the mode of action of chromium. Is the effect on insulin an increased receptor-binding, an increased receptor sensitivity or a post-receptor effect with regards to glucose metabolism?

ANDERSON: We certainly know that there is an increased receptor-binding to red blood cells due to Cr supplementation. We haven't calculated the data yet to determine whether this is due to receptor number or receptor affinity. It's certainly due to increased receptor-binding.

EKMAN: Is there any post-receptor effect also?

ANDERSON: I think there is, but you're talking very mechanistically as to how chromium functions. How chromium functions is related pretty much to how insulin functions. Even after all the time and effort were put into insulin mechanisms and insulin actions, these are still not fully understood. I don't think we'll understand chromium mechanisms until we have a very good handle on the mechanism of insulin action alone.

EKMAN: As a naive surgeon I would like to know if it is known whether the anabolic effects of insulin are potentiated by adding chromium? Does the increased binding of insulin to the cells have any positive impact on protein synthesis when it's known that insulin does stimulate the initiation of protein transfer?

ANDERSON: Yes, chromium affects amino acid transport. That's not an area that is studied as much although there have been studies done.

FELLSTRÖM: Dr Anderson, apparently there are mainly peripheral effects of chromium in carbohydrate metabolism. One would perhaps anticipate that chromium would be more important in Type 2 diabetes than in Type 1 because of this phenomenon. You haven't presented any data on chromium levels in your patients with diabetes. I'm very well aware of the analytical problems but do you have any data on chromium levels in patients with diabetes or do you know of any studies dealing with that?

Secondly, there have been some reports on diabetic patients being given fiber in their diet. On such a diet the need for insulin has apparently decreased. Do you know if by any chance the content of chromium or perhaps zinc in a fiber diet would be the reason for that?

ANDERSON: To answer your second question first as far as the relation to fiber, we certainly think that chromium may play a role in the fiber story. For example, Jim

Anderson in Kentucky has done a lot of that work. When you change the fiber of the diet basically you're certainly improving the trace element intake, because for the most part you're decreasing the fat and refined carbohydrates and replacing them with fiber food which would be high in trace elements. The effects that they see from fiber are certainly very similar to the effects we see from chromium.

As far as your first question about the concentration of chromium in Type 1 and Type 2 diabetics and your comment on the analytical problem, I think the analytical problems regarding urine in serum and even tissue with respect to chromium are basically solved. There are a lot of people doing inadequate analytical work with chromium, but there's really no excuse for that. The methodology is such now that you can routinely do chromium in serum and in urine, the values should be approximately .1 to .2 ppb whether it be urine or serum. As far as Type 1 diabetics, their chromium concentration is usually about 50% higher in urinary excretion than it is for control subjects. As far as the Type 2 diabetics, which most of our work deals with, it is very difficult to see that there is a difference in chromium excretion. The values are much closer to those of the controls than in the Type 1 diabetics. There are two very clearly defined groups in Type 1 diabetes. You can see this in autopsy samples, the diabetic versus the normal, you can also look at hair samples.

AGGETT: I'd just like to ask Dr Anderson what has happened to the "glucose tolerance factor" and what the general feeling about it is now; and if you think chromium has an effect on binding, does it have similar effects, say, on human growth hormone or with cortico-steroid effects?

ANDERSON: Concerning the first question as to what has happened to the glucose tolerance factor, I don't think anything has happened to it, it's still there as it was before. But what does glucose tolerance factor mean? I think that's the key question. For most of the people in this room the glucose tolerance factor is not needed in the diet to improve cholesterol levels or triglycerides, since most people can convert inorganic chromium to a usable form. If you want to call that usable form glucose tolerance factor or GTF, it's certainly still there. If you're going to isolate this so-called mysterious GTF and say this is a vitamin like B_{12} or something like that, then I don't know where GTF is and I don't know if GTF ever existed. But, on the other side of that, there is a certain group of people who do not respond to inorganic chromium and when we give these people brewer's yeast, which is high in insulinpotentiating chromium, these people often do respond. I haven't talked about any of those results because those aren't double-blind crossover studies. It's very hard to camouflage 10 to 15 g of brewer's yeast. It has a very distinct taste, a very distinct odor, etc. Still you do definitely see an improvement in some people with brewer's yeast and not with inorganic chromium. As far as the absorption being much better than inorganic chromium, we can't demonstrate that. For example, we grow yeast on radioactive chromium, extract the chromium and measure its potentiation activity, stomach-tube it to rats and we don't see very high levels of absorption, usually less than 1% not 10 to 25%. If you talk to other people you may get different opinions. All I can do is state what I feel the state of the field is now and what my interpretations of it are.

SHAMBERGER: In your experiments, did you look at HDL, LDL, insulin or other vital proteins?

ANDERSON: Absolutely. We look at the complete profile. We do it both by heparin-manganese precipitation for HDL and then we do it by ultracentrifugation, because as you know there's some controversy as to the different types of HDL.

Again, we do see changes in certain people but we can't predict a priori whom this is going to affect. In some it goes up, in some it goes down. As far as the specific chromium effect, we really can't say for sure. Other people have certainly seen, in double-blind crossover studies, an effect of chromium supplementation on HDL. The HDL goes up and the total cholesterol either remains the same or goes down. Therefore, the total HDL/cholesterol relationship is improved.

WEISMANN: I have just a short comment on the diabetics' chromium and zinc metabolism. The results seem to show a difference in the actions of chromium and zinc. Zinc seems to directly influence the stability of insulin. In chromium it seems that first a small peptide has to be formed to explain the effect of chromium in diabetics.

ANDERSON: I don't see why you say there has to be a small peptide. Perhaps when you say small peptide you mean GTF. Chromium has to be converted to a usable form. But I don't think zinc functions as zinc chloride or zinc sulphate. Zinc is going to bind to other proteins and *that* is going to be its usable form. I think in that respect they're the same. But, certainly, there are very big differences in the way zinc functions and the way chromium functions.

THEORELL: What is the possible contribution of cooking in stainless steel?

ANDERSON: The possible contribution of cooking in stainless steel is very substantial to chromium nutrition. I think this is really an important health problem. Now, at least it's true in the United States, when you cook your meals you cook in teflon, aluminum or some kind of coated cookware. This definitely decreases chromium intake. You say: Is this chromium that leaches from the stainless steel material usable? Certainly. We've done some studies and found that the absorption of chromium that leaches into beer from stainless steel, is basically the same as the absorption of chromium when it's endogenously incorporated in foods. It has a very definite effect. Again, with this in mind, there are all kinds of values for the chromium intake. The values I've shown are low. In all our studies we use either low-chromium steel or plastic. If you take a plastic blender with its stainless steel blender blade, blend up food and analyze for chromium, measuring chromium content after 30 seconds, one minute, two minutes, five minutes of blending, you see a linear relationship between time of blending and the chromium content of that food. That has absolutely nothing to do with the food you are eating, because you're not eating that food after it has been blended, you're just taking it from your plate. So it has a very definite effect. That explains why a lot of the older values are totally erroneous where they used a plastic blender but they used the stainless steel blender blades.

WRETLIND: My question is, if you have observed any correlation between the response to chromium and the previous chromium intake? I should also very much like to know the amount of chromium consumed by the patient before entering the study.

ANDERSON: The values we show as far as intake are concerned are roughly for a female 25 μg and for a male 30 μg of chromium. But, again it turns out that you excrete the amount of chromium taken in very quickly. If you take in 10, 20 or 40 μg of chromium in your diet, the amount that is actually absorbed is very similar because there are changes in the percent absorption. For example, if you take in 10 μg, absorption is about 2% which would give you about 0.2 μg. But if you take in 40 μg, your absorption is about 0.5%, and you're still absorbing about 0.2 μg. Therefor, when you look at urinary chromium excretion *below* 40 μg, it's going to be about constant. Once you get above 40 μg you see a linear relationship between chromium intake and chromium absorption.

BRUCE: Regarding the question about stainless steel, we analyzed a number of stainless steel pans for nickel and found that there was a large variation in the amount of release. A few released a lot but the majority only a little.

Dr Anderson, I think you mentioned that 20 individuals out of 76 showed an impaired glucose tolerance. That is quite a large number. Is that what you expect in your populations?

ANDERSON: I think that it depends on how you define impaired glucose tolerance. Keep in mind we defined people with glucose levels greater than 100 mg/dl 90 min after a glucose load as marginally impaired. For any medical criteria, that is not impaired glucose tolerance. This is why you get a higher percentage. But, from the nutrition standpoint, what we need to do, for example, is not to wait for someone to be classified as diabetic—having a fasting-glucose greater than 140 mg/dl—then intervene with nutrition and expect to help them. What we want to do is prevent this from ever happening and that's basically what our mission at Beltsville is: To keep the healthy people healthier. It's not to treat the people who already have diabetes, cardiovascular disease, etc.

BRUCE: Was there any correlation to overweight?

ANDERSON: The subjects in this study were not overweight. If they were over 30% above ideal body weight, they were not allowed to be in the study.

BRUCE: Do you think your findings indicated a marginal chromium deficiency or a disturbed metabolism which increased the requirement for chromium?

ANDERSON: I don't think there is anything unique about this group of subjects. The most unique thing about them would be that they would be healthier than most, because we excluded the people who are overweight or taking medications. I think this group is reasonably representative, certainly of the people in the Beltsville area.

BRUCE: How do you interpret the finding—as a marginal or biochemical deficiency or that they for some other reason have increased requirements?

ANDERSON: No, I think their intake is low based upon the suggested safe and adequate intake. As far as how you predict someone is chromium-deficient, I don't think you really can. You can't determine chromium deficiency from serum chromium, urine chromium or any other known variable. But what you have to do is supplement these people with chromium and determine the effects of supplemental chromium on glucose tolerance and serum lipids. I think their intake is suboptimal because after treatment—remembering that we're not giving them pharmacological doses, we're giving nutritional doses—we do see the effect. So we're looking at nutritional effect as opposed to pharmacological effect.

BRUCE: I have a last question about HDL. There is at least one study which has shown quite a substantial increase in HDL after chromium supplementation. Are there any other studies which confirm this finding?

ANDERSON: Yes, Riales and Albrink (*Amer. J. clin. Nutr.* 1981:34, 2670) were the first to come out with it. They had a group which consisted only of physicians. They saw an improvement in HDL, more so at two months than at three months. There is a fellow named Mossop down in Zimbabwe working with diabetics. He reported more than a 30% increase in HDL following chromium supplementation. We do not see such large effects but, again, part of our problem is that we selected people with lower total cholesterol and triglycerides. We've eliminated the people who possibly would respond the most, the ones who have the very low HDL or the very high cholesterol.

Cellular Stores of Macro- and Trace Elements in Peripheral Blood Cells Isolated from Patients with Inflammatory Connective-Tissue Diseases

By Roger Hällgren, Erland Johansson, Karin Svenson and Ulf Lindh

INTRODUCTION

The alterations of trace element metabolism in association with chronic inflammatory diseases has been a field beset with controversy but has during recent years come into focus partly due to the development of anti-rheumatic therapies which involve the manipulation of trace elements but also due to the discovery of the central role certain metals have in free radical generation. For a long time, a great number of studies have been performed on the more common connective-tissue diseases with regard to altered metabolism of essential metals. However, most of these studies are based upon analyses of single elements in serum/plasma or urine, while analyses of macro- and trace elements in isolated cells have been sparse, mainly due to analytical problems. The main purpose of this article is to briefly review the possible role of calcium, strontium, zinc and manganese in chronic inflammatory diseases in the light of our observations on the abnormal stores of these macro- and trace elements in peripheral blood cells isolated from patients with rheumatoid arthritis and other inflammatory connective-tissue diseases.

METHODS

In our studies we have applied the nuclear microprobe technique on isolated cells for elemental mapping. Erythrocytes, granulocytes and platelets were isolated from venous blood drawn into venoject tubes (Terumo, Tokyo, Japan) with K_3EDTA as anticoagulant (1). The isolated cell populations were put onto clean Formvar films (Formvar 1595 E; Merck, Darmstadt, W. Germany). After freezing to −80°C, the cells were freeze-dried. During the preparation and analysis, the cells were stored in desiccators over silica gel in darkness in a cooler. From the blood cell preparations 10 cells of each type were selected under the light microscope prior to microprobe analysis in the Studsvik Nuclear Microprobe. A technical account of the analytical instrument has been published elsewhere (2). The selected cells were irradiated with a 5 μm beam of 2.5 MeV protons from the Van de Graaf accelerator of the Natural Science Research Laboratory at Studsvik, Sweden. The induced spectra of characteristic X-rays were collected by a multichannel analyser. Handling of the registered data was performed as previously described (3). The conversion of X-ray counts to relative amounts was possible by registration of the continuous Brehmsstrahlung being proportional to the mass (2, 4).

Analysis of macro- and trace elements in isolated cells is faced by several problems. Compared with other techniques used—volumetry, flame emission spectrometry, neutron activation, solution absorption spectrometry and atomic absorption spectrometry—the nuclear microprobe technique demands a minimum of additives thereby reducing the risk of contamination. Incomplete separation of the blood cells is another possible source of error, which, however, is minimized by using the present technique with selection of cells through microscopy. Finally, by the preparation procedure using ultrathin sample supports, the contribution of the continuous background radiation from the support material has become negligible.

RESULTS AND DISCUSSION

Calcium

During the last decades there has been a growing awareness that changes of cellular calcium can play an important role in cell injury caused by, e.g., ischemia (5), biological toxins (6), and genetic abnormalities (7). Experimental studies also indicate that the extent of immunologically induced cell injury can be affected by an increase in intracellular calcium (8). A disturbance of the calcium balance might, therefore, be one of several ways by which immunological and inflammatory principles alter cell metabolism and function in chronic inflammatory connective-tissue diseases. We have recently reported conspicuous accumulation of calcium in erythrocytes and granulocytes isolated from patients with certain inflammatory connective-tissue diseases: rheumatoid arthritis, seronegative spondarthritis and scleroderma (1). The intensity of the inflammatory process seems to be linked to the abnormal calcium balance since we observed significant positive correlations between acute-phase plasma proteins and the granulocyte or erythrocyte content of calcium. During corticosteroid therapy of patients with inflammatory arthritides, no acute effects on the calcium stores in these cell types were observed, but after three months on such therapy a significant reduction of cellular calcium was evident.

At rest more than 99% of calcium in nucleated cells is bound to ligands as well as sequestered in organelles (9). In erythrocytes, the dominating part of cellular calcium seems to be associated with the membrane (10). The most important calcium ligands identified are a class of regulatory calcium-binding proteins called calmodulins (11). We have no data on the cellular amount of free calcium or the subcellular localization of calcium in the blood cells isolated from patients with inflammatory diseases but assume that the increased total cellular calcium reflects increased bound calcium. The cellular calcium-binding structures have a very potent buffering capacity. They rapidly remove free calcium when appearing in increased cytoplasmic concentrations.

A steady state normally exists between the cytoplasmic free calcium and the bound calcium in the cell. An increase of cytoplasmic calcium over a significant time period would, therefore, cause an increase in bound and hence total cell calcium. An increase in cytoplasmic free calcium can arise by a variety of pharmacological and physiological stimuli and toxic agents; either by increasing the passive membrane permeability to calcium or by mobilization of calcium stores in the cell (12). A cellular overload of calcium could also be a consequence of a defective calcium efflux. Cell tissue injury in chronic inflammatory tissue diseases may be provoked by a number of inflammatory or immunological principles: circulating immune complexes, activated complement components, autoantibodies against proteins or cell membranes. It is, therefore, of particular interest to note that antibodies to cell surface receptors (13) and activated complement (8) may increase intracellular calcium, evidently by a change of the permeability of the cell membrane for calcium.

The biological consequences of accumulation of calcium in granulocytes and erythrocytes in chronic inflammatory diseases are unknown. A calcium overload of granulocytes may result in an abnormal response of the cell to a stimulus, such as activated complement components or immune complexes, provided that the calcium stores are mobilized during the activation. One should in this situation expect an enhanced degranulation and an increased production of oxygen-radical products by polymorphs (14–16). Such possible consequences should be of central pathogenetic importance for inflammatory destructive processes in the connective tissue.

An overload of calcium in red cells is associated with changes of shape and membrane flexibility which reduces the life span of such cells (7, 17, 18). Previous studies have shown that the erythrocyte survival is shortened in, e.g., rheumatoid arthritis (19). However, the anaemia which frequently accompanies chronic inflammatory diseases has been attributed to impaired marrow response and defective iron mobilization. Our finding of a negative correlation between erythrocyte content of calcium and hemoglobin values supports the notion that calcium accumulation in erythrocytes may be another factor behind the anaemia in chronic inflammatory disorders.

Strontium

Strontium resembles calcium in its physiological and biochemical properties and appears in high concentration in the bone tissue in which it may have a structural function. Other functions of this alkaline earth metal in the human body remain uncertain. However, it may have a regulatory role in inflammatory processes since experimental *in vitro* studies have demonstrated that strontium stimulates degranulation of granulocytes, mast cells, platelets and large granular lymphocytes (20–23). Evidently, strontium may substitute calcium in its degranulation function and has, therefore, been used as a probe for intracellular calcium in *in vitro* situations (24). Its possible role for the degranulation process *in vivo* and its role in inflammatory diseases has until now not been considered. We have recently found considerable amounts of strontium in granulocytes isolated from patients with untreated rheumatoid arthritis and seronegative spondarthritides in spite of plasma strontium within the normal ranges (25). Granulocytes from healthy individuals did not contain measurable amounts of strontium. No data exist on the subcellular localization of strontium but there may exist a specific storage system in granulocytes since strontium was not detectable in erythrocytes or platelets isolated from the patients or healthy controls.

The cause of the granulocyte accumulation of strontium is not known but evidently linked to the intensity of the inflammatory process since total granulocyte strontium was strongly correlated to the acute-phase plasma proteins. The suspicion that inflammatory principles may govern the strontium overload was further strengthened by the conspicuous reduction of granulocyte strontium during corticosteroid therapy. Moreover, the individual reduction of granulocyte strontium was closely related to the individual reduction of the acute-phase reaction. Accumulation of strontium and calcium may be governed by similar principles since the granulocyte amounts of these elements were positively correlated to each other. Based on experimental studies, one may suspect that accumulation of strontium may be one way to induce enhanced degranulation of granulocytes triggered by various stimuli.

Zinc

There is a basic requirement for zinc in order for cells to function. Zinc is involved in nearly all aspects of cellular metabolism and has a key role in numerous essential processes: protein synthesis, DNA and RNA metabolism, carbohydrate and lipid metabolism. Zinc has also a central role in the regulation of cell function and activity. A number of cell types are inhibited by zinc, possibly by antagonism of calcium action. Examples of inflammatory cell activities inhibited by an excess of zinc are release of histamine by stimulated mast cells (26), granulocytic chemotaxis and phagocytosis (27), platelet release reaction and platelet aggregation (28). Zinc deficiency has been associated with lymphopenia and atrophy of lymphoid tissues (29). Both primary and secondary antibody responses to T-cell-dependent antigens are reduced (30). Zinc-deficient subjects have poor lymphocyte proliferation response to mitogens and wound healing is impaired (29). Based on these zinc-dependent effects, it is not surprising that considerable attention has been paid to zinc as an element of importance in inflammatory diseases. In most studies on rheumatoid arthritis, plasma zinc is reported to be reduced, but it is uncertain whether or not this really reflects a true deficiency of importance for the disease process. Clinical improvement in patients with rheumatoid arthritis treated with zinc sulphate has been reported (31), but other studies have failed to confirm such an effect (32). We have recently reported that patients with inflammatory connective-tissue diseases, scleroderma, rheumatoid arthritis and other inflammatory arthritides, not only have low plasma zinc values but also considerably reduced total zinc in isolated erythrocytes, granulocytes and platelets (33).

Reduced plasma zinc in rheumatoid arthritis and other inflammatory diseases has in part been attributed to decreased amounts of zinc-binding proteins. About 40% is firmly bound to α_2-macroglobulin, 50% is more loosely bound to primarily albumin and the rest, the biologically active fraction, circulates as a microligand with one of several aminoacids, in particular histidine. Intracellular zinc is largely soluble in the cytoplasm and bound to aminoacids and calmodulins (34) serving as ligands. Minor amounts of zinc may be located in organelles and granules. The decrease of intracellular zinc in chronic inflammatory diseases might, therefore, reflect a reduction of zinc-binding sites either due to reduced synthesis of ligands or as a result of competitive inhibition of common binding sites by other elements. Thus, it is possible that a reduction of cellular zinc is a secondary event to cellular accumulation of, e.g., calcium.

We observed in our study a relationship between plasma zinc and the acute-phase reaction suggesting that the inflammatory process to some extent governs the plasma zinc levels. This idea is in accordance with previous studies demonstrating that activated phagocytes release mediators which induce hypozincemia in experimental animals by redistribution of zinc from the plasma to the liver (35). It is also possible that such mediators may account for the observed decrease of cellular zinc in peripheral blood cells. However, we were unable to observe any connection between the acute-phase plasma proteins and cellular zinc content. Anyhow, it seems less plausible that reduced cellular zinc reflects a true deficiency but rather is a consequence of zinc redistribution since during corticosteroid treatment the cellular zinc amounts started to return towards normal values.

Based on experimental findings, it is reasonable to assume that the observed alterations in cellular zinc may influence the process of chronic inflammatory diseases. In the case of future therapeutical trials with zinc supplementation in rheumatoid arthritis it should be of great value to follow not only plasma zinc levels but also the cellular zinc concentrations.

Manganese

Cotzias et al. were the first to show that total serum and above all whole-blood manganese concentrations increased in rheumatoid arthritis (36). They also demonstrated that manganese has a slow turn-over rate in rheumatoid arthritis and that this can be accelerated by prednisone (37). Manganese is involved as an enzyme activation in synthesis and maturation of the connective-tissue components (38, 39). Manganese also occurs in one form of superoxide dismutase enzyme (40), related in part to the protection of the cell to the toxic effects of free superoxide radicals (41). Thus, alterations of manganese metabolism seem to have a potential role in chronic inflammatory diseases.

We have observed a significant increase of the manganese amounts in granulocytes isolated from patients with rheumatoid arthritis, other inflammatory arthritides and scleroderma, while erythrocytes and platelets contained normal amounts (42). The cause of the granulocyte manganese accumulation is not known, but evidently linked to the intensity of the inflammatory process defined by ESR and certain acute-phase plasma proteins. Strong positive correlations were found between granulocyte manganese and granulocyte stores of calcium and iron suggesting a close relationship in the cellular regulation of these elements in chronic inflammatory conditions. During corticosteroid therapy granulocyte manganese concentration started to return towards normal levels. Glucocorticoids might influence the manganese balance by reduction of the inflammatory activity but also, as demonstrated in healthy experimental animals, by redistribution of manganese (43).

SUMMARY

Isolated blood cells from patients with chronic inflammatory connective-tissue diseases—rheumatoid arthritis, other inflammatory arthritides and scleroderma—contain abnormal stores of certain macro- and trace elements; erythrocytes and granulocytes are overloaded with calcium but contain subnormal amounts of zinc as do platelets. Granulocytes, but not erythrocytes and platelets, contain increased amounts of strontium and manganese. These alterations seem to be linked to the production of an acute-phase plasma protein response and begin to normalize during corticosteroid treatment. Are these and other alterations of the mineral balance during chronic inflammation physiological changes which check the disease process and facilitate remission of the disease? Or are they pathological changes which overstimulate the inflammatory response or provoke defect synthesis and maturation of the connective-tissue components? No definite answer can be given at present. However, we should consider the marked alterations of macro- and trace elements as part of the multifaceted inflammatory response, which is of utmost importance in host defence and tissue repair, but which also can cause considerable harm to the connective tissue. One therapeutic aim in chronic inflammatory diseases is to reduce the intensity of the inflammatory reaction and it cannot be exluded that manipulation of the mineral balance inducing normalization of certain macro- and trace elements in inflammatory cells is one way to reduce the inflammatory response.

ACKNOWLEDGEMENT

This study was supported by the Swedish Medical Research Council, the Swedish National Science Research Council and Pharmacia AB, Sweden.

REFERENCES

1. HÄLLGREN, R., SVENSON, K., JOHANSSON, E. & LINDH, U. (1985). Abnormal calcium and magnesium stores in erythrocytes and granulocytes from patients with inflammatory connective tissue disease. *Arthr. and Rheum.* In press.
2. LINDH, U. (1982). Elemental characterization of individual glia and glioma cells in the nuclear microprobe. *Nucl. Instr. and Meth.* 193, 343.
3. LINDH, U. (1983). Elemental mapping of tissue sections by means of microparticle-induced X-ray emission spectroscopy and computer graphics. *Anal. Chim. Acta* 150, 223.
4. UEMURA, Y. J., KUNO, Y., KOYAMA, H., YAMAZAKI, T. & KIENLE, P. (1978). *A New Way of Determining Concentrations in P.I.X.E. Trace Element Analysis.* 153, 573.
5. SIEGAL, B. A., ENGEL, W. K. & DERRER, E. C. (1977). Localization of technetium-99 diphosphonate in acutely injured muscle. Relationship to calcium deposition. *Neurology* 27, 230.
6. OKAMOTO, M. & MAYER, M. M. (1978). Studies on the mechanism of action of guinea-pig lymphotoxin. II. Increase of calcium uptake rate in LT-damaged target cells. *J. Immunol.* 120, 279.
7. EATON, J. W., SKELTON, T. D., SWOFFORD, H. S., KOLPIA, C. E. & JACOB, H. S. (1973). Elevated erythrocyte calcium in sickle cell disease. *Nature (London)* 246, 105.
8. CAMPBELL, A. K., DAW, R. A., HALLET, M. B. & LUZIO, J. P. (1981). Direct measurement of the increase in intracellular free calcium ion concentration in response to the action of complement. *Biochem. J.* 194, 551.
9. ASHLEY, C. C. & CAMPBELL, A. K. (1979). *Detection and Measurement of Free Ca^{++} in Cells.* Elsevier/North Holland, Amsterdam.
10. LICHTMAN, M. A. & WEED, R. I. (1972). Divalent cation content of normal and ATP-depleted erythrocytes and erythrocyte membranes. *Nouv. Rev. franç. Hémat.* 12, 799.
11. KRETZINGER, R. H. (1976). Calcium binding proteins. *Ann. Rev. Biochem.* 45, 239.

12. CAMPBELL, A. K. (1983). *Intracellular Calcium. Its Universal Role as a Regulator.* John Wiley & Sons Ltd., Chichester, New York.
13. SHEARER, W. T., ATKINSON, J. P. & PARKER, C. W. (1976). Humoral immunostimulation. Increased calcium uptake by cells treated with antibody and complement. *J. Immunol.* 117, 973.
14. IGNARRO, L. J. & GEORGE, W. J. (1974). Mediation of immunologic discharge of lysosomal enzymes form human neutrophils by guanosine 3′, 5′-monophosphate. *J. exp. Med.* 140, 225.
15. WEISSMANN, G., SMOLEN, J. E. & KORCHAK, H. M. (1980). Release of inflammatory mediators from stimulated neutrophils. *New Engl. J. Med.* 303, 27.
16. HALLET, M. B., LUZIO, J. P. & CAMPBELL, A. K. (1981). Stimulation of Ca^{++}-dependent chemiluminscence in rat polymorphonuclear leukocytes by polystyrene beads and the non lytic action of complement. *Immunology* 44, 569.
17. LONG, C. & MONAT, B. (1973). The influx of calcium ions to human erythrocytes during cold storage. *Biochem. J.* 132, 559.
18. WHITE, J. G. (1974). Effects of an ionophore, A 23187, on the surface morphology of normal erythrocytes. *Amer. J. Pathol.* 77, 507.
19. CARTWRIGHT, G. E. (1966). The anemia of chronic disorders. *Semin. Hematol.* 3, 351.
20. FOREMAN, J. C., SOBOTKA, A. K. & LICHTENSTEIN, L. M. (1979). The action of strontium on basophil leukocytes and its use to prove the relationship between immunologic stimulus and secretory response. *J. Immunol.* 123, 153.
21. FOREMAN, J. C. (1977). Spontaneous histamine secretion from mast cells in the presence of strontium. *J. Physiol.* 217, 215.
22. BEST, L. C., BONE, E. A. & RUSSEL, G. G. (1981). Strontium ions induce production of thromboxane B_2 and secretion of 5-hydroxytryptamine in washed human platelets. *Biochem. Pharmacol.* 30, 635.
23. NEIGHBOUR, P. A. & HUBERMAN, H. S. (1982). Sr^{++}-induced inhibition of human natural killer (NK) cell-mediated cytotoxicity. *J. Immunol.* 128, 1236.
24. FOREMAN, J. C., HALLET, M. B. & MONGAR, J. L. (1977). Strontium ions as a probe for the role of alkaline earth metal ions in histamine secretion. *Biochem. Soc. Trans.* 5, 879.
25. HÄLLGREN, R., SVENSON, K., JOHANSSON, E. & LINDH, U. (1984). Elevated granulocyte strontium in inflammatory arthritides is related to the inflammatory activity. *J. Lab. clin. Med.* 84, 893.
26. KAZIMIERCZAK, W. & MASHINSKI, C. (1974). The effect of zinc ions on selective and nonselective histamine relase in vitro. *Agents Actions* 4, 1.
27. CHAPIL, M., STANKOVA, L., ZUKOSKI, C. & ZUKOSKI, C. F. (1977). Inhibition of some functions of polymorphonuclear leukocytes by in vitro zinc. *J. Lab. clin. Med.* 88, 135.
28. CHAPIL, M., WELDY, P. L., STANKOVA, L., CLARK, D. A. & ZUKOSKI, C. F. (1975). Inhibitory effects of zinc ions on platelet aggregation and serotonin release reaction. *Life Sci.* 16, 561.
29. CHANDRA, R. K. (1983). Nutrition, immunity and infection: present knowledge and future directions. *Lancet* 1, 688.
30. FERNANDES, G., NAIR, M., ONOE, K., TANAKA, T., FLOYD, R. & GOOD, R. A. (1979). Impairment of cell-mediated immunity functions by dietary zinc deficiency in mice. *Proc. Nat. Acad. Sci.* 75, 457.
31. SIMKIN, P. A. (1976). Oral zinc sulphate in rheumatoid arthritis. *Lancet* 2, 539.
32. JOB, C., MENKES, C. J. & DALBARRE, F. (1980). Zinc sulphate in the treatment of rheumatoid arthritis. *Arthr. and Rheum.* 23, 1408.

33. SVENSON, K., HÄLLGREN, R., JOHANSSON, E. & LINDH, U. (1985). Reduced zinc in peripheral blood cells from patients with inflammatory connective tissue diseases. *Inflammation*. In press.
34. BREWER, G. J. (1980). Calmodulin, zinc and calcium in cellular and membrane regulation, an interpretive review. *Amer. J. Hematol.* 8, 231.
35. PEKAREK, R. S. & BEISEL, W. R. (1971). Characterisation of the endogenous mediator(s) of serum zinc and iron depression during infection and other stresses. *Proc. Soc. Exp. Biol. Med.* 138, 728.
36. COTZIAS, G. C., MILLER, S. T. & EDWARDS, J. (1966). Neutron activation analysis: the stability of manganese concentrations in human blood and serum. *J. Lab. clin. Med.* 67, 836.
37. COTZIAS, G. C., PAPAVASILIOU, P. S., HUGHES, E. R., TANG, L. & BORG, D. C. (1968). Slow turnover of manganese in active rheumatoid arthritis accelerated by prednisone. *J. clin. Invest.* 47, 992.
38. TSAI, H. C. C. & EVERSON, G. J. (1967). Effect of manganese deficiency on the acid mucopolysaccharides in cartilage of guinea-pigs. *J. Nutr.* 9, 441.
39. LEACH, R. M. (1971). Role of manganese in mucopolysaccharide metabolism. *Fed. Proc.* 30, 991.
40. WEISIGER, R. A. & FRIDOVICH, I. (1973). Superoxide dismutase: organelle specificity. *J. biol. Chem.* 248, 3582.
41. MCCORD, J. B., KEELE, B. B. JR. & FRIDOVICH, I. (1971). An enzyme-based theory of obligate anaerobiosis: the physiological function of superoxide dismutase. *Proc. Nat. Acad. Sci.* 68, 1024.
42. HÄLLGREN, R., SVENSON, K., JOHANSSON, E. & LINDH, U. (1985). Elevated granulocyte manganese in rheumatoid arthritis, other inflammatory arthritides and scleroderma. Submitted for publication.
43. HUGHES, E. R. & COTZIAS, G. C. (1961). Adrenocorticosteroid hormones and manganese metabolism. *Amer. J. Physiol.* 201, 1061.

Trace Elements and Rheumatoid Arthritis

By JAN AASETH

INTRODUCTION

The discoveries of the essential roles for metal ions in biology and medicine have provided a rationale for metal supplementation therapy. For instance, the symptoms of acrodermatitis enteropathica can now be treated successfully with high doses of zinc given orally. Copper or selenium supplementations are also used clinically in various disorders with metal deficiencies. The opposite approach, metal-depletion therapy, can be obtained by use of metal chelating agents, which are important therapeutic agents, particularly the chelator D-penicillamine which is used in lead poisoning and also in copper deposition (Wilson's disease). It is surprising that active rheumatoid arthritis (R.A.) can also be ameliorated or brought to remission by treatment with D-penicillamine or with copper or gold complexes. The mode of action of these agents is not fully understood, and the involvement of trace elements in the pathogenesis of R.A. is still unclear.

It is probable that future research in the mechanisms of action of gold, copper and penicillamine can increase our understanding of the complicated pathogenesis of R.A. The hallmark of R.A. is persistent synovial inflammation. As a direct consequence, bone, cartilage and supporting structures of the joints undergo gradual destruction which ceases only if a remission occurs.

The persistency of the inflammation is a crucial clinical trait, and effective remission-inducing agents, in some way, must interrupt or interfere with the mechanisms behind this cronicity. Current evidence supports the view that an immunological mechanism is tightly involved in the pathogenesis of the disease. This view requires the postulation of an unknown "antigen", possessing affinity for synovial structures. The nature of this antigen is, however, obscure.

The present survey will try to elucidate how the uptake or redistribution of trace metals, induced by therapeutic agents, can influence the pathogenetic events of R.A.

TREATMENT WITH GOLD SALT

Clinical effect

The story of the empirical discovery of the therapeutic effect of gold is remarkable. The first clinical tests around 1925 were precipitated by *in vitro* studies of the bacteriostatic effect toward tubercle bacilli of gold and other metals. Since R.A. was assumed to be an infectious disease, some patients suffering from R.A. were included in a programme of clinical testing of the heavy metals. This led to the introduction of gold complexes as remission-inducing agents (Forestier 1929).

However, it was not until the report of the British Rheumatism Council in 1960 that chrysotherapy was shown to be clinically effective in a controlled study (Research Subcommittee 1960). Nevertheless, already from the early thirties to the early forties, during the original clinical adoption of the treatment, it was observed that the most applicable gold compounds consisted of gold and sulphur-containing complexing agents. The compound most used in clinical medicine has been gold thiomalate (Myocrisin), although gold thiosulphate (Fig. 1) and gold thioglucose have also been given to many patients.

Astonishingly, these gold (I) complexes have only a weak or negligible anti-inflammatory action in animal models, although their antirheumatic effect has now been amply demonstrated. This indicates that gold has a rather specific action in R.A., perhaps interfering with some basic mecha-

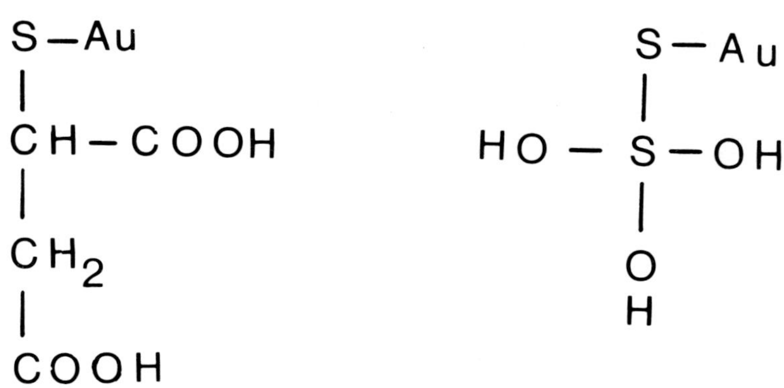

Gold thiomalate　　　Gold thiosulphate

Fig. 1　Chemical formula of gold thiomalate and gold thiosulphate

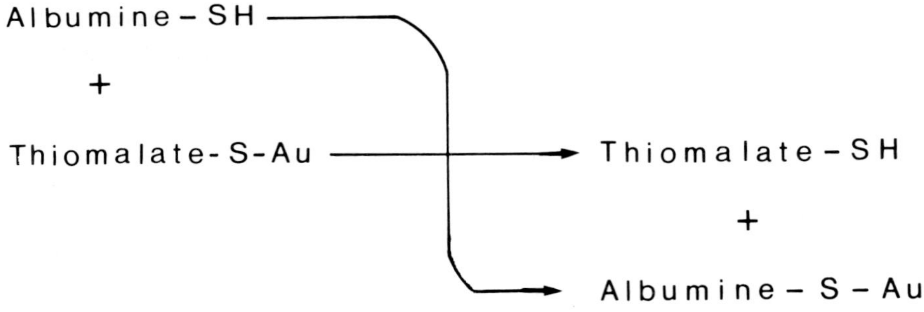

Fig. 2 Interaction of gold thiomalate with albumine-SH

nism underlying the perpetuating nature of the disease. However, the clinical use of gold has been limited, to some extent, by the toxic reactions it may provoke in the skin, blood-forming organs, liver and kidneys.

Pharmacokinetics

Goldthiomalate, as well as most other soluble gold compounds, is administered by intramuscular injection. After absorption, gold is bound to plasma proteins in the circulation, particularly to albumine.

We have found (Jellum et al. 1977) that gold (I) thiomalate complex is not stable in blood plasma: Au^+ and thiomalate is rapidly separated, gold being chelated by albumine while most of the thiomalate will be liberated in the free thiolate form (Fig. 2). *In vivo,* thiomalate and gold have different metabolic behaviour (Fig. 3), and it has been suggested that gold thiomalate

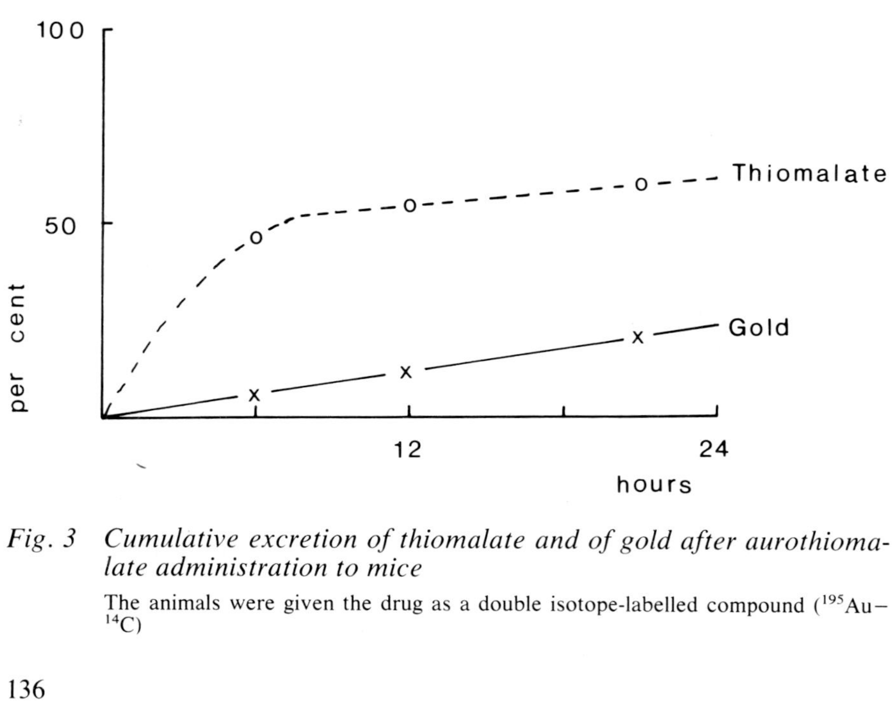

Fig. 3 Cumulative excretion of thiomalate and of gold after aurothiomalate administration to mice

The animals were given the drug as a double isotope-labelled compound (^{195}Au–^{14}C)

injections, in fact, involve simultaneous treatment with two different drugs, viz. the thiol mojety in addition to gold itself (Jellum et al. 1980). Possible therapeutic effects of thiomalate are discussed under the section on thiol-containing drugs (see also Fig. 6).

Gold concentrates chiefly in the kidney (Aaseth et al. 1980) and to a lesser extent in the liver (Kupffer cells and hepatocytes) and the spleen (macrophages) (Table 1).

Of particular interest is the fact that gold concentrates in articular tissues also, although the levels are lower than in the above-mentioned organs. Soluble gold compounds produce levels in the synovial fluid which are comparable to those in blood plasma (Johnsen et al. 1982). The synovial membrane has been shown to concentrate gold to a greater extent than synovial fluid, and this is especially prononunced if synovitis is present.

Ultrastructural studies, by electron microscopy with electron dispersive analysis, have shown that gold is deposited almost exclusively in the lysosomes, which will then undergo characteristic changes, justifying the term "aurosomes" which has been adopted to describe them (Ghadially 1979). The synovial membrane in R.A. is characterized by a remarkable increase in the number of lysosomes, and it is considered likely that gold enters and is sequestered by these preexisting lysosomes. This explains the gold accumulation in synovial intimal cells and subsynovial macrophages in R.A. (Nakamura & Garashi 1977).

Microanalysis of the lysosomal gold deposits has shown that the sulphur to gold ratio is higher than 1:1, namely as high as about 3:1 (Ghadially 1979). The excess of thiol groups has precipitated the suggestion that metallothionein-gold complexes may be present in the aurosomes.

Hypothetic mode of action

Important target cells for the therapeutic action of gold are presumed to be the peripheral blood monocytes and tissue macrophages (Davies 1981). In addition to their well-known phagocytic ability, these cells have been shown to have important functions in the mediation of cell-mediated immune responses. It has been reported by several authors that patients with R.A. show greater phagocytic activity by the macrophages than healthy

Table 1 *Concentration of Au (nmol/g, mean and range) in tissues from rats 7 days after an intramuscular injection of Myocrisin (35 μmol/kg)*

Blood	1.4	(1.1– 1.6)
Liver	20.4	(12.8–25.0)
Kidney	66.1	(29.7–93.9)
Brain	0.3	(0.3– 0.4)
Spleen	13.4	(9.0–17.2)

controls. The phagocytic activity of synovial macrophages of R.A. patients is significantly reduced in the presence of gold salt (Jessop & Wilkins 1975), and gold in appropriate concentrations can inhibit the chemotactic migration of the same cells. Furthermore, several investigators have shown that the gold salts can inhibit the cell-mediated immunity, as assessed by the degree of activation (transformation) of T-lymphocytes induced by incubation with suitable mitogens or antigens (see Førre et al. 1984). Thiomalate, without gold, could not bring about a comparable inhibition. An intact monocyte population is necessary to initiate the normal transformation response, and it has been claimed that the inhibition of gold salts is due primarily to an effect on monocytes rather then directly on T-lymphocytes (Lipsky & Ziff 1977).

The activated phagocytes characterizing R.A. are reported to generate superoxide and peroxides, which are discharged along with lysosomal enzymes (Fig. 4). Presumably, the immobilization of cells and lysosomes obtained by gold therapy can reduce this discharge of toxic oxygen and enzymes, and thus reduce the enzymatic joint destruction. It might also be speculated if the oxygen radicals can bring about structural rearrangements of IgG-molecules (Gerber 1974), thus provoking anti-IgG-production and immune complex formation. Gold treatment is supposed to extinguish such effects of increased macrophage activity.

ZINC

Clinical effects of zinc administration

According to Simkin (1982), four controlled studies of oral zinc therapy in patients with R.A. have been carried out (Table 2).

The first of these was conducted in Seattle (Simkin 1977) and included 21 patients. During a 12-week double-blind trial, the patients on oral zinc therapy showed significant improvement in joint swelling, severity of morning stiffness and overall impression of well-being.

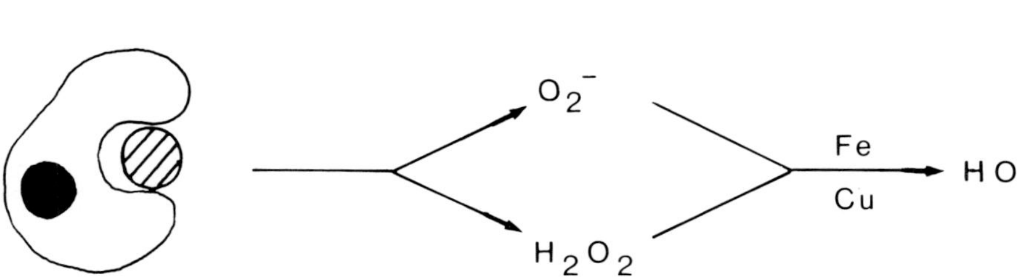

Fig. 4 Discharge of oxygen radicals from a macrophage during the consumption of immune complexes

Interaction of O_2^- and H_2O_2 in the presence of free iron or copper ions gives rise to the highly reactive hydroxyl radical

Table 2 Positive (+) and negative (–) results of clinical trials with zinc sulphate in R.A. patients (N=number) from various parts of the world

	Seattle	Poona	Paris	Oxford
N	21	18	35	24
Age (mean, in years)	54.3	42.5	59	51
Treatment duration (weeks)	12	12	16	26
Effect	+	+	–	–

A second trial was conducted in Poona, India by Desai and colleagues. Joint tenderness and global impression of general condition improved significantly within a 12-week period in this study. However, two other studies have shown negative results, one of them being carried out in Paris by Job and colleagues and another in Oxford by Mattingly and Mowat. The latter trial was conducted for a full 6-month period, but, as in the study from Paris, the investigators found no evidence that zinc sulphate was better than the placebo.

The principal hypothesis underlying the initial trial in Seattle was that some patients with R.A. may have an acquired zinc deficiency and that correction of the deficiency might ameliorate the disease process. Hypozincemia in R.A. patients has been reported by several investigators, but true zinc deficiency may in fact be rather inconstant. For example, in a Norwegian study we found the mean serum zinc only moderately decreased in a group of R.A. patients, to 77% of the average control value (Table 3), and this decrease could be ascribed to the lowering of serum albumine in our patients rather than to a true zinc deficiency.

As the absorption of zinc is known to be homeostatically regulated, it seems unlikely that orally-given zinc should lead to much more than a correction of a deficiency state. A reasonable assumption is, therefore, that oral zinc treatment leads to clinical improvement only in zinc-deficient R.A. patients. However, parenteral administration of zinc has not yet been tried clinically, although this mode of administration may lead to more extensive cellular and pharmacological effects of zinc. Such treatment would be a potent stimulus for the synthesis of the low molecular weight protein, metallothionein, in several organs. This protein can probably act as an oxygen radical scavenger, owing to its high content of thiol groups.

Table 3 Serum concentration (μmol/l) of trace metals in patients with R.A. (mean ± SD)

	Patients (N = 23)	Controls (N = 40)
Zn	10 ± 3	13 ± 3
Cu	28 ± 5	14 ± 3
Se	1.19 ± 0.32	1.53 ± 0.25
Fe	8 ± 4	23 ± 7

Cellular effects of zinc

By using peripheral lymphocytes incubated in the presence of both mitogens and high zinc concentrations (100–150 µmol/1) we could demonstrate induction of a metallothionein-like protein (Alexander et al. 1982). This metallothionein could not be detected when zinc without mitogens was added to the medium, and zinc alone did not stimulate the lymphocyte proliferation. We suggested that metallothionein might play a role for the inflammatory response *in vivo*. Similarly, carrageenan injection to mice induces metallothionein synthesis in the liver (Maitani & Suzuki 1981). In cultured liver cells, glucocorticoids could stimulate the cellular uptake of zinc and induce the synthesis of metallothionein (Failla & Cousins 1978). The established stabilization of lysosomes by glucocorticoids may be related to increased influx of Zn into the cell (Cox & Ruckenstein 1970), and the membrane-protecting properties of these agents may in part be related to the induced synthesis of metallothionein.

The activated macrophages characterizing R.A. are reported to produce toxic oxygen as a result of increased enzymatic activity of NADPH-oxidase (Figs 4 & 5). This enzyme will presumably be inhibited by zinc in appropriate concentrations (Chvapil et al. 1976). Furthermore, macrophages from mice injected intramuscularly with $ZnCl_2$ show significantly inhibited locomotion and phagocytosis and increased viability, as compared to control

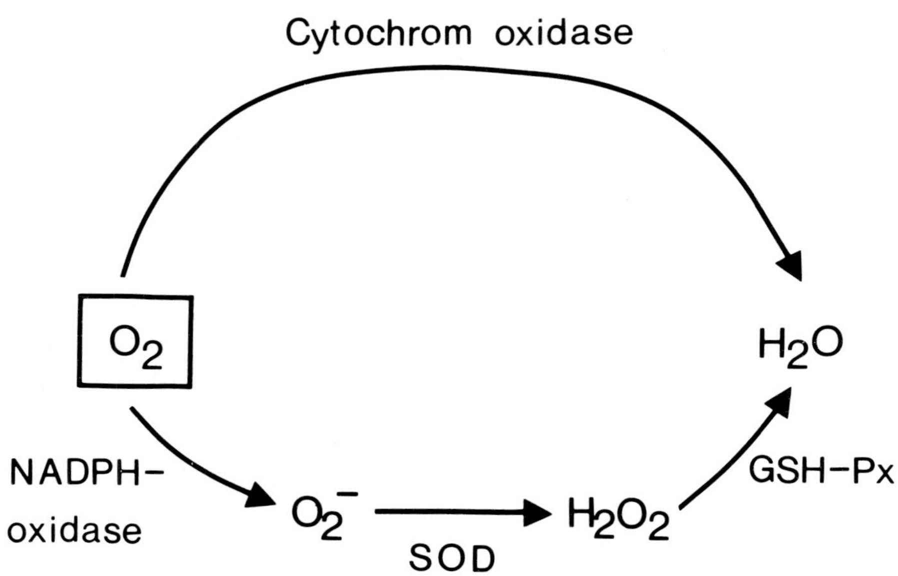

Fig. 5 Production and detoxification of oxygen radicals

Superoxide (O_2^-), formed by NADPH-oxidase, is converted to H_2O_2 by the action of SOD (superoxide dismutase). H_2O_2 is converted to H_2O by GSH-Px (glutathione peroxidase)

cells (Chvapil et al. 1976). It was proposed that Zn^{++} is involved in the regulation of the macrophage activity. A possible role of metallothionein in this respect is not fully evaluated.

Physiological changes of trace metal levels in R.A.

Several investigators have found that patients with R.A. have lower serum zinc and iron levels than healthy individuals. The values from a Norwegian study are given in Table 3.

This fall in serum zinc and iron is partially accounted for by an increase in iron and zinc in the liver, and probably also in synovial tissue (Sorenson 1978). It is known that corticosteroids can induce increased uptake of zinc by hepatocytes, but in addition it is found that a hormone-like substance liberated from leucocytes can induce increased transport of zinc, iron, copper and amino acids into liver cells, and probably into synovial cells, in patients with R.A.

Accelerated synthesis of metallothionein, ceruloplasmin and other acute phase proteins accompanies increased cellular uptake of trace metals, whereas the rate of synthesis of albumine and transferrin is low. It is supposed that the increased cellular uptake of Zn, as well as the increased ceruloplasmin synthesis and other parts of the acute phase response can serve tissue-protective functions (Sorenson 1978).

COPPER

Antiinflammatory effects of copper complexes

Forestier (1949) was among the first to report that a copper complex, Cupralene (3-allylcuprothio carbamido-benzoate), was effective in the treatment of rheumatoid arthritis. It is interesting to read the conclusions of Forestier (1949) 20 years after he had introduced gold, and six years after he had begun to try out copper compounds:

> "Copper salts are effective in the treatment of rheumatoid arthritis. They give better results than gold salts in the early stages of the disease. In cases of longer standing, they must be used if there is chryso-intolerance or chryso-resistance, but whenever gold salts are tolerated they are to be preferred."

These positive results with copper complexes were supported by the studies of Kuzell et al. (1951) and by Hangarter and Lübke (1952).

The latter investigators treated more than 600 patients suffering from R.A. with copper salicylate and reported that 65% became symptom-free, 23% improved and 12% of the patients remained unchanged. No serious toxic disturbances were recorded in association with the treatment. All the above clinical trials with copper complexes have made use of intramuscular or intravenous injections of the compounds. Controlled clinical studies are, however, still lacking, although extensive evaluation of copper complexes in animal models has been undertaken (see Sorenson 1982). The experimental models used include, i.a., carrageenan-induced paw edema and adjuvant arthritis in the rat. Whereas gold thiomalate is inactive in these models, copper thiomalate acts anti-inflammatorily (Whitehouse & Walker 1978). Copper complexes of salicylate or aspirin given by subcutaneous injection are five to six times more protective against carrageenan-induced edema than when tested by the oral route (Rainsford & Whitehouse 1976), presumably because orally-given copper is insufficiently absorbed, and the complexes are dissociated already in the stomach.

When discussing clinical treatment with copper-containing agents, the clinical use of the anti-inflammatory Cu-dependent metalloenzyme, superoxide dismutase (SOD), should also be commented upon. This drug, Orgotein, has now been shown to reduce inflammation when given intraarticularly into the joints of R.A. patients. The discovery and evaluation of this agent may provide insight into the biochemical mechanisms of actions for all copper compounds (Lund-Olesen & Menander 1974).

Proposed mechanism of action

It is found that rheumatoid arthritis is associated with decreased superoxide dismutase (SOD) activity (Rister et al. 1978). This is interesting since SOD has anti-inflammatory activity. It is known that the cytosolic SOD is a copper-/zinc-containing enzyme (see also Table 5).

Ceruloplasmin and therapeutic copper complexes have been shown to have SOD-like activity (see Sorenson 1982). Thus, the demonstrated physiological rise of ceruloplasmin in R.A. is suggested to be a protective response. Consistent to this, a lack of the rise of ceruloplasmin may increase the risk of chronic disease, as seen in copper-deficient animals with adjuvant arthritis (see Denko 1979, Sorenson 1982). Biochemically, SOD can act protectively by detoxifying superoxide radicals discharged from activated phagocytes. The less toxic product H_2O_2 thus formed can be further degraded by glutathione peroxidase in the presence of glutathione (Fig. 5).

COMPLEXING AGENTS

The idea that anti-inflammatory corticosteroids, salicylates and slow-acting drugs (penicillamine, levamisole, gold thiomalate) owe part of their pharmacological activity to interactions with metal ions *in vivo*, has been discussed previously by several authors (see Sorenson 1982). Before discussing this hypothesis some general principles of metal-binding will be briefly outlined.

Basic principles of metal chelation

A qualitative (or semiquantitative) indication of the chemical affinity between a metal ion, M, and a complexing agent, L, can be obtained from the principles developed by Pearson (1968), which are often referred to as the HSAB-theory or Hard-Soft-Acid-Base theory. According to this theory the metal ions can be classified into soft, hard and borderline, as shown in Table 4. So-called soft-metal cations have a large atomic radius and a high number of electrons in the outer shell, in contrast to the hard ions. Formation of a metal complex, ML, involves that the metal cation M coordinates or accepts free electron pairs from a ligand, L. Chelating drugs make use of sulphur, nitrogen or oxygen as electron donor atoms. Chemically, these groups are classified as soft, borderline or hard, as shown in Table 4. The general principle of the HSAB-theory is that soft metals (so-called sulphur-seekers) form the most stable complexes with soft ligands, and hard metals (so-called oxygen-seekers) form stable complexes with hard ligands. Most of the trace metals that are of interest as regards the therapy of R.A. belong to the soft class or the borderline class. For instance, iron, zinc and copper(II) are borderline, whereas gold and copper(I) are soft. The interaction between a chelating agent, L, and metal, M, can be described in a quantitative fashion by the use of stability constants (for a review, see Aaseth 1983).

When several complexing ligands are present in the same medium, e.g., blood plasma, the calculation of the molecular distribution of an exchangeable metal is possible, on the basis of the stability constants, by using a computer simulation programme. For example, computer simulation has shown that exchangeable copper in plasma is partly albumine-bound, but most of the low molecular weight Cu-complexes involve histidin (Agerwal

Table 4 Binding species of chelates classified according to the hard/soft theory
(Pearson 1968)

A) Three chemical classes of metal ions

Soft	Borderline	Hard
Hg^{2+}	Pb^{2+}	Na^{+}
Au^{+}	Cd^{2+}	K^{+}
Cu^{+}	Cu^{2+}	Mg^{2+}
Pt^{2+}	As^{3+}	Ca^{2+}
Tl^{+}	Zn^{2+}	Al^{3+}
Ag^{+}		Be^{2+}
		Sr^{2+}

B) Metal-binding electron donors in chelating agent (the free electron pair is indicated)

Soft	Borderline	Hard
$—S:^-$	$—\ddot{N}(H)_2:$ (H above and below N)	$—\overset{O}{\overset{\|\|}{C}}—O:^-$

& Perrin 1976). Being electrically neutral, these histidin-complexes are supposed to be responsible for the blood-to-tissue equilibration of Cu. Copper-histidin is found to possess SOD-activity and should, therefore, act anti-inflammatorily (Sorenson 1982). In contrast, free uncomplexed Cu^{++}-ions are injurious (Aaseth et al. 1984), being able to catalyze the formation of toxic hydroxyl radicals (see Fig. 4). In healthy humans, the concentrations of free Cu^{++} is therefore kept very low, namely around 10^{-15} mol/l (Agerwal & Perrin 1976). However, in R.A. patients the plasma-histidin concentration is reduced, while the low molecular weight copper fraction is increased (Sorenson 1978), involving the risk of raised concentrations of free cupric ions. It follows that copper supplementation may not be a treatment to be recommended without considering the intake of histidin or other chelators.

The drug D-penicillamine is one of the most effective agents in promoting reduction of the free cupric ion fraction. Furthermore, the Cu-penicillamine chelate formed has SOD-activity. Salisylic acid can also form a copper chelate with SOD-activity, but the stability of the latter chelate is relatively low (see Pearson 1968). The biological significance of the chelating properties of salicylate has been questioned, although the drug can also bind ferric ions. It is seen from Fig. 4 that uncomplexed iron, as well as copper, in the medium around activated phagocytes can catalyze the formation of injurious hydroxyl radicals, and some investigators have suggested that salicylic acid can inhibit this reaction.

It is apparent that the ratio of free to bound copper ions depends on the available complexing ligands. The ratio of Cu(II) to Cu(I) depends on the actual biological redox potential. Intracellularly, in the presence of excess glutathione, cuprous copper (Cu^{+}) will dominate, while the cupric form (Cu^{++}) dominates extracellularly in the absence of glutathione. Chronic arthritis is found to be associated with depletion of glutathione from liver cells (Bragt et al. 1980) and red blood cells (see Table 5), a depletion which should lead to increased free Cu^{++} concentration intracellularly. However, it is known that free copper ions, as well as zinc, can induce the synthesis of the sulphhydryl-rich protein metallothionein which is an endogenous metal chelator.

Table 5 Glutathione (GSH), GSH-Px and copper in red blood cells from R.A. patients (N = 13)

	Patients	Controls
GSH (mmol/l)	2.15 ± 0.13	2.60 ± 0.11
GSH-Px (% of control)	66 ± 15%	100 ± 14%
Cu (μmol/l)	14 ± 3	14 ± 4

Thiol-containing drugs

The well-controlled multicentre trial from the United Kingdom in 1973 laid the foundation for the increasing use of D-penicillamine in R.A. (Multicentre Trial Group 1973). Penicillamine is now recognized as a basic antirheumatic compound with a long latency of effect comparable to gold thiomalate. Like gold, penicillamine has little or no anti-inflammatory effect on adjuvant arthritis in rats (see Munthe et al. 1979b), and its effect is presumed to be specific for R.A.

Since penicillamine is metabolized to a small extent, the active form of the drug is supposed to be the intact molecule (Fig. 6). The thiol group is its most reactive group, and is responsible for several biological properties including the chelation of copper and zinc. In our clinical studies we found no significant changes, however, in the serum zinc concentrations during penicillamine treatment (Aaseth et al. 1978). Other investigators have found that penicillamine increases the uptake of zinc from the gut, and have also suggested that it increases the influx of Zn into cells (Salbu & Bibow, personal communication). As discussed above, the copper chelate of penicillamine has SOD-activity, but the significance of the chelating properties of penicillamine for its antirheumatic effects is still unclear.

Penicillamine, like several other thiols, can form mixed disulphides with sulphhydryl- or disulphide-containing proteins. Through these reactions, penicillamine can protect thiol groups against free radical attacks. This tendency of penicillamine to form mixed disulphides can also involve liberation of protein-bound glutathione within cells. Normally about 30% of the glutathione content in the body is bound to proteins as mixed disulphides. Thusly increased intracellular free glutathione levels will increase the effectiveness of the glutathione peroxidase system.

The cellular effects of penicillamine depend on to what extent the drug penetrates into or through the cellular membranes. Binderup and Arrigon-Martelli (1979) reported that penicillamine seems to diffuse passively throughout the lymphocyte, but is not retained there, in contrast to a specific binding to receptors in the macrophage membrane. Penicillamine is reported to inhibit granulocyte migration and to stabilize lysosomal membranes (Chvapil et al. 1972, Carevic 1979). Thus it resembles gold thiomalate as to its action on macrophages.

It is of great interest that penicillamine can reduce the *in vivo* concentrations of pathological immune complexes in R.A. The drug reduces complexes that cannot be split by its direct action *in vitro*, namely the intermediate 7–19S IgG complexes, which are the dominating ones in rheumatoid joint fluid and synovial tissue. Apparently, the drug is able to interfere with the *in vivo* production of these complexes. It is possible that penicillamine, through its mixed disulphide formation with IgG, can inhibit some molecular aggregation or rearrangement which stimulates anti-IgG production and immune complex formation (Gerber 1974).

Thiol-containing agents like penicillamine, thiomalate and a levamisole metabolite (Fig. 6) have been increasingly studied during recent years in order to develop more effective antirheumatic drugs.

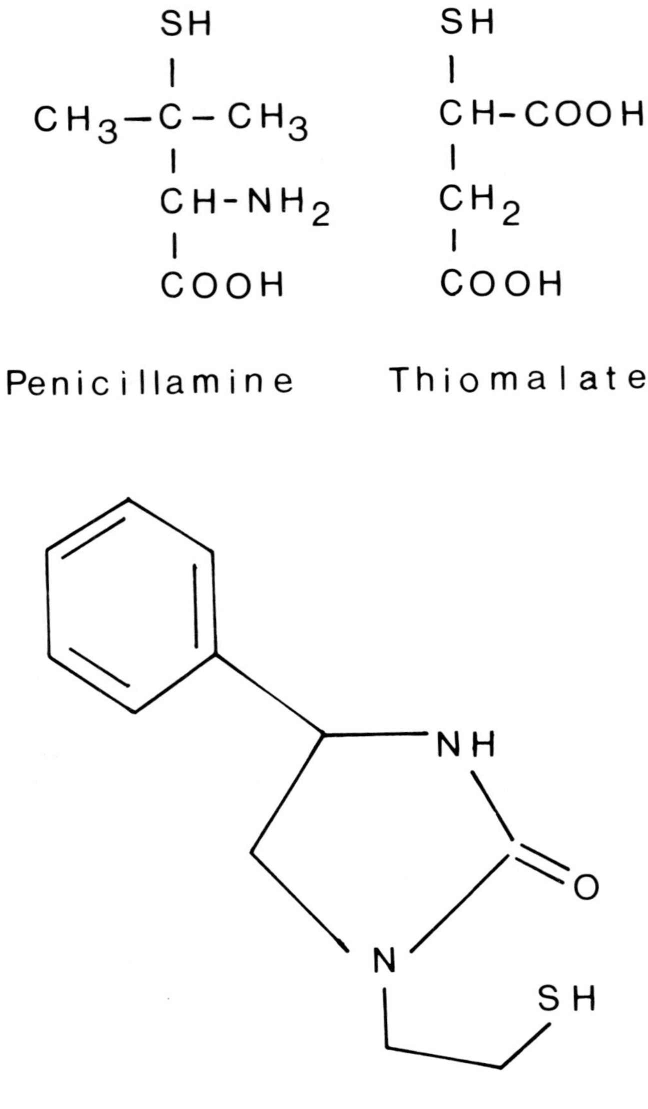

Fig. 6 Chemical formula of penicillamine, thiomalate and a levamisole metabolite

Note that all compounds are thiols

SELENIUM AND GLUTATHIONE

Selenium is an interesting trace element since it is known to act as a component of the membrane-protecting enzyme glutathione peroxidase (GSH-Px) (Fig. 7). In a group of R.A. patients we have found serum selenium lowered to a mean of 1.19 μmol/l as compared to 1.53 μmol/l in healthy controls (Table 3). GSH-Px in red blood cells was lowered to 66% ± 15% of control level (Table 5). GSH in red cells from R.A. patients was lowered to around 60–70% of the control levels.

The results reviewed here indicate that the *in vivo* activities of GSH-Px and of SOD are decreased in R.A. Such insufficient enzymatic activity, in combination with the increased discharge of superoxide anions from activated macrophages, is presumed to lead to lipoperoxidation of the rheumatic disease. Consistent to this, it is found that free radical scavengers have anti-inflammatory properties (Bragt et al. 1980).

Furthermore, increased intracellular levels of GSH are reported after treatment with penicillamine or gold thiomalate (Munthe et al. 1979a).

Selenium supplementation (Aaseth & Munthe 1983) has been tried clinically in a small group of patients (N=13), using sodium selenite (2 μmol/day) combined with tocopherol acetate (8 mg/day). After 12 weeks, serum selenium had increased from 1.19 to 1.60 μmol/l, and GSH-Px increased by 16%,

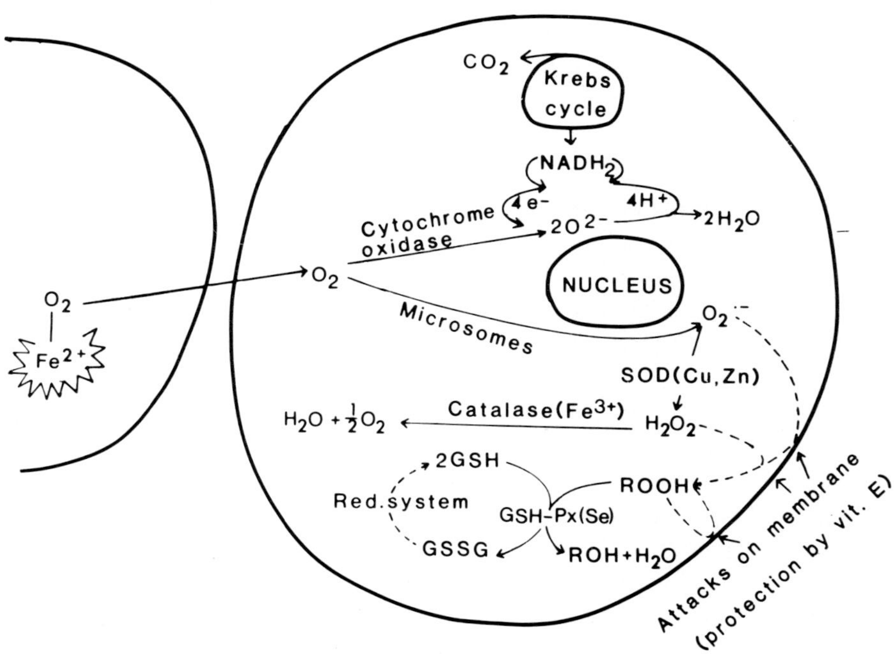

Fig. 7 The same reactions as in Fig. 5 usually take place intracellularly
It is indicated that SOD, GSH-Px and catalase are metalloenzymes

whereas glutathione remained unchanged. Forty per cent of R.A. patients improved in pain score and morning stiffness.

IRON AND MANGANESE

The serum iron concentration is decreased in R.A. patients (Table 3) whereas iron in synovial fluid and in the inflamed synovia are increased (see Sorenson 1978). Deposits of iron in synovial tissue are reported to be a constant feature of R.A. The relatively low transferrin values found in serum may be due to the changed protein synthesis in the liver. The synovial deposits of iron may be related to some unexplained lack of utilization. A possible role of GSH for the cellular iron utilization is suggested, as cellular GSH is found to increase in cases of iron deficiency. GSH may be involved in the reduction of trivalent iron before it can be incorporated into myoglobin or hemoglobin. R.A. is characterized by cellular GSH depletion, whereas the activated lymphocytes and macrophages have increased number of transferrin receptors, explaining the cellular uptake of trivalent iron.

Analyses of blood and its components for manganese in R.A. patients have demonstrated changed metabolism also for this element. Manganese in serum and red blood cells is reported to be increased (see Sorenson 1978). The patients have a retarded turnover of radiolabelled manganese, as compared to healthy controls. It is tempting to suggest that this is related to increased needs for intracellular SOD activity, since Mn is an essential component of the mitochondrial SOD.

CONCLUDING REMARKS

Rheumatoid arthritis is characterized by increased activity of macrophages, which in cooperation with other inflammatory cells infiltrates the synovial tissue. The activated macrophages generate reactive forms of oxygen which have been suggested as mediators of inflammation. Gold is accumulated in the lysosomes of the macrophages, which are thereby immobilized, causing an arrest of the proinflammatory signalation. Zinc in high doses can also immobilize macrophages. Gold and zinc as well as copper can induce synthesis of the sulphhydryl-rich protein metallothionein. Copper is a component of the cytosolic enzyme superoxide dismutase, and several copper-containing molecules including ceruloplasmin possess superoxide-dismutating activity.

The anti-inflammatory activity of Cu-complexes is attributed to their SOD activity. The therapeutic effect of penicillamine, as well, may be related to an antioxidative or membrane-protecting action. Increased intracellular levels of GSH and the selenium-containing enzyme GSH-Px can also accelerate the break-down of reactive oxygen. Future research is of interest to evaluate a possible therapeutic effect of selenium supplementation.

ACKNOWLEDGEMENT

Thanks are due to Det Norske Revmatismeråd for support to the research.

REFERENCES

AASETH, J. (1983). Recent advance in the therapy of metal poisonings with chelating agents. *Hum. Toxicol.* 2, 257–272.

AASETH, J. & MUNTHE, E. (1983). Treatment of rheumatoid arthritis with selenium and vitamin E. *Scand. J. Rheumatol.* Suppl. 49, 35.

AASETH, J., JELLUM, E. & MUNTHE, E. (1980). The effect of pencillamine and 2, 3-dimercaptosuccinic acid on urinary excretion and tissue distribution of gold. *Scand. J. Rheumatol.* 9, 157–160.

AASETH, J., MUNTHE, E., FØRRE, Ø. & STEINNES, E. (1978). Trace elements in serum and urine of patients with rheumatoid arthritis. *Scand. J. Rheumatol.* 7, 237–240.

AASETH, J., SKAUG, V. & ALEXANDER, J. (1984). Haemolytic activity of copper as influenced by chelating agents, albumine and chromium. *Acta pharmacol. toxicol.* 54, 304–310.

AGERWAL, R.P. & PERRIN, D.D. (1976). Computer-based approach to chelation therapy. *Agents and Actions* 6, 667–673.

ALEXANDER, J., FØRRE, Ø., AASETH, J. & ØVREBØ, S. (1982). Induction of a metallo-thionein protein in human lymphocytes. *Scand. J. Immunol.* 15, 217–220.

BINDERUP, L. & ARRIGONI-MARTELLI, E. (1979). (^{14}C) D-penicillamine uptake and distribution in rat lymphocytes and macrophages. *Biochem. Pharmacol.* 28, 189–192.

BRAGT, P.C., BANSBERG, J.L. & BONTA, I.L. (1980). Depletion of hepatic antioxidants during granulomatous inflammation in the rat and local anti-inflammatory effects of free radical scavengers. *Agents and Actions* Suppl. 7, 214–219.

CAREVIC, O. (1979). The effect of D-penicillamine on the release of acid hydrolases from rat liver lysosomes induced by gamma-hexachlor cyclohexane. *Biochem. Pharmacol.* 28, 2181–2185.

CHVAPIL, M., RYEN, J.N. & BRADA, Z. (1972). Effects of selected chelating agents and metals on the stability of liver lysosomes. *Biochem. Pharmacol.* 21, 1079–1105.

CHVAPIL, M., ZUKOSKI, C.F., HATTLER, B.G., STANKOVA, L., MONTGOMERY, D., CARLSON, E.C. & LUDWIG, J.C. (1976). In *Trace Elements in Human Health and Disease,* Vol. I, pp. 269–282. Ed. by A.S. Prasad. Academic Press, New York.

COX, R.P. & RUCKENSTEIN, A. (1970). Studies on the mechanism of hormonal stimulation of zinc uptake in human cell cultures. *J. Cell. Physiol.* 77, 71–82.

DAVIS, P. (1981). Effect of gold salts on periphereal blood monocytes and macrophages. In *Trace Elements in the Pathogenesis and Treatment of Inflammation,* pp. 477–485. Ed. by K.D. Rainsford, K. Brune and M.W. Whitehouse. Birkhaüser, Basel.

DENKO, C.W. (1979). Protective role of ceruloplasmin in inflammation. *Agents and Actions* 9, 333–336.

FAILLA, M.L. & COUSINS, R.J. (1978). Zinc accumulation and metabolism in primary cultures of adult rat liver cells. *Biochim. biophys. Acta* 543, 293–304.

FORESTIER, J. (1929). L'aurotherapy dans les rheumatismes chroniques. *Bull. Soc. Méd. Hôp. Paris.* 53, 323–327

— (1949). Comparative results of copper salts and gold salts in rheumatoid arthritis. *Ann. rheum. Dis.* 8, 132–134.

FØRRE, Ø., MELBYE, O.J. & AASETH, J. (1984). In vitro effects of gold salts and various thiol compounds on parameters in cellular and humoral immunity. In *Health Effects and Interactions of Trace Elements.* Ed. by M. Abdulla. *J. Nutr.* Suppl. In press.

GERBER, D.A. (1974). Copper-catalyzed thermal aggregation of human gamma-globulin. *Arthr. and Rheum.* 17, 85–91.

GHADIALLY, F.N. (1979). The technique of electron probe X-ray analysis and the atomic composition of aurosomes. *J. Rheumatol.* 6, Suppl. 5, 25–30.

HANGARTER, W. & LUBKE, A. (1952). Über die Behandling Rheumatischer Erkrankungen mit einer Kupfer Natrium Salicylate-Komplex-Verbindung. *Dtsch. med. Wschr.* 77, 870–872.

JELLUM, E., AASETH, J. & MUNTHE, E. (1977). Is the mechanism of action during treatment of rheumatoid arthritis with penicillamine and gold the same? *Proc. Roy. Soc. Med.* 70, Suppl. 3, 136–139.

JELLUM, E., MUNTHE, E., GULDAHL, G. & AASETH, J. (1980). Fate of gold and thiomalate part after intramuscular administration of aurothiomalate to mice. *Ann. rheum. Dis.* 39, 155–158.

JESSOP, J.D. & WILKINS, M. (1975). The effects of gold salts on the phagocytic activity of synovial macrophages in organ culture. *J. Rheumatol.* 6, Suppl. 5, 136–142.

JOHNSEN, A.C., WIBETOE, G., LANGMYHR, F.J. & AASETH, J. (1982). Atomic absorption spectrometric determination of the total contents and distribution of copper and gold in synovial fluid from patients with rheumatoid arthritis. *Anal. Chim. Acta.* 135, 243–248.

KUZELL, W.C., SCHAFFARZICK, R.W., MANKLE, E.A. & GARDNER, G.M. (1951). Copper treatment of experimental and clinical arthritis. *Ann. rheum. Dis.* 10, 336.

LIPSKY, P.E. & ZIFF, M. (1977). Inhibition of antigen and mitogen induced human lymphocyte proliferation by gold compounds. *J. clin. Invest.* 59, 455–456.

LUND-OLESEN, K. & MENANDER, K.B. (1974). Orgotein, a new antiinflammatory metalloprotein drug: Preliminary evaluation of clinical efficacy and safety in degenerative joint disease. *Curr. ther. Res.* 16, 707–717.

MAITANI, T. & SUZUKI, K.T. (1981). Alterations of essential metal levels and induction of metallothionein by corrageenan injection. *Biochem. Parmacol.* 30, 2353–2355.

Multicentre Trial Group. (1973). Controlled trial of D(-) penicillamine in severe rheumatoid arthritis. *Lancet* 1, 280–290.

MUNTHE, E., GULDAL, G. & JELLUM, E. (1979a). Increased intracellular glutathione during penicillamine treatment for rheumatoid arthritis. *Lancet* 2, 1126–1127.

MUNTHE, E., JELLUM, E. & AASETH, J. (1979b). Some aspects of the mechanism of action of penicillamine in rheumatoid arthritis. *Scand. J. Rheumatol.* Suppl. 28, 6–12.

NAKAMURA, H. & GARASHI, M.I. (1977). Localization of gold in synovial membrane of rheumatoid arthritis treated with sodium aurothiomalate. *Ann. rheum. Dis.* 36, 209–215.

PEARSON, R.G. (1968). Hard and soft acids and bases-HSAB. *J. Chem. Educ.* 45, 643–648.

RAINSFORD, K.D. & WHITEHOUSE, M.W. (1976). Concerning the merits of copper aspirin as a potential antiinflammatory drug. *J. Pharm. Pharmacol.* 28, 83–86.
Research Subcommittee (1960). Gold therapy in rheumatoid arthritis. *Ann. rheum. Dis.* 19, 55–119.
RISTER, M., BAUERMEISTER, K., GRAVERT, U. & GLADTKE, E. (1978). Superoxide-dismutase deficiency in rheumatoid arthritis. *Lancet* 1, 1094.
SALBU, B. & BIBOW, K. (1983). Personal communication.
SIMKIN, P.A. (1977). Oral zinc-sulphate in rheumatoid arthritis. *Lancet* 2, 539–542.
— (1982). Treatment of rheumatoid arthritis with zinc sulphate. In *Inflammatory Diseases and Copper,* pp. 483–490. Ed. by J.R.J. Sorenson. Humana Press, Clifton, New Jersey.
SORENSON, J.R.J. (1978). An evaluation of the altered copper, iron, magnesium, manganese and zinc concentrations in rheumatoid arthritis. *Inorg. Persp. Biol. Med.* 2, 1–26.
— Editor (1982). *Inflammatory Diseases and Copper.* Humana Press, Clifton, New Jersey.
WHITEHOUSE, M.W. & WALKER, W.R. (1978). Copper and inflammation. *Agents and Actions* 8, 85–95.

Discussion (the papers by Hällgren and Aaseth)

Chairman: BOSTRÖM

HURLEY: I'd like to ask Dr Hällgren a question first. You mentioned that giving glucocorticoids increases the zinc in the red blood cells, but giving these adrenal cortical hormones also produces an increased rate of bone breakdown which releases zinc from the bone. That may be where the zinc is coming from that goes to the red blood cells. But, eventually, is it going to be a good or a bad thing for the patient to have this bone breakdown?

HÄLLGREN: Yes, of course I don't find a breakdown of the skeleton as something good. Corticosteroids may certainly induce osteoporosis when given at higher dosages and for longer time periods. Our patients had high inflammatory activity and were initially treated with 20 mg prednisone per day. The dosage was then gradually reduced and after three months, i.e. at the end of the study, the average daily dosage was 7.5 mg, and the risk for development of osteoporosis is rather small at prednisone dosages between 5 and 7.5 mg per day. I cannot exclude that giving corticosteroids induced an increased mobilization of zinc from the skeleton. However, if there was a substantial efflux of zinc to the circulation, you should expect an increase in plasma zinc levels, but plasma zinc remained unchanged in our patients. I find your hypothesis of zinc released from the skeleton intriguing but not the most likely explanation to our findings.

HURLEY: I also have a question for Dr Aaseth. I just wonder what evidence you have for your statement that metallothioneine is a scavenger of oxygen-free radicals?

AASETH: We have no concluding evidence, but in Oslo a group has worked with metallothioneine and radio protection and found that metallothioneine is a radio-protective agent. Their hypothesis is that it is a scavenger of toxic oxygen as are many other thiols. It is a hypothesis rather than a conclusion.

HURLEY: I'd like to ask you another question as to how you visualize the action of penicillamine. We know that penicillamine combines with copper. It also causes release of copper from the body. Therefore, one would suspect, and we have some evidence from animal experiments, that if this continues for a long enough period of time the activity of copper-zinc-superoxide dismutase declines. That would seem to be in conflict with the idea that in the case of rheumatoid arthritis part of the pathology of the disease may be related to the depressed activity of SOD. In that connection, also, I'd like to mention that, as you know I'm sure, manganese deficiency also produces a depression of the activity of the manganese SOD enzyme. How do you relate all this to the effects of this drug and the copper and manganese status of the patients?

AASETH: I think the most important effect of penicillamine is the formation of mixed diasulphides with the sulphur-containing proteins. So in fact it will protect the proteins against free-radical attacks even if it may reduce copper-containing enzymes. This reduction of superoxide dismutase appeared according to one publication after more than one year. The positive effects reported are usually related to six months or twelve months. Perhaps after long-term studies penicillamine may turn out to have a lower effect. But, in rheumatoid arthritis the levels of manganese are rather high and not low. Perhaps penicillamine may interfere with manganese too.

AGGETT: I'd like to ask Dr Hällgren something which would help me interpret his results. It's really relating to the erythrocyte population you're looking at, to the 3-month period. Are you looking at all the erythrocytes or are you looking at a subpopulation of erythrocytes? What I'm really asking is, what happens to erythrocytes in three months of treatment for rheumatoid arthritis? I'm wondering if you could outline it in terms of reticulocyte production, the maturity of the cells, whether they're normocytic, microcytic, etc.

HÄLLGREN: Your question is, what happens with the erythrocyte if I give glucocorticoids for three months to patients with rheumatoid arthritis? The normocytic anaemia is corrected more or less, provided that it is inflammatory-mediated and that the patient is not suffering from a true iron deficiency. Serum iron will start to return towards normal levels and we may suspect that we induce an increase of the marrow release of erythrocytes. The survival rate of erythrocytes in rheumatoid arthitis has been reported to be moderately reduced and is perhaps normalized during potent anti-inflammatory treatment. Did you also ask if we had studied subpopulations of erythrocytes?

AGGETT: Yes, because you're not comparing the same populations of cells, are you?

HÄLLGREN: That's true. The erythrocyte population has changed during a 3-month period due to the turn-over of erythrocytes and the influence of corticosteroids. The erythrocytes which were isolated before and after treatment were selected under the light microscope before microprobe analysis and were normal-sized.

BOSTRÖM: You more or less asked for one question and this is: What happens with your calcium-loaded, zinc-low, strontium-loaded granulocyte? I suppose it explodes sooner or later. And what happens then?

HÄLLGREN: If we stimulate a granulocyte membrane by, e.g., immune complexes or activated complement components, the granulocytes respond by the generation of free radicals and the release of lysosomal enzymes. This activation of the cell is evidently governed by an immediate increase of cytoplasmic ionized calcium which arises by mobilization of calcium stored within the cell and also by increasing the passive permeability to caliçum of the cell membrane. If we postulate a relationship between the amount of ligand-bound calcium and the amount of ionized calcium mobilized after stimulation, we may speculate that a certain stimulus to a granulocyte with normal total calcium will induce a weak inflammatory response when compared with a granulocyte loaded with calcium.

We are now testing the idea that the calcium-loaded granulocyte in rheumatoid arthritis is an aggressive cell, more apt to react to inflammatory stimuli. If this hypothesis proves to be correct, then perhaps a lot of therapeutical effects with steroids, penicillamine, gold, etc. can be explained by manipulation of cellular calcium. Recently, Gerald Weissman presented data supporting the idea that non-steroidal anti-inflammatory drugs exert their clinical effect in rheumatoid arthritis not only by inhibition of prostaglandin synthesis but also by preventing the mobilization of ionized calcium. I think that these data have not been published yet but they were presented at the International Congress of Inflammation in Paris about two months ago.

A stimulated generation of free radicals and an enhanced degranulation will induce a more severe inflammatory reaction. In rheumatoid arthritis we have a very pronounced release of lysosomal enzymes at least in the inflamed joint cavity. However, I don't think the granulocyte accumulation of calcium is the primary event of the inflammatory reaction in rheumatoid arthritis. I think that this abnormality may occur as a physiological response to a chronic inflammatory stimulatory agent which perhaps may be a virus. We have not cured until now one single patient with rheumatoid arthritis, but we have been able to reduce the inflammatory activity of the disease more or less successfully. This we do in different ways and perhaps most anti-inflammatory principles have in common an effect on calcium mobilization.

WESTER: I wonder if there is any experience of calcium entry blockers on the inflammatory response in rheumatoid arthritis and, also, if there is any experience of calcium antagonizers such as magnesium?

HÄLLGREN: I am not aware of any clinical studies on calcium-blocking agents and antagonizers in rheumatoid arthritis, but there are animal experimental studies which claim that calcium-blocking agents may reduce the inflammatory reaction. I doubt that magnesium has been given to patients with rheumatoid arthritis. However, it's not excluded that an increased magnesium intake is one way to reduce the inflammatory activity. Supplementation with zinc and selenium may be other ways. So, my idea is that we should not discuss the possible beneficial effect of one element at a time. I think that we should consider the cellular elements as part of an interdependent system of importance for the behaviour of the cell. Since many elements are competing for common binding sites, it is likely that the cellular element stores may be influenced by either chelating agents or increased intake of, e.g., zinc, selenium or magenesium.

SHAMBERGER: I have a question for Dr Hällgren. Because strontium had an effect on granulocytes which was equal to the effect by calcium and greater even than the effect of magnesium, do you perhaps think strontium may be an essential element?

HÄLLGREN: In what respect do you mean "essential element"?

SHAMBERGER: Essential just for granulocyte production.

HÄLLGREN: I don't think that strontium is essential in that respect, since we can't detect strontium in normal granulocytes. Perhaps strontium is "essential" as one way to create aggressive granulocytes of importance when we are threatened by invading microorganisms.

Antioxidation and Trace Elements in Cancer

Epidemiologic Review

By Raymond J. Shamberger

During the past two decades there has been a growing interest in the effect of trace elements such as selenium on human health. World-wide geographic variability in selenium concentrations has been observed in foods, forage crops, milk, and human blood. These variations are a result of geological action and climatic effects, particularly rainfall. Although selenium was once considered to be a toxic, undesirable, and a possibly carcinogenic element, it is now recognized as an essential element for the life of mammals and birds and an essential cofactor of glutathione peroxidase, an important scavenger of peroxides. Selenium has anticarcinogenic properties in animals, perhaps through its peroxide scavenging effect. Epidemiological studies in the United States have shown an inverse relationship between selenium intake and certain forms of cancer in humans. Neither the dietary amount of selenium essential for human life, nor the amount of selenium required to prevent cancer are known. The present paper summarizes some of the anticarcinogenic and antimutagenic properties of selenium and the epidemiological studies relating selenium to cancer.

ANTICARCINOGENIC EFFECT

There have been several reported anticarcinogenic effects of selenium against carcinogen-induced carcinoma of several organs. Some of these effects are summarized in Table 1. The organs mainly affected are the skin, liver, colon, and the breast.

Table 1 Influence of selenium on chemical carcinogens in mammary glands, lungs, and intestine in small animals as reported by various investigators

Level in diet		Species of anmial	Chemical carcinogen	Tissue of tumors	% Tumor[a] reduction by selenium	Reference
Se	Diet					
.0005%[b]	commercial	mice	3-methylcholanthrene	skin	22	Shamberger (1970)
1.0 ppm	torula yeast	mice	benzopyrene	skin	40	Shamberger (1970)
5 ppm	casein-based	rat	3-methyl-4-dimethyl-aminoazobenzene	liver	48	Clayton and Baumann (1949)
6 ppm	commercial	rat	3-methyl-4-dimethyl-aminoazobenzene	liver	40	Griffin and Jacobs (1977)
0.5 ppm	torula yeast	rat	2-acetylaminofluorene	liver	83	Harr et al. (1972)
4 ppm	commercial	rat	2-acetylaminofluorene	liver	48	Marshall et al. (1979)
1.0 ppm	?	rat	aflatoxin B_1	liver	80	Grant et al. (1977)
5 ppm	commercial	hamster	1 methyl-1-nitro-sourea	trachea	23	Thompson and Becci (1979)
6 ppm	commercial	mice	7,12-dimethylbenz-anthracene	mammary gland	62	Medina and Shepherd (1981)
1 ppm	torula yeast (5% unsat. fat)	rat	7,12-dimethylbenz-anthracene	mammary gland	25	Ip and Sinha (1981)
1 ppm	torula yeast (25% unsat. fat)	rat	7,12-dimethylbenz-anthracene	mammary gland	38	Ip and Sinha (1981)
1 ppm	torula yeast (25% unsat. fat)	rat	7,12-dimethylbenz-anthracene	mammary gland	17	Ip and Sinha (1981)
1.5 ppm	torula yeast (5% oil)	rat	7,12-dimethylbenz-anthracene	mammary gland	28	Ip (1981a)
1.5 ppm	torula yeast (25% oil)	rat	7,12-dimethylbenz-anthracene	mammary gland	21	Ip (1981a)
0.1 ppm	torula yeast (25% oil)	rat	7,12-dimethylbenz-anthracene	mammary gland	38	Ip (1981b)
5 ppm	commercial	rat	N-methyl-N-nitrosourea	mammary gland	11	Thompson and Becci (1980)
1.0 ppm	torula yeast	rat	N-methyl-N-nitrosourea	mammary gland	0	Thompson and Becci (1980)
4 ppm[c]	commercial	mice	7,12-dimethylbenz-anthracene	mammary gland	52	Welsch et al. (1981)
4 ppm[c]	commercial	rat	1,2-dimethylhydrazine	colon	54	Jacobs et al. (1977[a])
4 ppm[c]	commercial	rat	dimethylhydrazine	colon	56	Jacobs et al. (1981)
4 ppm[c]	commercial	rat	dimethylhydrazine	colon	43	Jacobs et al. (1981)
4 ppm[c]	commercial	rat	dimethylhydrazine	colon	18	Ankerst and Sjogren (1982)
1.0 ppm	casein-based	rat	bis(2-oxopropyl)nitro-samine	colon	45	Birt et al. (1982)
1.0 ppm	casein-based	rat	bis(2-oxopropyl)nitro-samine	lungs	100	Birt et al. (1982)
2 ppm[c]	casein-based	rat	azoxymethane	large & small bowel	15	Soullier et al. (1981)
2 ppm[c]	casein-based	rat	azoxymethane	large & small bowel	7	Nigro et al. (1982)

[a] Calculated as percentage reduction of tumors in animals receiving selenium plus the carcinogen in comparison to those receiving the carcinogen without selenium (controls).
[b] Selenium and the carcinogen were applied to the skin as a mixture in solution.
[c] Selenium was present in the drinking water.

Skin cancer

Sodium selenide and other antioxidants such as vitamin E were applied at the same time as croton oil to the backs of mice who had been initiated with 7,12-dimethylbenzanthracene (DMBA). In the first experiment, sodium selenide significantly reduced the number of mice with skin lesions (Shamberger & Rudolph 1966). Riley (1968) also has observed a similar effect when mice were treated with DMBA-phorbol ester (the active component of croton oil). In five of six additional nondietary tumor-promotion experiments, sodium selenide also significantly reduced the number of mice with tumors (Shamberger 1970). Dietary selenium significantly inhibited the number of mice with lesions induced by DMBA-croton oil and benzopyrene. The subsequent number of cancers formed in the benzopyrene experiments was also reduced in the mice fed 1.0 ppm of sodium selenite.

Liver cancer

Dietary selenium at 5 ppm (Clayton & Baumann 1949) and selenium added to the drinking water (Griffin & Jacobs 1977) have reduced the incidence of liver tumors induced by dimethylaminobenzene (DAB). However, the anti-tumor effect at 5 ppm may have been due to selenium toxicity as 3 ppm levels of selenium are considered borderline toxic. The rats on the 5 ppm selenium diet showed a slower weight gain and a decreased food intake. Dietary selenium (Harr et al. 1973) and selenium added to the drinking water (Marshall et al. 1979) have also reduced the incidence of liver tumors.

Balanski and Hadsiolov (1979) have fed diethylnitrosamine to rats on selenium diets containing 1, 5, or 10 ppm. There was not a significant difference between the number of animals with tumors, but there was a decrease in the number of tumors in the rats fed selenium. Dzhioev (1978) has also added selenium to the diets and found that the percentage of rats with tumors was reduced from 100% to 27%. In another experiment, dietary selenium reduced the percentage of mice with DEN-induced lung tumors from 76% to 54%. LeBoeuf et al. (1983) have reported that dietary selenium has significantly decreased the development of gamma-glutamyltranspeptidase-positive liver foci (GGTP foci) induced by DEN in rats. GGTP foci induced by aflatoxin in rats has also been decreased by dietary selenium (Baldwin et al. 1983).

Colon cancer

Jacobs et al. (1977a) have found that selenium added to the drinking water reduced the total number of tumors induced by 1,2-dimethylhydrazine (DMH) or methylazoxymethanol acetate. Selenium reduced the incidence of DMH-induced colon tumors by more than 50%, but the incidence of MAM-induced tumors was about the same. Jacobs et al. (1981) have reported significant reductions in the percentage of selenium-supplemented rats with tumors induced by DMH when the supplement was added to the drinking water before, during, and after 20 weekly injections of DMH. Ankerst and Sjogren (1982) have also observed that dietary selenium has reduced the number of tumors by DMH.

Soullier et al. (1981) have found that selenium added to the drinking water reduced the incidence of azoxymethane-induced cancer in rats fed a 30% beef fat diet. In addition, a significant reduction was observed in the tumor incidence in the proximal half of the colon in these rats. Birt et al. (1982) have also reported that there was a reduction of colon cancer induced by bis(2-oxopropyl)nitrosamine in rats which were fed dietary selenium.

Breast cancer

Selenium has been shown to inhibit both viral and chemically induced breast cancer. Schrauzer and Ishmael (1974) have observed that by adding 2 ppm of selenium to the drinking water the incidence of spontaneous mammary tumors induced by the Bittner milk virus was reduced from 82% to 10% in the selenium-treated mice. In addition, Schrauzer et al. (1980) have also reported that by feeding mice a torula yeast diet containing 1 ppm of organically bound selenium, a significant decrease was also observed in the percentage of mice with spontaneous mammary tumors.

Thompson and Tagliaferro (1980) and Ip and Sinha (1981) have reported that dietary selenium has reduced the incidence of rat mammary tumors induced by 7,12-dimethylbenzanthracene. Antineoplastic activity was dependent on the amount of selenium that was ingested. Thompson et al. (1984) have observed that sodium selenite was more effective than selenomethionine in reducing DMBA carcinogenesis. Vitamin E was found to have a synergistic effect on selenium in the chemoprevention of mammary carcinogenesis in rats (Horvath & Ip 1983).

In rats given an adequate amount of selenium, an increased amount of an unsaturated fat such as corn oil was added to the diet. The rats had an increased tumor incidence (Ip & Sinha 1981). By increasing the amount of dietary selenium, the tumor yields were correspondingly decreased (Ip 1981c).

Ip et al. (1981) have studied the effect of varying the timing of selenium supplementation of DMBA-induced mammary carcinogenesis in rats fed a high selenium diet. The experimental groups were supplemented with 5 ppm of selenium for various periods of time: −2 to 24 weeks; −2 to +2; +2 to +24; +2 to +12; +12 to +24; and −2 to +12. Control animals were fed 0.1 ppm of sodium selenite. The time of DMBA administration was taken as zero. Selenium again inhibited tumorigenesis to various degrees. Ip (1981c) concluded from these experiments: (1) selenium is able to inhibit both the initiation and the promotion phase of carcinogenesis; (2) a continuous intake of selenium is necessary to achieve a maximum inhibition of carcinogenesis (Schrauzer et al. (1980) had previously made a similar observation in his experiments with viral-induced mammary cancer); (3) the inhibitory effect of selenium is probably reversible in the early promotion phase; and (4) there is reduced efficacy of selenium when it is given long after carcinogenic injury.

Medina and Shephard (1981) have found that SeO_2 added to the drinking water inhibited DMBA-induced mammary carcinogenesis in BALB/c, C3H/StWi, and BD2F mice. Similarly, selenium also markedly reduced the induction of mammary preneoplastic dysplasias. The later stages of mammary tumorigenesis (preneoplastic to neoplastic transformation and tumor growth) were not as sensitive to selenium-mediated inhibition as the early stages—i.e., the induction and/or expression of mammary preneoplastic lesions (Medina & Lane 1983). There is a possibility that in both the rat and mouse experiments, the DMBA not only attacks the cellular target but is also dissolved in fat and slowly releases to attack the cellular target. In this case, selenium might actually be blocking the initiation phase rather than the apparent later promotion phase.

Sodium selenite has also reduced the transformation of mammary cells in organ culture of the whole mammary glands from BALB/c mice. Transformation was determined by the presence of nodule-like alveolar lesions (NLAL) induced by DMBA in the glands *in vitro*. This organ culture model system may be an important *in vitro* model for future studies on the mechanism of selenium's chemoprevention of the neoplastic process.

Pancreatic cancer

Dietary selenium has reduced the incidence of azaserine-induced preneoplastic abnormal acinar cell nodules in rat pancreas (O'Conner et al. 1983).

ANTIMUTAGENIC EFFECT

Both antimutagenic and mutagenic effects of selenium have been observed. The average blood selenium level in the United States is about 20 μg Se/100 ml or 2.53×10^{-6} M. In blood, concentrations greater than this amount seem to have a mutagenic effect, but selenium additions at less than physiological concentrations have been antimutagenic. In general, additions of selenium to the Ames Salmonella test system usually reduced mutagenesis.

Effect on DNA

Russel et al. (1980) have observed that selenium compounds are able to induce DNA repair synthesis as indicated by uptake of (^{3}H) thymidine-isolated rat liver cells. Williams (1978) has previously reported that (^{3}H) thymidine uptake by whole liver cells may be a measure of DNA repair synthesis. The repair of N-nitrosobis(2-oxopropyl)amine (BOP)-induced pancreatic DNA damage as measured by an alkaline sucrose gradient has been studied by Lawson and Birt (1981) when hamsters were pretreated with selenium. In the hamsters fed 5.0 ppm of selenium, the DNA damage was repaired quicker so that by 24 hours all of the DNA sedimented at the same density as the pancreatic DNA from control hamsters. Fewer single strand breaks were also observed in the selenium-fed animals. There was a small statistically significant increase in pancreatic DNA synthesis, but autoradiographic analysis indicated that this was a repair synthesis rather than a *de novo* DNA synthesis.

Effect on bacterial mutagenesis

Several investigators have reported that selenium added to the test system or selenium derived from microsomes (S-9 mix) prevents mutagenesis induced by several mutagenes in the Salmonella test system of Ames (Table 2). In most cases S-9 mix was used; however, the use of rat liver extracts will introduce some natural antioxidants, such as vitamin E and selenium

Table 2 The antimutagenic effect of selenium on Salmonella tester strains

Mutagen	Investigator	–	Year
2-Acetylaminofluorene	Jacobs et al.	–	1977b
N-hydroxy-2-acetylaminofluorene	Jacobs et al.	–	1977b
N-hydroxyaminofluorene	Jacobs et al.	–	1977b
Malonaldehyde	Shamberger et al.	–	1979
Beta-Propiolactone	Shamberger et al.	–	1979
N-metyl-N^1-nitro-N-nitrosoguanidine	Rosin and Stich	–	1979
N-acetoxy-2-acetylaminofluorene	Rosin and Stich	–	1979
Azoxymethane	Moriya et al.	–	1979
1,2-Dimethylhydrazine	Moriya et al.	–	1979
7,12-Dimethylbenzanthracene	Adams et al.	–	1980
7,12-Dimethylbenzanthracene	Martin et al.	–	1981
7,12-Dimethylbenzanthracene	Schillaci et al.	–	1982
7,12-Dimethylbenzanthracene	Arciszewska et al.	–	1982
Sodium nitrite	Adams et al.	–	1980
Acridine orange	Martin et al.	–	1981
7-Hydroxylmethyl-12-methylbenzanthracene	Arciszewska et al.	–	1982
12-Hydroxymethyl-7-methylbenzanthracene	Arciszewska et al.	–	1982
3-Hydroxy-7,12-dimethylbenzanthracene	Arciszewska et al.	–	1982
2-Aminofluorene	Gairola and Chow	–	1982
2-Aminoanthracene	Gairola and Chow	–	1982
Benzopyrene	Calle and Sullivan	–	1982
Benzopyrene	Teel	–	1984
3,2-Dimethyl-4-aminobiphenyl	Reddy et al.	–	1983

which may complicate interpretation of the experiment. The inhibition of mutagenicity by selenium could be related to the numerous reports of the anticarcinogenicity of selenium. If so, the Ames system might also be used to help elucidate some of the early steps of carcinogenesis. However, selenium has also reduced the direct mutagenic effect of malonaldehyde and beta-propiolactone using several strains of Salmonella bacteria (Shamberger et al. 1979). Selenium as well as other antioxidants such as vitamin C, vitamin E, and butylated hydroxytoluene reduced malonaldehyde-induced mutagenesis in those variants that mutated by a frameshift mechanism.

Effect on mammalian chromosomes

Selenium also has been shown to reduce the mutagenicity of known mutagens in human leukocyte cultures (Shamberger et al. 1973, Ray et al. 1978). Shamberger et al. (1973) have incubated blood leukocyte cultures with DMBA and then either with or without the antioxidants: ascorbic acid, BHT, sodium selenite and D,L-tocopherol. All of the antioxidants decreased the percentage of human chromosomal breaks induced by DMBA.

Sodium selenite (Morimoto et al. 1982) and selenous acid (Sayato & Nakamuro 1980) both have protected against the cytogenetic toxicity of methyl mercury and mercuric chloride in human whole-blood cultures in regard to their ability to induce sister-chromatid exchanges (SCE). The formation of bis(methylmercuric) selenide or a high molecular complex consisting of glutathione-Se-Hg which involves glutathione in red blood cells might be important intermediates. Sweins (1983) has studied the combined effects of sodium selenite and sodium arsenite on the chromosomes of cultured human lymphocytes. Selenium was found to reduce the frequency of gaps and chromatid breaks induced by arsenic.

Parshad et al. (1980) have studied the exposure of human fetal lung fibroblasts to fluorescent light which causes chromatid breaks and exchanges. Production of H_2O_2 likely causes the chromatid damage because the addition of catalase almost prevents damage, and H_2O_2 is able to induce chromatid breaks. If selenite is added to the cultures during light exposure, chromatid damage is decreased in a dose-dependent manner and may be necessary to maintain glutathione peroxidase activity. In these experiments, mannitol which scavenges $^{\cdot}OH$ also significantly reduced chromatid damage. The OH can be generated through interaction of H_2O_2 with divalent cations such as Fe^{2+} or Cu^{2+} in the cell. There is likely less $^{\cdot}OH$ in the selenite-treated group because glutathione peroxidase directly uses H_2O_2 thereby indirectly reducing $^{\cdot}OH$ because less H_2O_2 is available for conversion to $^{\cdot}OH$. The mutagenicity of dimethylnitrosamine (DMN) in Chinese hamster V79 cells after metabolic activation by the isolated perfused rat liver, was about doubled when selenium-deficient livers were used in comparison to the selenium-supplemented livers (Olsson et al. 1984).

Effect on yeast and plant mutagenesis

Rosin (1981) has observed that sodium selenite has completely suppressed spontaneous mutagenesis at two dependent genetic loci in nine mutator strains of *Saccharomyces cerevisiae*. Walker and Ting (1967) have found that sodium selenate interferes with the genetic crossing-over in barley. As a result of selenium treatment there was a deformation of the chromatin content of the meiocyte. This observation suggests that selenium might reduce crossing-over by a relaxation of the chromosomal protein which might relax the chromosomal fibril. Differences in bond strengths and distances between selenohydryl groups and sulfhydryl groups might cause alterations in the physiochemical properties of selenosubstituted proteins. Agabeyli et al. (1980) have found that low concentrations of sodium selenite decrease chromosome mutations induced by chemicals and radiation. This protective effect of selenite against wheat chromosome breakage was enhanced by vitamin E. Medzhidov (1982) has reported that sodium selenite at low concentrations showed antimutagenic activity in the meristemic cells of *Allium Fistulosum*.

Effect on drosophilia melanogaster

Selenocystine and selenomethionine are able to reduce crossover distribution along the X chromosome of *Drosophilia melanogaster* (Ahmed & Walker 1975). Their study also supports a mechanism of DNA damage induced by stress in an associated chromosomal fibril.

EPIDEMIOLOGICAL RELATIONSHIPS

There have been two large epidemiological studies showing an inverse relationship between environmental selenium and the incidence of cancer. One showed an inverse relationship of cancer mortality to selenium bioavailability in forage crops, and the other related the level of selenium in blood from different countries to cancer mortality.

ENVIRONMENTAL SELENIUM AND CANCER

Kubota et al. (1967) measured the selenium content of various forage crops such as alfalfa, soybeans, and corn, which take up selenium representative of the amounts bioavailable in the soil, and then constructed a map showing the generalized regional distribution pattern of selenium (Fig. 1). In the epidemiological studies of Shamberger and Willis (1971) and Shamberger et al. (1976), states were divided into three groups by the amount of selenium that Kubota et al. (1967) found in their forage crops: 0.02 to 0.05 ppm; 0.06 to 0.10 ppm; and 0.11 ppm or more. Alaska was not included in

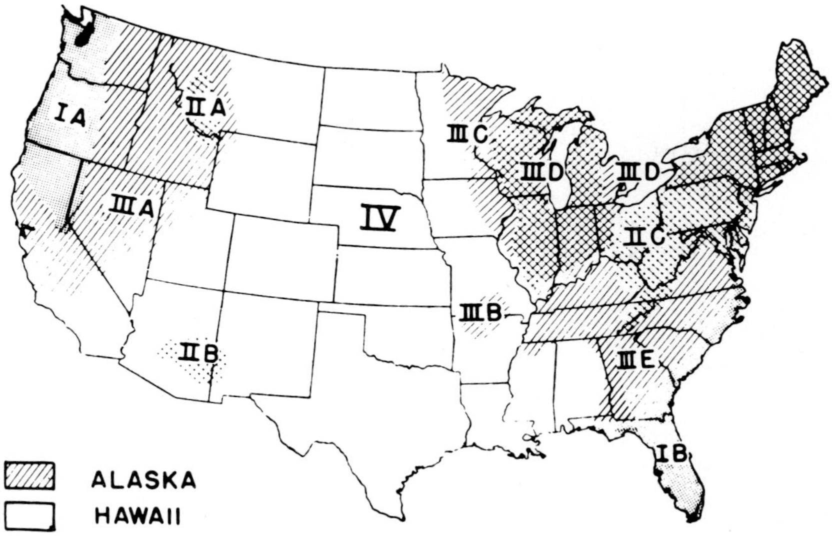

Fig.1 Selenium in forages and grains of the United States

Median concentration of selenium (ppm). IA 0.03; IB 0.02; IIA, IIB, IIC, IIIB 0.05; IIIA, IIIC 0.09; IIID 0.10; IIIE 0.06; and IV 0.26.

Reprinted with permission from *Ag. Food Chem.* 15, 448–453, 1967, by American Chemical Society.

the study and the District of Colombia was encluded in the low-selenium group.

The classification of cancer mortality is by state or political boundaries and does not always correspond to the agricultural boundaries. The transitional states, for the most part, appear in the intermediate classification. The high-selenium states had the greatest levels of forage selenium as well as frequent occurrence of plants that concentrate selenium (selenium indicator plants). The states that are considered to have very high selenium are separated for comparative purposes. These very high selenium states include: Colorado, Kansas, Nebraska, North Dakota, South Dakota and Wyoming. Selenium indicator plants containing more than 50 ppm have been frequently encountered in these states.

The 1968 age-specific cancer death rate for white males, for states located in different regions where selenium is found, is illustrated in Fig. 2. The 55- to 64-year age-specific cancer death rate in 1968 in the 19 states with high selenium levels was 429.7 ± 12.8 (Table 3). Highly significant differences were observed among the states with high, medium and low selenium levels. The six states with very high selenium levels showed the smallest age-specific cancer death rate (392.0 ± 11.6). The Chi square test value using the average mortality of 484.0 for the United States is 28.08 ($P<.001$).

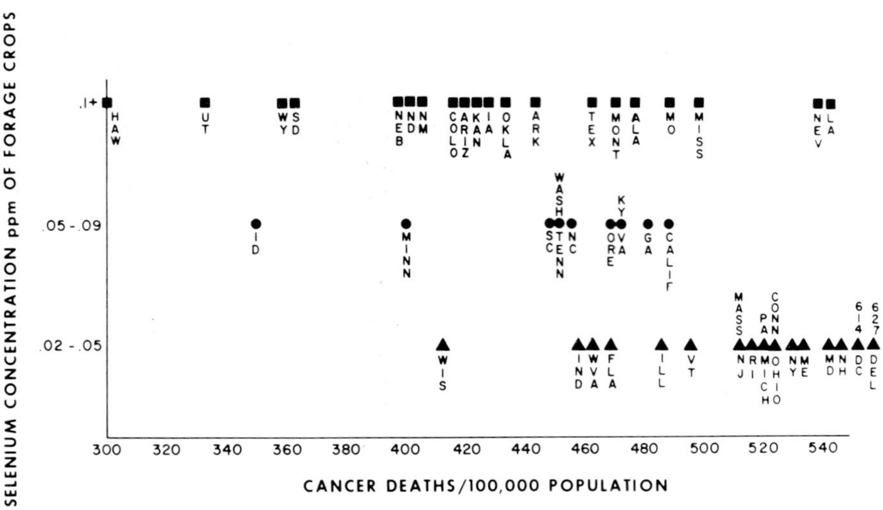

Fig. 2 *The 1968 age-specific (55- to 64-year-old group) cancer death rates for white males, for states located in different regions where selenium is found.*

For white males, significantly lower cancer death rates from neoplasms at sites such as the tongue, the esophagus, the stomach, the intestine, the rectum, the liver, the pancreas, the larynx, the lungs, the kidneys, and the bladder were observed in the states with high selenium levels (Table 4). In addition, lower death rates for subjects with Hodgin's disease and lymphoma were found.

For white females in the states with high selenium levels, significantly lower cancer death rates were found from neoplasms of the esophagus, stomach, intestine, rectum, liver, pancreas, larynx, lungs, bladder, and the thyroid gland. In addition, death rates for subjects with Hodgkin's disease, lymphoma, breast and uterine carcinoma were lower in the states with the high selenium levels.

Table 3 *Age-specific (55- to 64-year group) cancer death rates in 1968 for white males in states where selenium is found*

No. of states	Selenium level (ppm)		Cancer death rates/100,000 (mean ± SE)	Probability
6	Very high	0.26+	392.0±11.6	<.001
19	High	0.10+	429.7±12.8	<.001
11	Medium	0.06–0.09	450.0±12.2	<.001
20	Low	0.01–0.05	516.0±10.17	...

NOTE: Each value was compared individually to the low value by Student's *t*-test. Using the United States average mortality figure 484.0, the X^2 test value is 28.08 ($P<.001$)

Table 4 Age-adjusted cancer death rate by site and sex in states located in high-, intermediate-, and low-selenium areas

Site or Type of Cancer	ICD[a]	Male			Female		
		High	Medium	Low	High	Medium	Low
Lip	140	0.41±0.02	0.38±0.04	0.32±0.02	....	....	....
Tongue	148	3.27±0.25	3.73±0.39	5.20±0.34	1.02±0.08	1.29±0.15	1.06±0.04
Esophagus	150	2.63±0.12	3.00±0.28	4.73±0.28	0.78±0.05	1.07±0.10	1.06±0.04
Stomach	151	9.17±1.43	12.72±1.25	15.81±0.63	7.13±1.35	6.47±1.55	8.00±0.33
Intestine	153	12.39±0.45	12.42±0.81	18.50±0.64	14.11±0.62	15.36±1.45	15.88±0.76
Rectum	154	4.93±0.26	5.17±0.64	9.00±0.43	3.73±0.24	4.57±0.69	4.62±0.26
Liver, biliary tree	155	4.74±0.15	4.41±0.26	5.31±0.13	4.91±0.18	4.69±0.44	5.49±0.19
Pancreas	157	9.19±0.20	9.35±0.26	9.61±0.14	5.47±0.10	5.61±0.13	5.99±0.11
Larynx	161	1.85±0.13	1.95±0.20	2.95±0.16	0.20±0.02	0.23±0.02	0.27±0.02
Lung, trachea, bronchus	163	33.27±1.86	33.25±2.54	40.06±1.18	5.45±1.26	5.73±0.41	6.33±0.16
Breast	170	0.25±0.01	0.24±0.02	0.30±0.02	21.66±0.54	22.18±1.26	27.02±0.74
Uterus							
Cervix	171	....	....	....	7.43±0.33	8.25±0.75	8.28±0.40
Corpus	174	....	....	....	5.43±0.16	5.42±0.20	6.57±0.18
Ovary, fallopian	175	....	....	....	7.55±0.24	7.56±0.46	8.91±0.21
Kidney	180	3.50±0.11	3.40±0.24	4.09±0.10	1.94±0.10	1.87±0.11	2.06±0.04
Bladder	181	5.42±0.22	5.17±0.47	7.62±0.27	1.92±0.07	2.15±0.10	2.63±0.08
Hodgkin's disease	201	2.22±0.05	2.21±0.10	2.38±0.07	1.20±0.05	1.21±0.09	1.43±0.05
Lymphoma	202	4.43±0.14	4.44±0.24	4.96±0.09	3.04±0.09	2.94±0.22	3.27±0.07

NOTE: Data presented as mean ± SE
[a] ICD is the classification number

The greater differences found in males might be anticipated because in the United States, which is a highly industrialized country, males are more likely to be exposed to carcinogen-containing industrial fumes and air pollution. Men are also known to be heavier smokers than women. The protective effect of selenium observed in animal experiments would be expected to be greater in males.

If selenium protects humans against environmental carcinogens in the same way that it protects mice or rats, then one would expect a lower mortality from cancer of the organ systems concerned with assimilation metabolism and excretion of selenium. Selenium is concentrated by the kidneys, the liver, and the pancreas. Lower cancer mortality was observed for each type of cancer for both males and females in the high-selenium areas.

Environmental marker types of cancer (i. e., esophageal, stomach, intestinal, and rectal cancer death rates) were especially decreased in the areas of high selenium levels for both males and females. Cowgill (1983) re-examined the study of Shamberger and Willis (1971) for the years 1969–1971 and found lower cancer mortality of the digestive organs (ICD 150–159), respiratory organs (ICD 160–163), and the breast (ICD 174) in the high-selenium areas. In the provinces of Canada with high selenium levels, lower age-adjusted rates for gastrointestinal cancer have been observed (Shamberger & Frost 1969). From selenium tracer studies, it is known that the entire gastrointestinal and urinary tracts of man and animals are exposed to selenium. Selenium would then be available to protect against cancer of these sites. However, there was greater cancer mortality from cancer of the lip, skin, and eyes as well as leukemia in the high-selenium states. This may be due to a greater amount of solar or other type of radiation in the Southwestern states, many of which are included in the high-selenium areas.

Because food is widely distributed throughout the United States, geographic variations in blood or breast milk selenium levels may be difficult to explain. There are some variations of selenium content in locally grown food and milk and also in local drinking water. Large amounts of selenium may be inhaled and absorbed from breathing the dust of the area. This might explain why mortality from cancer of the larynx and of the lungs appears to be lower in the high-selenium states. However, the states with high selenium levels in this study are more rural and have less air pollution. For some types of cancer, the lower cancer mortality in the high-selenium areas might be caused by factors other than selenium bioavailability. Attempts to compensate for the degree of urbanization were made by matching 17 high-selenium and 17 low-selenium large cities based on the ratio of the observed to the expected cancer death rate by site and sex (Table 5). The cities in the

Table 5 The ratio of the observed to the expected cancer death rate by site and sex in 17 paired large cities occurring in high- or low-selenium areas

Standard errors are indicated. M = Male; F = Female. Parentheses = a high-selenium area; no parentheses = low-selenium area

Cancer	M	(M)	F	(F)
Pharynx	1.86±0.150	1.58±0.128	---	---
Esophagus	1.51±0.073	0.90±0.065	---	---
Small intestine[a]	1.05±0.104	0.79±0.082	---	---
Stomach	1.68±0.100	0.99±0.042	0.68±0.036	0.50±0.024
Large intestine	1.08±0.032	0.80±0.077	1.03±0.036	0.81±0.014
Rectum	1.39±0.060	0.89±0.060	0.80±0.040	0.56±0.030
Liver	1.17±0.068	1.07±0.068	0.74±0.052	0.59±0.048
Pancreas	1.27±0.092	1.27±0.053	0.73±0.011	0.74±0.030
Bladder, urinary organs	1.65±0.082	1.35±0.063	0.54±0.026	0.47±0.030
Kidney	1.49±0.084	1.23±0.058	0.69±0.038	0.59±0.050
Bronchus, lung	1.78±0.053	1.85±0.082	---	---
Leukemia	1.23±0.045	1.28±0.028	0.81±0.039	0.86±0.027
Lymphatic	1.26±0.031	1.22±0.036	0.78±0.028	0.76±0.010
Prostate	2.09±0.072	2.19±0.068	---	---
Ovary	---	---	1.92±0.073	1.66±0.054
Cervix, uteri	---	---	1.94±0.089	1.59±0.057
Breast	---	---	1.88±0.039	1.60±0.039

[a] M and F

high-selenium states had a lower gastrointestinal, liver, and bladder cancer death rate. However, there did not seem to be much difference in the amount of lung cancer in the 17 sets of cities. This may indicate that the differences in lung cancer in the high- and low-selenium areas in Table 1 may be due to the degree of urbanization rather than differences in the environmental levels of selenium.

Schrauzer et al. (1977) have correlated the age-adjusted mortality from cancer at 17 body sites with the apparent dietary selenium intakes estimated from food consumption data in 27 countries. Even though there is some variance in the selenium content of food grown in one place compared to another, the contributions of fruits and vegetables to the overall amount of selenium intake would be small compared to the contribution of selenium in beef or seafood where the selenium content is comparatively large and fairly constant. Schrauzer et al. (1977) observed significant inverse correlations for cancers of the large intestine, rectum, prostate, breast, ovary, and lung and for leukemia; weaker inverse associations were found for cancers of the pancreas, skin and the bladder.

In another part of the study, similar inverse correlations were observed between cancer mortalities at the above sites, and the selenium concentrations in whole blood which had been collected from healthy human donors in the United States and several other countries (Schrauzer er al. 1977). Schrauzer et al. (1977) have postulated that the cancer mortalities observed in the United States as well as other Western industrialized nations would markedly decline if the dietary selenium intakes were increased to about twice the average amount in the U.S. diet. Willet et al. (1983) and Salonen et al. (1984) have measured blood selenium in several thousand people in the United States and Finland and then followed their cancer rate for several years. Higher blood selenium was associated with a two-fold reduction (Willet et al. 1983) and a three-fold reduction of the subsequent cancer mortality.

CONCLUSIONS

Selenium inhibits many types of carcinogen-induced cancer in animals including skin, liver, and the fat-sensitive breast and colon cancer. In addition, selenium inhibits mutagenesis in bacterial test systems and reduces human chromosome breakage. Epidemiological studies seem to indicate that where selenium occurs in the environment or in large amounts in the blood, there is a decreased cancer mortality, especially of the fat-sensitive cancers such as breast and colon cancer. More epidemiological studies would be desirable in this regard.

REFERENCES

ADAMS, G., MARTIN, S. & MILNER, J. (1980). Effects of selenium on the Salmonella/microsome mutagen test system. *Fed. Proc.* 39, 790.

AGABELYI, R. A., MEKHTIEV, N. K. & MELIKOVA, N. K. (1980). Influence of sodium selenite on ethylene imine and gamma-rays induced wheat chromosome mutations. *Genetika* 16, 2226–2228.

AHMED, Z. U. & WALKER, G. W. R. (1975). The effects of urethane, sodium monohydrogen arsenate and selenocystine on crossing-over in Drosophila melanogaster. *Canad. J. Genet. Cytol.* 17, 55–66.

ANKERST, J. & SJOGREN, H. O. (1982). Effect of selenium on the induction of breast fibroadenomas by adenovirus type 9 and 1,2-dimethylhydrazine-induced bowel carcinogenesis in rats. *Int. J. Cancer* 29, 707–710.

ARCISZEWSKA, L. K., MARTIN, S. E. & MILNER, J. A. (1982). The antimutagenic effect of selenium on 7,2-dimethylbenzanthracene and metabolites in the Ames *Salmonella*/microsome system. *Biol. Tr. Element* 4, 259–267.

BALANSKI, R. M. & HADSIOLOV, D. H. (1979). Influence of sodium selenite on the hepatocarcinogenic action of diethylnitrosamine in rats. *C. R. Acad. Bulg. Sci.* 32, 697–698.

BALDWIN, S., PARKER, R. S. & MISSELBECK, N. (1983). Effect of dietary fat and selenium on the development of preneoplastic lesions in rat liver. *Fed. Proc.* 42, 1312.

BIRT, D. F., LAWSON, T. A., JULIUS, A. D., KUNICE, C. E. & SALMASI, S. (1982). Inhibition by dietary selenium of colon cancer induced in the rat by bis-(2-oxopropyl)nitrosamine. *Cancer Res.* 42, 4456–4459.

CALLE, L. M. & SULLIVAN, P. D. (1982). Screening of antioxidants and other compounds for antimutagenic properties towards benzopyrene-induced mutagenicity in strain TA 98 of *Salmonella typhimurium*. *Mutation Res.* 101, 99–114.

CLAYTON, C. C. & BAUMANN, C. A. (1949). Diet and azo dye tumors. Effect of diet during a period when the dye is not fed. *Cancer Res.* 9, 575–582.

COWGILL, U. M. (1983). The distribution of selenium and cancer mortality in the continental United States. *Biol. Tr. Elem. Res.* 5, 345–361.

DZHIOEV, F. D. (1978). Effect of selenium, phenobarbital, teturam, and carbon tetrachloride on the carcinogenic effect of diethylnitrosamine and 1,2-dimethylhydrazine. In *Kantserog N-Nitrozonsoedin: Desitvie, Obraz., Opred., Mater Simp.*, 3rd Ed., pp. 51–53. Ed. by G. O. Looga. Tallinn, USSR

GAIROLA, C. & CHOW, C. K. (1982). Dietary selenium, hepatic arylhydrocarbon hydroxylase and mutagenic activation of benzopyrene, 2-aminoanthracene and 2-aminofluorene. *Toxicol. Letters* 11, 281–287.

GRANT, K. E., CONNER, M. W. & NEWBERNE, P. M. (1977). Effect of dietary sodium selenite upon lesions induced by repeated small doses of aflatoxin B_1. *Toxicol. appl. Pharmacol.* 41, 166.

GRIFFIN, A. C. & JACOBS, M. M. (1977). Effects of selenium on azo dye hepatocarcinogenesis. *Cancer Lett.* 3, 177–181.

HARR, J. R., EXON, J. H., WESWIG, P. H. & WHANGER, P. D. (1973). Relationship of dietary selenium concentration; chemical cancer induction; and tissue concentration of selenium in rats. *Clin. Toxicol.* 8, 487–495.

HORVATH, P. M. & IP, C. (1983). Synergistic effect of vitamin E and selenium in the chemoprevention of mammary carcinogenesis in rats. *Cancer Res.* 43, 5335–5341.

IP, C. (1981a). Factors influencing the anticarcinogenic efficacy of selenium in dimethylbenzanthracene-induced mammary tumorigenesis in rats. *Cancer Res.* 41, 2683–2686.

— (1981b). Modification of mammary carcinogenesis and tissue peroxidation by selenium deficiency and dietary fat. *Nutr. Cancer* 2, 136–142.

— (1981c). Prophylaxis of mammary neoplasia by selenium supplementation in the initiation and promotion phases of chemical carcinogenesis. *Cancer Res.* 41, 4386–4390.

IP, C. & SINHA, D. K. (1981). Enhancement of mammary tumorigenesis by dietary selenium deficiency in rats with a high polyunsaturated diet. *Cancer Res.* 41, 31–34.

IP, C., IP, M. M. & KIM, U. (1981). Dietary selenium intake and growth of MT-W9B transplantable rat mammary tumor. *Cancer Lett.* 14, 101–107.

JACOBS, M. M., JANSSON, B. & GRIFFIN, A. C. (1977a). Inhibitory effects of selenium on 1,2-dimethylhydrazine and methylazoxymethanol acetate induction of colon tumors. *Cancer Lett.* 2, 133–138.

JACOBS, M. M., MATNEY, T. S. & GRIFFIN, A. C. (1977b). Inhibitory effects of selenium on the mutagenicity of 2-acetylaminofluorene (AAF) and AAF metabolites. *Cancer Lett.* 2, 319–322.

JACOBS, M. M., FORST, C. F. & BEAMS, F. A. (1981). Biochemical and clinical effects of selenium on dimethylhydrazine-induced colon cancer in rats. *Cancer Res.* 41, 4458–4465.

KUBOTA, J., ALLAWAY, W. H., CARTER, D. L., CARY, E. E. & Lazar, V. A. (1967). Selenium in crops in the United States in relation to selenium-responsive diseases of livestock. *J. Agric. Food Chem.* 15, 448–453.

LAWSON, T. & BIRT, D. (1981). BOP induced damage of pancreas DNA and its repair in hamsters pretreated with selenium. *Proc. Amer. Ass. Cancer Res.* 22, 94.

LEBOEUF, R. A., LAISHES, B. A. & HOEKSTRA, W. C. (1983). Effect of dietary selenium concentration on early post-initiation stages of hepatocarcinogenesis. *Fed. Proc.* 42, 669.

MARSHALL, M. V., ARNOTT, M. S., JACOBS, M. M. & GRIFFIN, A. C. (1979). Selenium effects on the carcinogenicity and metabolism of 2-acetylaminofluorene. *Cancer Lett.* 7, 331–338.

MARTIN, S. E., ADAMS, G. H., SCHILLACI, M. & MILNER, J. A. (1981). Antimutagenic effects of selenium on acridine orange and 7,12-dimethylbezanthracene in the Ames Salmonella/microsomal system. *Mutation Res.* 82, 41–46.

MEDINA, D. & LANE, H. W. (1983). Stage specificities of selenium-mediated inhibition of mouse mammary tumorigenesis. *Biol. Tr. Elem. Res.* 5, 297–306.

MEDINA, D. & SHEPHARD, F. (1981). Selenium-mediated inhibition of 7,12-dimethylbenzathracene-induced mouse mammary tumorigenesis. *Carcinogenesis* 2, 451–455.

MEDZHIDOV, M. M. (1982). Features of the effect of several selenium-containing compounds on the experimentally induced mutation process. In *K. Izuch, Rezist. Rast. Ekstremalnykh Vozdiestv. Sredy.* Ed. N. A. Kasumov. Izd. Azerb. Gos. Univ., Baku, USSR.

MORIMOTO, K., Iijima, S. & KOIZUMI, A. (1982). Selenite prevents the induction of sister-chromatid exchanges by methyl mercury and mercuric chloride in human whole-blood cultures. *Mutation Res.* 102, 183–192.

MORIYA, M., OHTA, T:, WATANABE, K., WATANABE, Y., SUGIYAMA, F., MIYAZAWA, T. & SHIRASU, Y. (1979). Inhibitors for the mutagenicities of colon carcinogens, 1,2-dimethylhydrazine and azoxymethane in the host-mediated assay. *Cancer Lett.* 7, 325–330.

NIGRO, N. D., BULL, A. W., WILSON, P. S., SOULLIER, B. K. & ALOUSI, M. A. (1982). Combined inhibitors of carcinogenesis: Effect on azoxymethane-induced intestinal cancer in rats. *J. Nat. Cancer Inst.* 69, 103–107.

O'CONNER, T. P., YOUNGMAN, L. D. & CAMPBELL, T. C. (1983). Effect of selenium on development L-azaserine (Aza) induced preneoplastic abnormal acinar cell nodules (AACN) in rat pancreas. *Fed. Proc.* 42, 670.

OLSSON, U., ONFELT, A. & B.EIJE, B. (1984). Dietary selenium deficiency causes decreased N-oxygenation of N, N-dimethylaniline and increased mutagenicity of dimethylnitrosamine in the isolated rat liver/cell culture system. *Mutation Res.* 100, 73–80.

PARSHAD, R., TAYLOR, W. G., SANFORD, K. K., CAMALIER, R. F., GANTT, R. & TARONE, R. E. (1980). Fluorescent light-induced chromosome damage in human IRM-90 fibroblasts. Role of hydrogen peroxide and related free radicals. *Mutation Res.* 73, 115–124,

RAY, J. H., ALTENBURG, J. L. & JACOBS, M. M. (1978). Effects of sodium selenite and methyl methanesulphonate or N-hydroxy-2-acetylaminofluorene co-exposure on sister chromatid exhange production in human whole blood cultures. *Mutation Res.* 57, 359–368.

REDDY, B. S., HANSON, D., MATHEWS, L. & SARMA, C. (1983). Effect of micronutrients, antioxidants, and related compounds on the mutagenicity of 3,2′-dimethyl-4-aminobiphenyl, a colon and breast carcinogen. *Food Chem. Toxicol.* 21, 129–132.

RILEY, J. F. (1968). Mast cells, cocarcinogenesis and anticarcinogenesis in the skin of mice. *Experimentia* 15, 1237–1238.

ROSIN, M. P. (1981). Inhibition of spontaneous mutagenesis in yeast cultures by selenite, selenate, and selenide. *Cancer Lett.* 10, 75–81.

ROSIN, M. P. & STICH, H. F. (1979). Assessment of the use of the Salmonella mutagenesis assay to determine the influence of antioxidants on carcinogen-induced mutagenicity. *Int. J. Cancer* 23, 722–727.

RUSSELL, G. R., NADER, C. J. & PATRICK, E. J. (1980). Induction of DNA repair by some selenium compounds. *Cancer Lett.* 10, 75–81.

SALONEN, J. T., ALFTHAN, G., HUTTUNEN, J. K. & PUSKA, P. (1984). Association between serum selenium and the risk of cancer. *Amer. J. Epidem.* 120, 342–349.

SAYATO, Y. & NAKAMURO, K. (1980). Chromosomal aberrations in cultured human lymphocytes induced by simultaneous treatment with mercury compounds and selenium compounds. *Eisei Kagaku* 26, 99–102.

SCHILLACI, M., MARTIN, S. E. & MILNER, J. A. (1982). The effects of dietary selenium on the biotransformation of 7,12-dimethylbenzathracene. *Mutation Res.* 101, 31–37.

SCHRAUZER, G. N. & ISHMAEL, D. (1974). Effects of selenium and of arsenic on the genesis of spontaneous mammary tumors in inbred C_3H mice. *Ann. clin. Lab. Sci.* 4, 411–417.

SCHRAUZER, G. N., WHITE, D. A. & SCHNEIDER, C. J. (1977). Cancer mortality correlation studies—III: Statistical associations with dietary selenium intakes. *Bioinorg. Chem.* 7, 23–34.

SCHRAUZER, G. N., MCGINNESS, J. E. & KUEHN, K. (1980). The effects of temporary selenium supplementation on the genesis of spontaneous mammary tumors in inbred female C_3H/S-mice. *Carcinogenesis* 1, 199–201.

SHAMBERGER, R. J. (1970). Relationship of selenium to cancer. I. Inhibitory effect of selenium on carcinogenesis. *J. Nat. Cancer Inst.* 44, 931–936.

SHAMBERGER, R. J. & FROST, D. V. (1969). Possible inhibitory effect of selenium on human cancer. *Canad. Med. Ass. J.* 100, 682.

SHAMBERGER, R. J. & RUDOLPH, G. (1966). Protection against carcinogenesis by antioxidants. *Experientia* 22, 116.

SHAMBERGER, R. J. & WILLIS, C. E. (1971). Selenium distribution and human cancer mortality. *CRC Crit. Rev. Clin. Lab. Sci.* 2, 211–221.

SHAMBERGER, R. J., BAUGHMAN, F. F., KALCHERT, S. L., WILLIS, C. E. & HOFFMAN, G. C. (1973). Carcinogen-induced chromosomal breakage decreased by antioxidants. *Proc. Nat. Acad. Sci.* 70, 1461–1463.

SHAMBERGER, R. J., TYTKO, S. A & WILLIS, C. E. (1976). Antioxidants and cancer. VI. Selenium and age-adjusted human cancer mortality. *Arch. Environm. Hlth* 31, 231–235.

SHAMBERGER, R. J., CORLETT, C. L., BEAMON, K. D. & KASTEN, B. L. (1979). Antioxidants reduce the mutagenic effect of malonaldehyde and beta-propiolactone. Part IX. Antioxidants and cancer. *Mutation Res.* 66, 349–355.

SOULLIER, B. K., WILSON, P. S. & NIGRO, N. D. (1981). Effect of selenium on azoxymethane-induced intestinal cancer. *Cancer Lett.* 12, 343–348.

SWEINS, A. (1983). Protective effect of selenium against arsenic-induced chromosomal damage in cultured human lymphocytes. *Heriditas* 98, 249–252.

TEEL, R. W. (1984). Selenium modified mutagenicity of benzopyrene in an S9-dependent system. *Mutation Res.* 127, 9–14.

THOMPSON, H. J. & BECCI, P. J. (1979). Effect of graded dietary levels of selenium on tracheal carcinomas induced by 1-methyl-1-nitrosourea. *Cancer Lett.* 7, 215–219.

— (1980). Selenium inhibition of N-methyl-N-nitrosourea-induced mammary carcinogenesis in the rat. *J. Nat. Cancer Inst.* 65, 1299–1301.

THOMPSON, H. J. & TAGLIAFERRO, A. R. (1980). Effect of selenium on 7,12-dimethylbenzanthracene-induced mammary tumorigenesis. *Fed. Proc.* 39, 1117.

THOMPSON, H. J., MEEKER, L. D. & KOKOSKA, S. (1984). Effect of an inorganic and organic form of dietary selenium on the promotional stage of mammary carcinogenesis in the rat. *Cancer Res.* 44, 2803–2806.

WALKER, G. W. R. & TING, K. P. (1967). Effect of selenium on recombination in barley. *Canad. J. Genet. Cytol.* 9, 314–320.

WELSCH, C. W., GOODRICH-SMITH, M., BROWN, C. K., GREENE, H. D. & HAMEL, E. J. (1981). Selenium and the genesis of murine mammary tumors. *Carcinogenesis* 2, 519–522.

WILLET, W. C., POLK, B. F., MORRIS, J. S., STAMPFER, M. J., PRESSEL, S., ROSNER, B., TAYLOR, J. O., SCHNEIDER, K. & HAMES, C. G. (1983). Prediagnostic serum selenium and risk of cancer. *Lancet* 2, 130–134.

WILLIAMS, G. M. (1978). Further improvements in the hepatocyte primary culture DNA repair test for carcinogens: detection of carcinogenic biphenyl derivatives. *Cancer Lett.* 4, 69–75.

Selenium in Cardiovascular Diseases and Cancer

Epidemiologic Findings from Finland

By Jukka T. Salonen

INTRODUCTION

The content of selenium in the soil is very low in Finland (Koljonen 1975). Consequently, the selenium content in Finnish foodstuffs is very low (Koivistoinen 1980, Varo et al. 1980, Varo & Koivistoinen 1981). The relative lack of selenium is particularly pronounced in cereal grains (Mutanen & Koivistoinen 1983), and the intake of selenium by Finns from grains is determined by the ratio of imported to domestic grain. The concentration of selenium of 100–200 μg/kg in the former is about ten times greater than in the latter. The crops in Finland were rather plentiful during the 1970's so foreign imports of cereal grains were small (Varo et al. 1980). The proportion of imported grains started to increase in the late 1970's. The limited dietary intake of selenium in the 1970's was reflected in the low average blood and serum concentrations of selenium in the Finns (Westermarck et al. 1977, Kumpulainen & Koivistoinen 1981).

The function of selenium in the human body was elucidated when Hoekstra and co-workers (see Hoekstra 1974) discovered that selenium is a constituent of glutathione peroxidase in erythrocytes. Mills showed later that this enzyme is present in liver, lung, kidney, and other tissues (1960). The possible role of selenium in the development of cardiovascular disease (CVD) is not clear (Lancet editorial 1983). The most probable hypothetical mechanisms are listed in Table 1. Salmon et al. (1978) showed that the enzyme responsible for the formation of prostacyclin, prostacyclin synthetase, is strongly inhibited by lipid peroxides. The assumed role of selenium in arachidonic acid metabolism is presented in Fig. 1.

Increases in platelet glutathione peroxidase activity were obtained by giving dietary selenium to depleted animals (Levander et al. 1983a) or humans (Levander et al. 1983b). Increased aggregability of platelets was

Table 1 Hypothetical mechanisms for increased risk of IHD due to selenium deficiency

1. Increased intimal damage by lipid peroxides
2. Reduction of prostacyclin synthesis and subsequently
2.1 Increased thrombocyte aggregability
2.2 Elevated blood pressure
2.3 Increased risk of coronary spasm
(3. Impaired calcium transport)

reported in selenium-deficient rats (Masukawa et al. 1983). Moreover, a decreased prostacyclin production in aortas (Masukawa et al. 1983) and increased thromboxane A_2 production after collagen stimulation in platelets (Schoene et al. 1983) was found in rats after selenium depletion compared with control rats. An altered ratio of prostacyclin and thromboxane could be important in the etiology of both cancer (Menter et al. 1984) and cardiovascular diseases (Whittle & Moncada 1983).

After Hoekstra (1975) had shown that a selenium-dependent enzyme destroys lipid hydroperoxides and other peroxides, it was postulated that selenium may be involved in the inhibition of carcinogenesis by reducing the mutagenicity of cancer-causing chemicals, by effecting carcinogen metabolism or by protecting cellular membranes against oxidative damages (Griffin 1979).

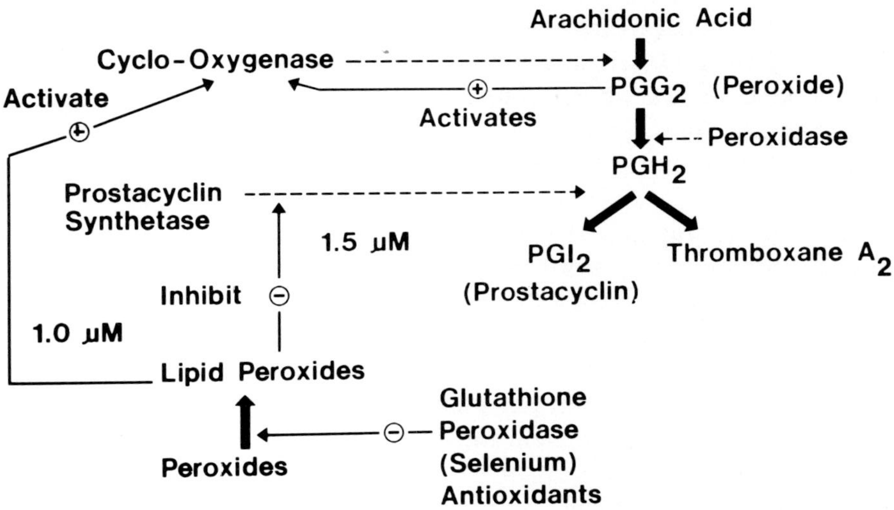

Fig. 1 Role of selenium in arachidonic acid metabolism

SELENIUM AND THE RISK OF CARDIOVASCULAR DISEASES

Epidemiologic findings

The first observational indications of an inverse association of ischaemic heart disease (IHD) and cerebrovascular disease mortality with the selenium content of forage crops, drinking water and pooled blood-bank blood came from ecologic between-area comparisons (Bostrom & Wester 1967, Frost 1972, Shamberger et al. 1975, 1978, 1979, Shamberger 1981). Ecologic studies are, however, subject to biases arising from the multicollinearity of various risk factors and nutrients between populations—the ecological fallacy—and no causal inferences can thus be drawn on the basis of cross-population data.

In Finland, indeed, higher serum selenium levels were observed in the eastern parts with the highest known rates of cardiovascular diseases (Keys et al. 1980) than in the southwest of Finland (Virtamo et al. 1984).

So far, four epidemiologic studies on the role of selenium in CVD have been completed in Finland. All these are based on a prospective follow-up of a cohort from which serum had been sampled from individual persons before the follow-up (Salonen et al. 1982, 1984a, Miettinen et al. 1983, Virtamo et al. 1984). In all these studies selenium determinations were made from frozen serum samples after storage at −20°C for six to ten years. At the start of the follow-up, measurements of the IHD history and the major established risk factors for IHD were done in all four studies. The follow-up period varied between five and seven years, during which the cardiovascular deaths in the cohort were identified by means of the National Death Certificate Register, which records all deaths of Finnish citizens. Admissions to hospital due to an acute myocardial infarction (AMI) were obtained from the National Hospital Discharge Data Register. In Finland, patients who receive medical attention for an AMI are customarily hospitalized. Concentrations of serum selenium were determined in all four studies by a graphite furnace atomic absorption spectrometric method (Alfthan & Kumpulainen 1982).

The first and the largest study so far was based on the cohort of the baseline survey of the North Karelia project (Salonen et al. 1982). The baseline survey was conducted in 1972 in two provinces of eastern Finland, North Karelia and Kuopio. A random 6.7% population sample was drawn from the people aged 25 to 59 years. Altogether approximately 11,000 persons were studied with a participation rate of 90%. A semi-fasting (at least for 4 hours) blood sample was drawn from each survey participant (Salonen et al. 1981).

There were 8,113 men and women aged 35 to 59 years who reported no history of AMI or cerebrovascular stroke in the 12 months preceding the baseline survey. Among those who had a sufficient serum sample, 131 died of CVD, 95 of whom died from IHD, and 252 had either non-fatal AMI or died of acute IHD during a seven-year follow-up. For each of these cases, an event-free control was matched for sex, age, tobacco consumption, serum total cholesterol, diastolic blood pressure, and history of angina pectoris.

The mean serum selenium concentration for all cases was 52 µg/1 and for all controls 55 µg/1 ($p < 0.01$ for difference in paired t-test). Serum selenium concentration was classified into more categories using the lowest (35 µg/1) and third (45 µg/1) deciles as the cut-off points. The relation between serum selenium and the risk of death from IHD was significant in the Mantel's extension test for a linear trend (Chi 3.15, $p < 0.01$).

Serum selenium concentration of 35 µg/1 or less was associated with a 6.9-fold (95% Confidence Interval (CI), 2.4–23.6) risk of IHD death compared with persons with serum selenium of 45 µg/1 or more. The respective relative risk for serum selenium levels of 35–44 µg/1 was 2.2 (95% CI, 1.1–6.5). The respective relative risks for death from CVD were slightly lower: 6.2 and 1.5 (Fig. 2).

The association of serum selenium level, broken down into two categories, with the risk of death from IHD and CVD, was also tested separately for men and women in multivariate logistic models, which allowed for the matching, and additionally controlled for six other possible confounding variables (Salonen et al. 1982). The adjusted relative risk of death for men from IHD associated with levels of serum selenium lower than 45 µg/1 was 3.6 (95% CI, 1.4–9.2), and that of death from CVD was 2.7 (95% CI, 1.2–5.9) for men (Table 2).

The second eastern Finnish study was based on another random 6.7% population sample from the same two provinces, examined in 1977 in the same time of year as previously (Salonen et al. 1984a). The survey was conducted in an identical way, but comprised persons aged 30 to 64 years (Salonen et al. 1981). This cohort was followed for five years during which

Table 2 Relative risk (RR) of coronary and cardiovascular death and myocardial infarction associated with levels of selenium lower than 45 µg/l in men and women in eastern Finland in 1972

Based on multiple logistic models allowing for history of angina pectoris, congestive heart disease and valvular heart defect, antihypertensive drug treatment, history of MI or AP in either parent, dietary saturated fats, intake of strong alcoholic beverages, and study area (province)

(From Salonen et al. 1982)

	Men		Women	
	RR	95% CI	RR	95% CI
Coronary death	3.6	1.4–9.2	—[1]	—
Cardiovascular death	2.7	1.2–5.9	—[1]	—
Myocardial infarction	2.2	1.2–3.4	2.1	0.8–5.4

[1] Not analyzed because number of pairs insufficient

Fig. 2 Relative risk of coronary death, cardiovascular death, and myocardial infarction according to concentration of serum selenium in eastern Finland in 1972

(From Salonen et al. 1982)

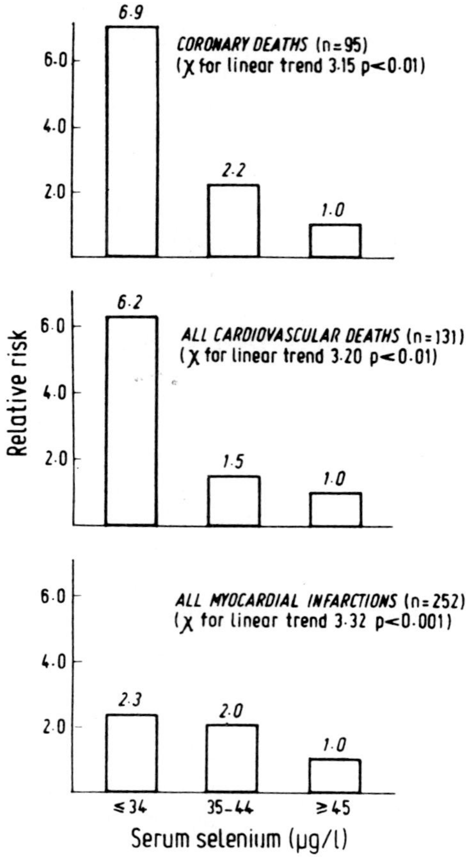

all deaths were collected. There were 92 deaths from IHD among persons with no history of myocardial infarction in the previous five years. One control was matched for each of these cases for sex, age, tobacco consumption, serum total cholesterol, mean arterial pressure, and reported history of CVD.

The mean serum selenium concentration was 62 µg/l for the cases (IHD deaths only) and 68 µg/l for the controls. The difference was not statistically significant. The respective mean for 54 cases with no chest pain on effort by Rose's interview was 60 µg/l and for similar controls 74 µg/l. This difference did not reach statistical significance due to a relatively large variation in individual serum selenium values. A serum selenium level of less than 45 µg/l was associated with a 3.2-fold (95% CI, 0.6–6.7, n.s.) risk of death from IHD in a multivariate logistic model allowing for matching as well as for polyunsaturated to saturated fatty acid ratio (P/S ratio) and serum apolipoprotein AI concentration in persons with no chest pain on effort, but only 0.9 (95% CI, 0.3–2.3) in all 92 pairs (Salonen et al. 1984a).

Serum selenium concentration correlated positively with serum esterified arachidonic acid concentration in both the cases (r = 0.19) and the controls (r = 0.63) and weakly (n.s.) with serum esterified eicosapentaenoic acid (r = 0.13 and 0.08, respectively). Selenium had a positive correlation with serum fatty acid P/S ratio in the controls (r = 0.36) but not in the cases (r = −0.11). It had almost no correlations with either serum saturated fatty acids or serum apolipoprotein AI concentration (Salonen et al. 1984a).

Miettinen and co-workers (1983) analyzed the association between serum selenium concentration and the risk of myocardial infarction and sudden death in data based on a cohort of 1,222 men who participated in a multifactorial primary IHD prevention trial in Helsinki, southern Finland (Naukkarinen 1982). The cohort consisted of men aged 40 to 55 years from the upper social class. They were free of IHD and had one or more of the following risk factors: hypertension, hypercholesterolaemia, hypertriglyceridaemia, smoking, obesity, or abnormal oral glucose tolerance (Miettinen et al. 1983). The case-control design was used to study the impact of selenium, as in the previous study in eastern Finland. During a five- to seven-year follow-up, 33 men died suddenly or experienced fatal or non-fatal myocardial infarction. For these cases, 64 controls were sampled so that the two groups were comparable for age, blood pressure, serum cholesterol and triglyceride concentrations, smoking, obesity, and glucose tolerance at the start of the follow-up (Miettinen et al. 1983).

The serum selenium concentration of the subjects ranged from 50 μg/l to 105 μg/l. Thus, there were no persons with serum selenium below 45 μg/l, which was used as the cut-off point in eastern Finnish studies. The mean serum selenium concentration was 72 μg/l in cases who had myocardial infarction, 75 μg/l in fatal cases, 71 μg/l in non-fatal cases and 73 μg/l in the controls (Miettinen et al. 1983). Serum selenium correlated somewhat with both saturated (palmitic) and polyunsaturated (arachidonic and eicosapentaenoic) fatty acids of serum cholesterol esters and phospholipids among the controls. In the cases with myocardial infarction, serum selenium correlated only with serum eicosapentaeoic acid (Miettinen et al. 1983, Table I). No results in terms of relative risks have so far been published from the study of Miettinen et al.

As a part of the Seven Countries study (Keys et al. 1980), a sample of 1,710 men from rural areas in eastern and southwestern Finland were examined to investigate the role of various factors for the risk of IHD. The 15-year re-examination of this cohort was conducted in 1974. The survivors of the original cohort were then 55–74 years of age. The serum samples from the 1974 survey were kept frozen at −20°C and the selenium concentration was determined in 1982 for 1,110 men (Virtamo et al. 1984). Of these men,

141 died from CVD, 105 from IHD, during a five-year follow-up. These were 621 men who were defined to be free of IHD in the 1974 survey. Of these men, 42 died from CVD and 30 from IHD. Twenty men with no previous stroke in 1974 died from cerebrovascular stroke during the follow-up.

The overall mean of serum selenium concentration in the 1974 serum samples was 55 µg/1. Serum selenium of 45 µg/1 or less was associated with a 1.7-fold risk of CVD death (95% CI, 1.2–2.4) and a 1.3-fold risk of IHD death (95% CI, 0.9–2.0, n.s.) among all men of the east-west cohort and 2.0-fold (95% CI, 0.9–4.2) risk of IHD death in men free of previous IHD (Virtamo et al. 1984). The relative risk for serum selenium 45 µg/1 or less of death from cerebrovascular stroke in men with no previous stroke was 3.7 (95% CI, 1.0–13.1) when adjusting for blood pressure and six other possible risk factors. Relative risks for lower serum selenium levels than 45 µg/1 have not been presented. A summary of the epidemiologic prospective studies conducted so far concerning the association of serum selenium concentration with the risk of IHD is presented in Table 3.

Interpretation of results

If one just lists the findings of the four Finnish studies on selenium and the risk of death from IHD, one study found an unequivocally inverse association (Salonen et al. 1982), in two studies the results were uncertain but indicated an inverse association among persons free of previous IHD (Salonen et al. 1984a, Virtamo et al. 1984), and in one study no association whatsoever was seen (Miettinen et al. 1983).

Table 3 Summary of epidemiologic studies on serum selenium and the risk of IHD

Study	Subjects	Relative risk of IHD death associated with S-selenium below 45 mg/l: All	Relative risk of IHD death associated with S-selenium below 45 mg/l: No history of IHD (or MI)
Salonen et al. Lancet 1982: 2, 175–9	Men and women 35–59 years	Not studied	2.9 (1.4–6.0)[a]
Miettinen et al. B.M.J. 1983: 287, 517	Men 40–55 years upper social class elevated IHD risk factors	No difference in mean S-selenium between cases and controls	
Salonen et al. Submitted, 1984	Men and women 30–64 years	0.9[a] (0.3–2.3)	3.2 (0.6–16.7)
Virtamo et al. Manuscript	Men 55–74 years rural 69% of sample drawn 15 years before baseline	1.3 (0.9–2.0)	2.0 (0.9–4.2)

[a] with no history of MI

As explained above, all four studies were based on a prospective follow-up. The cohort was examined and blood samples were taken before the follow-up. In three studies selenium determinations were done only on the serums of the persons who died or experienced an AMI during the follow-up and on a group of control persons, selected from the cohort members who remained event-free for the follow-up period. In one study serum selenium concentrations were determined for all subjects in the cohort (Virtamo et al. 1984). It seems likely that differences in the pre-follow-up characteristics of the subjects examined in each study most often explain the differences between the results of these studies.

Both eastern Finnish studies (Salonen et al. 1982, 1984a) were based on random population samples that included unselected young and middle-aged men and women (25 to 64 years). The samples came from a population with exceptionally high IHD mortality (among men), high dietary intake of saturated fats, and very high average serum cholesterol levels (7.1 mmol/l for men and 7.0 mmol/l for women in 1972 and 6.7 mmol/l for men and 6.6 mmol/l for women in 1977, Salonen et al. 1981). Thus, the limitation of these two studies is that the results might not be generalizable to other kinds of populations.

The east-west study cohort in 1974 consisted of middle-aged and old men (55–74 years), who had possibly been representative of their sampling frame in 1959 but not any more in 1974. Reportedly, 31% of the original cohort men had died in the meantime (Virtamo et al. 1984). Those who died had presumably had higher IHD risk factor levels than those who survived. This survival bias tends to weaken the associations between the observed IHD risk and risk factors, including low serum selenium. Given the absence of any association of serum cholesterol and blood pressure with the risk of IHD in the 1974 survey survivors (Virtamo et al. 1984), one could speculate that the impact of serum selenium on the IHD risk could have been greater than that of serum cholesterol and blood pressure in an unbiased sample of the same age range.

The differential correlations between serum selenium and serum fatty acid concentrations in the cases compared to the controls in the studies of both Miettinen et al. (1983) and Salonen et al. (1984a) suggest that the cases (who experienced an IHD event during the follow-up) were not perfectly free of IHD at the start of the follow-up. The association of serum selenium level with the risk of IHD was stronger among the subjects with neither a history of myocardial infarction nor chest pain on effort than those with a history of IHD in both studies (Salonen et al. 1984a, Virtamo et al. 1984), in which these groups were analyzed separately. The possible mixture of persons with and without previous IHD among the cases of Miettinen et al. could have obscured the impact of selenium.

In the studies of Miettinen et al. (1983) and Salonen et al. (1984a) in the 1977 survey cohort there does not seem to be any survival bias. In these studies in the late 1970's the mean serum selenium level is higher than in the earlier studies. This is especially true for the study among upper-class voluntary participants in the primary prevention trial from Helsinki, whose mean serum selenium concentration was 73 μg/l (Miettinen et al. 1983). The mean serum selenium in the 1977 study in eastern Finland was 65 μg/l (Salonen et al. 1984a), compared with 54 μg/l in the 1972 study (Salonen et al. 1982) and 55 μg/l in the 1974 east-west cohort (Virtamo et al. 1984). On the basis of these findings, there has been an increase in the general serum selenium level during the second half of the 1970's in Finland. This is consistent with the increase in the estimated dietary intake of selenium resulting from a rise in the proportion of imported wheat grains during the late 1970's (Varo & Koivistoinen 1980, Mutanen & Koivistoinen 1983).

If a threshold value exists in the relationship of selenium intake with the risk of IHD as suggested by the 1972 eastern Finnish study (Salonen et al. 1982), no association could possibly be observed at higher selenium levels. Then, the high average serum selenium levels would explain the lack of association in the study by Miettinen et al. (1983). The threshold assumption receives some support by the experimental observations, which show that selenium supplementation increases the activity of glutathione peroxidase in platelets in selenium-deficient rats (Levander et al. 1983a) and humans (Levander et al. 1983b) and this increase levels off when a plasma selenium level of about 100–135 μg/l is achieved (Thomson et al. 1977, Levander et al. 1983b). If this finding holds in different populations, increased platelet aggregability possibly produced by depressed glutathione peroxidase activity is likely to manifest only at low serum selenium levels resulting from dietary selenium deficiency.

An almost linear inverse relationship was seen in cross-area comparisons between blood-bank blood concentration of selenium and CVD mortality over a wide range of selenium levels: 120 μg/l to 235 μg/l in whole blood, corresponding to 90–80 μg/l in serum (Shamberger et al. 1979). Within-population epidemiologic studies have, however, observed an inverse association only at very low serum selenium levels, although different ranges have been tested in different studies. Thus, the apparent association in cross-area studies at higher selenium levels might have been biased by cross-area covariation of other nutrients or risk factors with selenium. It must be noted, though, that all individual-based studies have so far been conducted in Finland, where the population generally has a low intake of polyunsaturated and a high intake of saturated fatty acids and a low intake of vitamin C, another antioxidant (Vartiainen et al. 1983). These and other dietary factors may modify the selenium–IHD relationship.

Setting the peculiarities of the study subjects aside, the studies of Miettinen et al. (1983) and Virtamo et al. (1984) suffer from an insufficient number of IHD events and consequently a low power to detect any associations of IHD risk with risk factors. For example, the *a priori* power of the study of Virtamo et al. (1984) to detect a relative risk of 2.0 for IHD death among men free of previous IHD, significant at alpha-level of 0.05, is only 45%.

In non-experimental epidemiologic studies, there is always the possibility that the observed association is biased due to covariation of the exposure and disease with some uncontrolled or unmeasured factors. For example, a selenium-poor diet usually lacks fish and mushrooms. Thus, a low serum selenium concentration might also be a marker for a generally unhealthy diet. Other nutrients that interact with selenium in food might additionally contribute to the excess risk related to selenium deficiency. A summary of the frequently observed correlations between selected nutrients is shown in Table 4.

Miettinen et al. (1983) have proposed that the association between a low serum selenium concentration and an excessive risk of IHD death would be a spurious one, introduced by the covariation of selenium and polyunsaturated fatty acids in foodstuffs and the resulting intercorrelations in serum levels. If this were the case, the association of serum selenium with the risk of IHD death should weaken or disappear when polyunsaturated fatty acid variables are added in a multivariate model including also selenium as an explanatory variable. However, in spite of the correlation of serum selenium with both serum arachidonic acid content ($r = 0.63$) and P/S ratio ($r = 0.36$) in the control persons of Salonen et al. (1984a), the partial impact of selenium did not decrease in the data set of the 1977 eastern Finnish study, in which the serum fatty acids were measured from the same serum samples as selenium (Salonen et al. 1984a).

An association observed in epidemiologic studies is considered causal if it is strong, graded, has the right temporal sequence, is consistent between studies, independent of other associations, is able to predict findings in other data sets and populations, and is coherent with findings from other research methods so that reasonable pathogenetic mechanisms are known (Smoking & Health 1964). Clearly, on the basis of these criteria, no causal relationship between dietary selenium intake or tissue selenium concentra-

Table 4 Frequently observed within-population intercorrelations of selected nutrients.

	SAT	P,n-3	P,n-6	Se	ANT	K,Mg	Na	ALC	Fiber
Energy	++			+	+	+	+	+	+
Saturated FA					++		+	+	
Poly FA n-3					++	++			+
Poly FA n-6				++	+	+			
Selenium									
Antioxidative vitamins									++
Potassium, magnesium									
Sodium								+	
Alcohol									

tion and the risk of IHD has been established. The four Finnish studies completed so far do, however, lend support to the assumption of an inverse association between serum selenium concentration and the risk of IHD in conditions of low selenium intake (reflected as a mean serum selenium of less than 60 μg/l or blood selenium of less than 90 μg/l) and low ratio of polyunsaturated to saturated fatty acids in diet.

SELENIUM AND THE RISK OF CANCER

As for cardiovascular diseases, the first observations on a possible inverse association between selenium intake and the risk of cancer came from ecological comparisons (Shamberger et al. 1971, 1976, Shamberger 1981, Schrauzer et al. 1977a, 1977b, Jansson 1981). At present, three individual-based prospective studies have confirmed this relationship (Willet et al. 1983, Salonen et al. 1984b, 1984c). One of these studies was based on the data set of the Hypertension Detection and Follow-up Program (HDFP) in 14 areas in the United States (Willet et al. 1983). In the HDFP cohort, the risk of cancer was 2.0-fold in the lowest serum selenium quintile (below 115 μg/l) compared with the highest quintile. In these data, selenium remained significantly associated with cancer risk when the effects of serum retinol, vitamin E, and lipid levels as well as age, sex, and race were taken into account in a multivariate logistic model (Willet et al. 1983). The relative risk of cancer for the lowest selenium tertile increased to 6.2 in comparison with the highest selenium tertile in the subgroup of the lowest tertiles of serum vitamin A and E concentrations.

Two other epidemiologic studies on selenium and cancer are based on the same survey cohorts in two eastern provinces of Finland, examined in 1972 and 1977 as those on cardiovascular disease. In the earlier study (Salonen et al. 1984b), deaths and hospital admission due to cancer were followed during a seven-year period. Only deaths in the last five years and hospitalization in the last six years were accepted for the analysis. Out of persons aged 31 to 59 years who reported no previous cancer in the 12 months preceding the baseline survey in 1972, there were 43 deaths from cancer and 85 other persons were admitted to hospital because of cancer. For each of these 128 cases, a control was matched for sex, age, consumption of tobacco products, and serum total cholesterol.

The mean concentration of serum selenium was 51 μg/l for all cases and 54 μg/l for all controls ($p < 0.05$ for difference). The means for cases who developed cancer in the last four follow-up years and their controls were 50 μg/l and 54 μg/l, respectively ($p < 0.05$) and for cases who died of cancer and their controls 48 μg/l and 55μg/l, respectively ($p < 0.05$) (Salonen et al. 1984b). When broken down from the approximate lowest and third decile, the overall relationship between serum selenium and the risk of cancer was statistically significant (Mantel's extension Chi 2.89, $p < 0.01$). In the multiple logistic model allowing for matching and additionally for consumption of tobacco, beer, dietary saturated fats, years of education, and province, serum selenium of less than 45 μg/l was associated with an adjusted relative risk of cancer of 3.1 (95% CI, 1.5–7.7) in all pairs and 3.6 (95% CI, 1.4–9.1) in pairs for which the cancer manifasted three or more years after the collection of serum samples (Salonen et al. 1984b).

In the study of the 1977 survey cohort in eastern Finland, 51 persons with serum samples taken in 1977 died of cancer during a four-year follow-up (Salonen et al. 1984c). One control was matched for each case for sex, age and tobacco consumption at the 1977 survey. The mean serum selenium concentration among the cases was 54 μg/l and among the controls 61 μg/l ($p < 0.05$ for difference). The respective means for persons who died after the first follow-up year and their controls were 54 μg/l and 61 μg/l ($p < 0.05$). In these data, the case-control difference in selenium was seen only in men but not in women and among men the difference was much greater in smokers than non-smokers (49 μg/l vs. 64 μg/l, $p < 0.05$ for smoking men, 50 μg/l vs. 58 μg/l, n.s. for non-smoking men). All women were non-smokers in these data. Serum selenium concentration had a significant partial inverse association with the risk of death from cancer also in a multivariate logistic model allowing for matching and serum retinol, vitamin E, and total cholesterol concentrations, years of smoking and number of drugs for chronic diseases. Selenium also had a strong positive interaction with serum vitamin E concentration, indicating a synergism of low serum levels (Salonen et al. 1984c).

In the 1972 cohort, the case-control difference in serum selenium was greatest for gastrointestinal, respiratory, hematologic and miscellaneous cancers and not seen for either skin, skeletal or urogenital cancers. In the 1977 data dealing only with cancer deaths, there was a difference for all of the three categories analyzed: gastrointestinal, respiratory, and other, and the difference was slightly greater for respiratory than for other cancers.

All three epidemiologic studies on the association of serum selenium concentration with the risk of cancer have consistently found an inverse relationship, which is seen over a wider range of selenium levels than for CVD. This finding is also in agreement with cross-population comparisons and animal experiments (Schrauzer et al. 1977a, 1977b, Ip & Sinha 1981, Welsch et al. 1981, Birt et al. 1982). It is still unclear whether the relationship exists in women, and which and how other nutrients and risk factors modify the association.

CONCLUSION

Epidemiologic studies in the 1980's have provided consistent evidence of an association between low serum selenium resulting from dietary selenium deficiency and the risk of cancer whereas the evidence of the relationship of dietary selenium with the risk of ischaemic heart disease is still inconclusive although indicative of an inverse relationship in certain conditions. New epidemiologic studies on the role of selenium in IHD are still needed to confirm or negate the previous findings. These should consider confounding and effect modification by other nutrients, especially fatty acids and other antioxidants, and other risk factors. The mechanisms through which selenium deficiency could increase the risk of IHD need to be established in experiments in animals and humans.

REFERENCES

ALFTHAN, G. & KUMPULAINEN, J. (1982). Determination of selenium in small volumes of blood plasma and serum by graphite furnace atomic absorption spectrometry. *Anal. Chim. Acta*. 140, 221–227.

BIRT, D. F., LAWSON, T. A., JULIUS, A. D., RUNICE, C. E. & SALMASI, S. (1982). Inhibition by dietary selenium of colon cancer induced in the rat by bis(2-oxopropyl)-nitrosamine. *Cancer Res*. 42, 4455–4459.

BOSTROM, H. J. & WESTER, P. O. (1967). Trace elements in drinking water and death rates of cardiovascular disease. *Acta med. scand*. 181, 465.

Editorial (1983). Selenium perspective. *The Lancet 1,* 685.

FROST, D. V. (1972). The two faces of selenium—can selenophobia be cured. *C.R.C. Crit. Rev. Toxicol*. 1, 467.

GRIFFIN, A. C. (1979). Role of selenium in the chemoprevention of cancer. *Adv. Cancer Res*. 29, 419–442.

HOEKSTRA, W. G. (1974). Biochemical role of selenium. In *Trace Element Metabolism in Animals,* 2, 61. Ed. by W. G. Hoekstra, J. W. Suttie, H. G. Ganther and W. Mentz. University Park Press, Baltimore.

— (1975). Biochemical function of selenium and its relation to vitamin E. *Fed. Proc*. 34, 2083–2089.

IP, C. & SINHA, D. K. (1981). Anticarcinogenic effect of selenium in rats treated with dimethylbenz (alpha)anthracene and fed different levels and types of fat. *Carcinogenesis* 2, 435–438.

JANSSON, B. (1981). Seneca County, New York: an area with low cancer mortality rates. *Cancer* 48, 2542–2546.

KARPPANEN, H. (1982). Mita seleenista ja kromista tiedetaan (What is known of selenium and chromium, in Finnish). *Suom. Lääk.-L*. 35, 3183–3187.

KEYS, A. (Ed.) (1980). *Seven Countries. A Multivariate Analysis of Death and Coronary Heart Disease*. Harvard University Press, Cambridge, Massachusetts and London.

KOIVISTOINEN, P. (Ed.) (1980). Mineral element composition of Finnish foods. I–XII. *Acta agr. scand*. Suppl. 22, 1–171.

KOLJONEN, T. (1975). The behavior of selenium in Finnish soils. *Ann. Agri. Fenn*. 14, 240–247.

KUMPULAINEN, J. & KOIVISTOINEN, P. (1981). Inter-laboratory comparison of selenium levels in human serum. *Kemia-Kemi* 8, 372–373.

LEVANDER, O. A., ALFTHAN, G., ARVILOMMI, H., GREF, C. G., HUTTUNEN, J. K., KATAJA, M., KOIVISTOINEN, P. & PIKKARAINEN, J. (1983b). Bioavailability of selenium to Finnish men as assessed by platelet glutathione peroxidase activity and other blood parameters. *Amer. J. clin. Nutr*. 37, 887–897.

LEVANDER, O. A., DELOACH, D. P., MORRIS, V. C. & MOSER, P. B. (1983a). Platelet glutathione peroxidase activity as an index of selenium status in rats. *J. Nutr.* 113, 55–63.

MASUKAWA, T., GOTO, J. & IWATA, H. (1983). Impaired metabolism of arrachidonate in selenium-deficient animals. *Experimentia* 39, 405–406.

MENTER, D. G., ONODA, J. M., TAYLOR, J. D. & HONN, K. V. (1984). Effects of prostacyclin on tumor cell-induced platelet aggregation. *Cancer Res.* 44, 450–456.

MIETTINEN, T. A., ALFTHAN, G., HUTTUNEN, J. K., PIKKARAINEN, J., NAUKKARINEN, V., MATTILA, S. & KUMLIN, T. (1983). Serum selenium concentration related to myocardial infarction and fatty acid content of serum lipids. *Brit. med. J.* 287, 517–519.

MILLS, G. C. (1960). Glutathione peroxidase and the destruction of hydrogen peroxide in animal tissues. *Arch. Biochem. Biophys.* 86, 1–5.

MUTANEN, M. & KOIVISTOINEN, P. (1983). The role of imported grain on the selenium intake of Finnish population 1941–1981. *Int. J. Vit. Nutr. Res.* 53, 34–38.

NAUKKARINEN, V. (1982). *The Feasibility of Administering Preventive Treatment for Coronary Heart Disease to Middle-Aged Men.* University of Helsinki, Helsinki, Finland.

SALMON, J. A., SMITH, D. R., FLOWER, R. J., MONCADA, S. & VANE, J. R. (1978). Further studies on the ensymatic conversion of prostaglandin andoperoxide into prostacyclin by porcine aorta microsomes. *Biochim. biophys. Acta.* 523, 250–262.

SALONEN, J. T., ALFTHAN, G., HUTTUNEN, J. K., PIKKARAINEN, J. & PUSKA, P. (1982). Association between cardiovascular death and myocardial infarction and serum selenium in a matched-pair longitudinal study. *The Lancet* 2, 175–179.

SALONEN, J. T., ALFTHAN, G., HUTTUNEN, J. K. & PUSKA, P. (1984b). Association between serum selenium and the risk of cancer. *Amer. J. Epidemiol.* 120, 342–349.

SALONEN, J. T., PUSKA, P., KOTTKE, T. E. & TUOMILEHTO, J. (1981). Changes in smoking, serum cholesterol and blood pressure levels during a community-based cardiovascular disease prevention program—the North Karelia Project. *Amer. J. Epidemiol.* 114, 81–93.

SALONEN, J. T., SALONEN, R., LAPPETELÄINEN, R., MÄENPÄÄ, P., ALFTHAN, G. & PUSKA, P. (1984c). Risk of cancer in relation to serum concentrations of selenium and vitamins A and E: Matched case-control analysis of prospective data. *Brit. med. J.* 290, 417–420.

SALONEN, J. T., SALONEN, R., PENTTILÄ, I., HERRANEN, J., JAUHIAINEN, J., KANTOLA, M., KAURANEN, P., LAPPETELÄINEN, R., MÄENPÄÄ, P. & PUSKA, P. (1984a). Serum fatty acids, apolipoproteins, selenium and vitamin antioxidants and the risk of death from ischaemic heart disease. Submitted for publication.

SCHOENE, N. W., MORRIS, V. C. & LEVANDER O. A. (1984). Effects of selenium deficiency on aggregation and thromboxane formation in rat platelets. *Fed. Proc.* 43, 477.

SCHRAUZER, G. N., WHITE, D. A. & SCHNEIDER, C. J. (1977a). Cancer mortality correlation studies. III. Statistical associations with dietary selenium intakes. *Bioinorg. Chem.* 7, 23–34.

— (1977b). Cancer mortality correlation studies. IV. Associations with dietary intakes and blood levels of certain trace elements, notably se-antagonists. *Bioinorg. Chem.* 7, 35–56.

SHAMBERGER, R. J. (1981). Selenium in health and disease. *Proceedings of a Nordic Symposium on Mineral Elements 80.* Helsinki, 501–509.

SHAMBERGER, R. J., GUNSCH, M. S., WILLIS, C. E. & MCCORMACK, L. J. (1978). Selenium and heart disease. II. Selenium and other trace metal intakes and heart disease in 25 countries. In *Trace Substances in Environmental Health — XII*, pp. 48–52. Ed. by D. D. Hemphill. University of Missouri, Columbia.

SHAMBERGER, R. J., TYTKO, S. A. & WILLIS, C. E. (1975). Selenium and heart disease. In *Trace Substances in Environmental Health — IX*, pp.15–22. Ed. by D. D. Hemphill. University of Missouri, Columbia.

— (1976). Antioxidants and cancer. VI. Selenium and adjusted human cancer mortality. *Arch. environm. Hlth* 31, 231–235.

SHAMBERGER, R. & WILLIS, C. (1971). Selenium distribution and human cancer mortality. *Clin. Lab. Sci.* 2, 211–221.

SHAMBERGER, R. J., WILLIS, C. E. & MCCORMACK, L. J. (1979). Selenium and heart disease. III. Blood selenium and heart mortality in 19 states. In *Trace Substances in Environmental Health — XIII*, pp. 59–63. Ed. by D. D. Hemphill. University of Missouri, Columbia.

Smoking and Health (1964). Report of the Advisory Committee to the Surgeon General of the Public Health Service, U.S. Department of Health, Education and Welfare. Public Health Service Publication No. 1103, United States Government Printing Office, Washington, D.C.

THOMSON, C. D., REA, H. M., DOESBURG, U. M. & ROBINSON, M. F. (1977). Selenium concentrations and glutathione peroxidase activities in whole blood of New Zealand residents. *Brit. J. Nutr.* 37, 457–460.

VARO, P. & KOIVISTOINEN, P. (1981). Annual variations in the average selenium intake in Finland: Cereal products and milk as sources of selenium in 1979/80. *Int. J. Vit. Nutr. Res.* 51, 62–65.

VARO, P., NUURTAMO, M., SAARI, E. & KOIVISTOINEN, P. (1980). Mineral element composition of Finnish foods. III. Annual variations in the mineral element composition of cereal grains. *Acta agr. scand.* Suppl. 22, 27–35.

VARTIAINEN, E., PUSKA, P., HUTTUNEN, J. K., KARPPANEN, H. & GEY, F. (1983). Vitamiinit ja sepelvaltimotauti. (Vitamins and coronary heart disease, in Finnish.) *Suom. Lääk.-L.* 38, 3146–3150.

VIRTAMO, J., VAKELA, E., ALFTHAN, G., PUNSAR, S., HUTTUNEN, J. K. & KARVONEN, M. (1984). Serum selenium and the risk of coronary heart disease and stroke in elderly Finnish men. Submitted for publication.

WELSCH, C. W., GOODRICH-SMITH, M., BROWN, C. K., GREENE, H. D. & HAMEL, E. J. (1981). Selenium and the genesis of murine mammary tumors. *Carcinogenesis 2*, 519–522.

WESTERMARCK, T., RAUNU, P., KIRJARINTA, M. & LAPPALAINEN, L. (1977). Selenium content of whole blood and serum in adults and children of different ages from different parts of Finland. *Acta pharmacol. toxicol.* 40, 465–475.

WHITTLE, B. JR. & MONCADA, S. (1983). Pharmacological interactions between prostacyclin and thromboxanes. *Brit. med. Bull.* 39, 232–238.

WILLET, W. C., POLK, F., MORRIS, J. S., STAMPFLER, M. J., PRESSER, S., ROSNER, B., TAYLOR, J. O., SCHNEIDER, K. & HAMES, C. G. (1983). Prediagnostic serum selenium and risk of cancer. *The Lancet* 2, 130.

Discussion (the papers by Shamberger and Salonen)

Chairman: WESTER

WESTER: Before opening this presentation for discussion I should like myself to give you some very recent data which we have from smelter workers in the northern part of Sweden. These data are not published yet, but I think they fit in very well with what we have been talking about. We have studied about 25 trace elements from deceased smelter workers in liver, kidney and lung tissue. A lot of these toxic and carcinogenic elements were highly accumulated in the lungs. There is a very high frequency of lung cancer in smelter workers in the Rönnskär smelter. Eight per cent of the deaths are from lung cancer in a very big study which has just been done. In the material we have now, out of 76 deceased smelter workers seven died from lung cancer, which fits in very well with the figure of 8% in the big study.

In Table 1 at the lower end there are the controls called 3A and 3B. There are 15 control cases from a rural area and 10 control cases from an urban area. Groups 1A, 1B and 1C are smelter workers deceased from different forms of cancer; groups 2A, 2B and 2C are workers deceased from cardiovascular disease (50%), cerebrovascular disease (about 15%) and from other causes. We can see that antimony is about 10 times enriched in the lung tissues of smelter workers. Arsenic, cadmium, chromium, cobalt and lanthanum are also enriched. The levels are very high both if the workers had died from cancer and from cardiovascular disease.

If we now look at selenium, we can see that the selenium value is the lowest in those who have died from lung cancer, which differs from all groups, even from the controls. If we then make a quotient between the different toxic elements and selenium, we will see that in group 1A, the lung cancer cases, they always have the highest quotient (Table 2). I think that these data also fit in with the assumption that selenium may be protective in cancer.

Table 1 Median values of selenium, antimony, arsenic, cadmium, chromium, cobalt, lanthanum, lead and zinc in lung tissue in smelter workers (groups 1 A–2 B) and controls (groups 3 A–3 B)

nd = not detected. Zinc in ppm (μg/g wet weight) all the others in ppb (μg/kg wet weight)

Group	Element								
	Se	Sb	As	Cd	Cr	Co	La	Pb	Zn
1 A	71	450	40	390	330	15	6.5	320	13.6
1 B	123	376	51	76	470	23	8.4	140	9.6
1 C	175	480	49	63	650	21	12.8	197	11.0
2 A	159	181	34	246	400	16	11.0	141	12.4
2 B	142	355	40	114	455	16	8.4	151	12.3
2 C	215	100	29	108	400	15	6.2	130	10.3
All workers	151	280	38	162	410	16	10.1	140	12.1
3 A	110	32	7	39	110	7	5.0	55	9.6
3 B	136	19	5	79	199	11	10.0	39	nd

Table 2 Median values of the quotients in lung tissue in smelter workers (groups 1 A–2 C) and controls (groups 3 A–3 B)

na = not analysed

Group	Quotient							
	Sb/Se	As/Se	Cd/Se	Cr/Se	Co/Se	La/Se	Pb/Se	Zn/Se
1 A	4.53	0.87	2.28	5.15	0.21	0.21	8.09	100
1 B	3.27	0.38	1.10	4.09	0.20	0.07	0.76	80
1 C	2.43	0.26	0.79	3.20	0.09	0.07	0.51	70
2 A	1.06	0.19	0.81	1.66	0.10	0.06	1.40	80
2 B	1.92	0.25	0.83	4.82	0.11	0.04	0.85	90
2 C	0.47	0.12	0.56	1.86	0.08	0.03	0.61	60
All workers	1.59	0.23	0.83	2.41	0.10	0.07	1.30	80
3 A	0.29	0.05	0.58	0.88	0.05	0.05	0.34	100
3 B	0.20	0.04	0.25	1.65	0.09	0.08	0.70	na

HURLEY: The speakers have both shown us some very impressive data which suggest that low selenium levels in the blood of people make them much more susceptible to cancer. This, I'm sure, is a question occurring to many of the members of this audience: Do you have any explanation for the apparent lack of high incidence of cancer in New Zealand?

SALONEN: I don't have the answer, but I make a suggestion. As estimated in several studies of all cancers, smoking contributes to more than half. Smoking rates in New Zealand are much lower than, for instance, in Finland or the United States. Secondly, I don't know but I suspect that other nutritional factors, especially antioxidants, haven't been taken into account when the lack of association from New Zealand has been mentioned. These might be at least partial explanations for that phenomenon.

HURLEY: In either your studies or Dr Shamberger's, were they controlled for smoking?

SALONEN: In all epidemiological studies about cancer, smoking needs always to be controlled for, because it is the most important risk factor for cancer. It would be nonsense to study cancer without a control for smoking. In cross-area comparisons, that is sometimes difficult but, of course, the mean smoking rates can be used there. But in all these three individual-based studies, smoking was controlled for in either matching or multivariate analysis.

HURLEY: Then I don't understand what you're saying about New Zealand. If the people in your study didn't smoke and they don't smoke in New Zealand, then what is the difference? Maybe I'm misunderstanding you.

SALONEN: "Controlling for" is a statistical term. Please excuse me. Prevalence of smoking is low in New Zealand. That might be protective of cancer in spite of the fact that the intake of selenium is probably the lowest in the world.

HURLEY: You're suggesting that there may be an interaction there?

SALONEN: Yes, as shown in all the studies and, as I pointed out, the association of selenium with the risk of cancer was stronger among smokers than among non-smokers.

SHAMBERGER: I think the question Dr Hurley is trying to get at is a question we don't know the answer to. But, we do have some ideas in that regard. The cancer and the heart disease rate in New Zealand is about the same as in the United States, yet one would expect them to be about three times as much. For 40–60 other countries the correlation works out pretty well. Something is happening in New Zealand we really don't understand. Now, there is a possibility that it could be due to the lack of pollution and, possibly, the lesser smoking. I cannot prove this, but I think that probably, at some point, selenium-independent glutathione peroxidase takes over and protects against carcinogenic damage. As soon as I'm able to, I'm going to try and get some blood from New Zealand and measure selenium-independent glutathione peroxidase.

SÖDERHJELM: I would like to comment on your findings in the smelters in Rönnskär, which is the biggest producer of selenium in Europe. I would think that the workers there might be protected instead of being damaged by the exposure to selenium every day. They have quite a lot of selenium there. I expect the lung cancer would have a higher content of selenium. Didn't they work there at the same place or how can you explain the low figure for lung cancer?

WESTER: If you compare with the controls, workers in general at the smeltery had in fact higher selenium values. Selenium was low just in the group that developed lung cancer and they had also been exposed to selenium as much as the others. So I don't know why the lung cancer patients had low selenium in their lung tissue.

SALONEN: I want to comment on the question that was made about your data on the case control study. I think, as Dr Shamberger also pointed out, that it's very dangerous to draw any causal conclusions about case control studies concerning cancer. Especially here I would suggest that it may be the course of disease that affects either the intake of selenium, or selenium metabolism or both. So, in this case, as it was specific for lung cancer, it might be cachexia or something associated with cancer that produced the selenium levels.

JOHANSSON: I have a question for Dr Shamberger. I think it's important to stress the chemical form of selenium. You mentioned that in your studies you have used sodium selenide and sodium selenite and I would like to hear which chemical form you consider most suitable in cancer prevention.

Secondly, you mentioned skin cancer in which selenium was protecting through glutathione peroxidase. In clinical studies you used croton oil and sodium selenide. Do you think that glutathione peroxidase is the only protecting agent in cancer prevention?

SHAMBERGER: First of all in regard to your first question, my initial experiment was done with sodium selenide. I found that sodium selenide was not unusually stable. So I switched to sodium selenite which I highly recommend. In fact, most of the cancer investigators subsequently did use sodium selenite, as it seems to be very effective. But, because of this I cannot extrapolate to sodium selenate, because I don't know of experiments with sodium selenate. I suspect you would need to use a lot more, because it's obviously not as effective, although it is less toxic.

Certainly other antioxidants besides selenium prevent cancer. Of the type we saw in animals, BHA and BHT dramatically will affect carcinogenesis in animals. Vitamin C and vitamin E in large amounts will also prevent some tumors in animals. So sodium selenite, working through glutathione peroxidase, is certainly not the only antioxidation reaction that prevents cancer.

CHRISTOPHERSEN: I think we should discuss the public health implications for all these epidemiological findings. I myself some years ago calculated various selenium intakes in Norway and it is clear that the Norwegian intake is much higher than in northern Finland and in Sweden because of higher average fish consumption and also because of higher consumption of cereals of North American origin. In the last year these differences have even increased. If we take blood analyses, there are two studies, one by Aaseth and collaborators and one more recent, about 1980, and if we compare blood analyses from Norway with the blood bank samples used by Schrauzer and Shamberger in their epidemiological studies, we find the situation in Norway about 1980 comparable to the highest selenium states in the United States. Still the situation in Norway is much better than it is in Sweden. In most of western and northern Europe the situation may either be compared to the most selenium-deficient areas in the United States or it is much worse.

I'd like to ask a question of Dr Bruce. When we have these data, if you just extrapolate from American studies, we can reduce the risk of cancer by increasing the selenium intake to the level of the highest selenium states in the United States. And we can probably also reduce the cardiovascular mortality. As far as I know there are no studies indicating any negative effects, if we do these in close intervals. Why isn't this considered in countries like Sweden and Finland, where the situation is definitely worse than in Norway?

BRUCE: Many of these findings have been reported during the last years and they have to be confirmed. For example, we have learned about the Finnish findings at very low serum selenium levels. There is a study going on just now, where serum samples are sent to Århus from various European countries. They will be analysed by Thorling in order to find out if there are any major variations in serum selenium levels between different European countries and, thus, form the basis for future epidemiologic studies.

AGGETT: I've just got a point of discussion along with one or two comments which I'd like to address to both of the speakers. The thing that we have of interest in Scotland is both a high incidence of ischaemic heart disease and of colorectal cancer. We are particularly impressed, of course, by the cutoff point which Dr Salonen suggests, because this, in fact, is very near the mean which we would calculate for the serum selenium of children in the northeast of Scotland. Obviously, this does have public health implications. What I was wondering was if Dr Salonen would like to comment on the data from Willet et al., who, I think, really pooled all their data for the incidence of cancer, whereas, in fact, their incidence of correlation with low seleniums for breast cancer was rather poor in contrast to the experimental evidence with mice. But, it was particularly high in relation to gastrointestinal cancer, or more precisely that of the large bowel. In this context I was under the impression, in fact, that New Zealand enjoyed the second or third highest incidence of large-bowel cancer, second only to Scotland and I think one area of Scandinavia, whereas Finland is about 9th in that league table. Therefore, in terms of possible carcinogenic factors I was wondering, if I could induce either Dr Shamberger or Dr Salonen to comment on the work that Wendel has been doing in Tubingen, showing that microsomal mixed function oxidase systems are defective before discernible changes in glutathione peroxidase activities in selenium-deficient animals, and the possible effects this type of defect may have on the metabolism of potentially carcinogenic xenobiotics.

SHAMBERGER: I would like to comment on the mixed function oxidase point. I wasn't totally aware of Wendel's work; however, the mixed function oxidase theory is an important cancer theory. Enzymes like benzpyrene hydroxylase or mixed function hydroxylases will change a carcinogen into non-toxic form and the animal will excrete it much better. So this is one of perhaps six to ten possible mechanisms of the way selenium might inhibit cancer. I know of a couple of experiments where one was positive and one was negative, but I was not aware of Wendel's work. But it is an important cancer theory and selenium might be working in this way.

SALONEN: I can take up the first part of the question. It was very interesting to hear that the serum level of selenium in Scottish children is so awfully low. I have to point out that the cutoff points that I've shown and that are in our publications, 35 and 45 μg/l, are very arbitrary. They are taken from the distribution of serum selenium in those specific study data. It is customary to use fractiles of the distribution to enable a statistical estimation and test of these relative risks that were calculated. Secondly, I think that the levels of other antioxidants and also exposures or carcinogens between countries vary and that the level of selenium below which there is an elevated risk of cancer, probably is different for different populations. For Finland, the only thing we know is that the intake of vitamin C, ascorbic acid, is extremely low, especially for men. That might be an aggravating factor. You know that rates of smoking are high, again especially for men. That's another factor since there seems to be a synergism between smoking and lack of selenium. We showed that there is a synergism between the lack of tocopherol and lack of selenium concerning the relationship of cancer. All these factors modify the association between selenium concentration in serum and the risk of cancer so that the cutoff points from one data set cannot be applied to any other population.

ANDERSON: I have a question regarding the dietary intake of selenium. It can either be to both of you or primarily to Dr Shamberger. In all of the studies that I am aware of, and we've just discussed this, dietary intake of selenium in the U.S. appears to meet or exceed the suggested safe and adequate intake. Therefore, when you make comparisons between a low-selenium area and a high-selenium area, for example South Dakota, since the food we eat isn't necessarily the food grown in our backyard, unless the selenium comes from the water, I don't see how these differences should affect the incidence of cancer.

SHAMBERGER: This is an interesting point. In the United States food is distributed rather well but, for whatever reason, selenium in the blood is higher in the high-selenium areas, especially North and South Dakota and Wyoming. In addition, there has been still another study by Shearer who studied the breast milk of women from these areas and found the breast milk selenium to be considerably higher in the high-selenium areas than in the so-called low-selenium areas.

ANDERSON: What is the overall difference in dietary intake from a high-selenium area to a low-selenium area?

SHAMBERGER: I would rather go on blood levels, because we don't really know exactly what the dietary intake is. In the United States it's probably somewhere around 100 μg a day on the average. I would think in the high-selenium areas it's perhaps 130 or 140, in the low-selenium areas maybe around 80 μg. But in this particular study we compared the population with about 250 μg of selenium per liter of blood to a population with 150 μg per litre. The study of Willet compared 150 approximately to 100 and, in Dr Salonen's study, a low of 45 to a high of 80. Effects were seen in all three studies. I really can't tell you exactly what is the maximum or best amount to have in the blood or as intake, but I do know in Japan they take in about 180 μg per day and they have low incidences of both colon and breast cancer which seem to be affected by selenium. Their heart rate is considerably lower than in the United States. Of course there certainly could be other factors involved there.

SALONEN: I have just a short remark on the example of Japan. There are extreme differences in diet and also in other respects, such as the intake of saturated fats which is extremely low as are smoking rates. I'd like to make a small methodological point and suggest that all the cross-area comparisons of disease rates and exposure levels are potentially confounded. Theoretical work concerning this "ecological fallacy" has been done for years. In the case of selenium and the risk of disease, if there is a threshold so that above a certain level there wouldn't be any association, such an association can still be seen in cross-area comparisons if there are differences in population means in certain directions. This phenomenon can introduce a completely biased association. This is especially true for ischaemic heart disease. For example, in the study by Virtamo and others actually the mean selenium level in serum was found to be higher in the east of Finland, with higher rates of ischaemic heart disease than in the southwest of Finland, in spite of the fact that, within the areas, there was an inverse relationship.

BRUCE: Breast cancer and colon cancer were mentioned. At another conference we have just discussed breast cancer and colon cancer. Breast cancer was related to the fat intake and colon cancer to dietary fibre. I think that for breast cancer epidemiology the relations to the fat intake and to the selenium intake are very similar. Perhaps there is some possibility to join these two. That is one question.

SHAMBERGER: Mutants and carcinogens are certainly in our diet. We take in an unusually large amount of chemicals that can cause mutations. In fact, I suspect we could take in 30 or 40 different kinds of chemicals that cause mutations. If we can extrapolate from our bacterial experiments to these human mutants, selenium probably blocks some of them but I don't know how many. The carcinogens also can react with DNA and cause mutants, and selenium does block that reaction. So in general I suspect selenium is blocking carcinogenic reactions of DNA and some of the mutant reactions with DNA, but specifically I couldn't tell you which ones it is blocking.

SALONEN: I think breast cancer is a good example where the cross-area comparison would give wrong or biased results, because we know that selenium intake correlates well with the fatty acid ratio and intakes of other antioxidants. Thus, the cross-national correlation between breast cancer mortality and selenium intake doesn't necessarily tell the truth.

Cardiovascular Disease: The Effect of Hard and Soft Water

By H. Mitchell Perry, Jr. and Elizabeth F. Perry

INTRODUCTION

In 1960, a report by Schroeder relating cardiovascular mortality to hardness of drinking water received a great deal of attention. Since then the topic has been the subject of extensive investigation. With few exceptions, the approximately 25 studies dealing with large geographic areas, i.e. whole countries, support a negative correlation between cardiovascular mortality and water hardness; however, despite intensive investigation, the mechanism of the "hard water–soft arteries" effect, or more simply the "hard water effect", remains obscure. Thus, the correlation is apparently real, but many questions have to be answered before the specific relationship is established, perhaps first: what are the critical characteristics of drinking water that evoke the effect and what specific types of cardiovascular death are involved? Since an understanding of this effect might provide a major lead to the pathogenesis of cardiovascular disease, the subject warrants enthusiastic investigation, including any new and different approaches that are available.

Because this relationship has been very adequately reviewed from several points of view (1–7), I shall use my limited time to outline what seem to be the salient facts, and then progress to several topics which are rarely considered in depth and which might provide new insight: (1) Could the "excess deaths" in the Multiple Risk Factor Intervention Trial be a manifestation of the "hard water effect"? (2) What is the likelihood that cadmium, lead, or some other trace substance is responsible for the effect? (3) Could chronic metal-binding by the antihypertensive drug hydralazine leading to remission of hypertension be a related process?

DESCRIPTION OF THE EFFECT

In 1957, the first evidence of a correlation between human health and water composition was reported by Kobayashi from the Far East. He observed that death rates from cerebral hemorrhage were directly correlated with the ratio of sulfate concentration to carbonate concentration of river water (8). In 1960, Schroeder recalled this observation when he reported a relationship between cardiovascular death rate and the hardness of drinking water in the United States (9). He observed a highly significant negative correlation between the average hardness of potable water to which a population was exposed and the statewide, age-adjusted, cardiovascular mortality rate of the population. Schroeder found the same relationship for deaths from both ischemic heart disease and cerebral vascular disease (Table 1) (10). He suggested that the effect might be mediated by hypertension, i.e. that blood pressure might be increased by soft water and then be responsible for excess strokes and heart attacks. His "hypertension hypothesis" has proved to be a frequently recurring theme; however, at least partly because of methodologic difficulties in determining usual diastolic pressure, there is little evidence for or against it. A strong negative correlation for deaths from "hypertensive heart disease" and hard water has often been cited as supportive of the hypothesis, but that rubric is poorly defined and includes only a few deaths. Except for the currently very rare malignant stage of hypertension, blood pressure *per se* seldom causes death; instead it has its effect by increasing the rate of progression of arteriosclerosis and hence the number of arteriosclerotic complications, including ischemic heart and cerebrovascular disease.

Morris and his coworkers in Great Britain quickly confirmed Schroeder's basic observations (11). Although the pattern varied slightly, they found similar correlations for mortality from all cardiovascular disease and for mortality due to ischemic heart and cerebrovascular disease. In both studies, there were some non-cardiovascular correlations (10,11), but they

Table 1 Correlations in the United States during 1950 between hardness of water and death rates

(From ref. 10)

Cause of death	Annual rate ($/10^5$)	Correlation coefficient (r)
All	844	−0.36
All non-cardiovascular	420	+0.02
All cardiovascular	424	−0.56
Cerebrovascular disease (whites 55–64)	170	−0.34
Ischemic heart disease (whites 55–64)		
Male	812	−0.50
Female	267	−0.46

seemed to be of secondary importance. In seeking other significant relationships to cardiovascular mortality, Morris' group examined 60 "socio-economic variables" besides hardness of water, including income, education, social class, population density, cigarette smoking, domestic overcrowding, motor vehicle accidents, and industrial air pollution, but found no comparably strong correlations (11).

Many other reports have confirmed an inverse correlation between cardiovascular death rates and water hardness. The negative association has been reported in a World Health Organization Study of 15 European cities (12) and in preliminary results from an ongoing survey by the United States Environmental Protection Agency (13). One interesting study by Masironi et al. reported that in Europe myocardial infarction increased as the latitude increased with attack rates doubling for each 15 degrees of northernly movement; these investigators observed a concomitant decrease in water hardness as one went north (14). A survey of the currently available data indicates that the inverse correlation has been consistent in those studies that covered wide geographical areas and involved large ranges in hardness. As noted by Marier, smaller studies, on the other hand, comparing a few cities, counties within the same state or province, different districts of the same town, or small differences in hardness, have sometimes revealed no association at all and occasionally even the reverse correlation. Negative findings have also occurred when the experimental design was inadequate, e.g. when authors used crude death rates without adjustments even for age and sex (15).

APPROACHES TO MECHANISM

The most convincing confirmatory evidence of a relationship between cardiovascular mortality and water hardness comes from the report by Crawford et al. of eleven British towns where water hardness changed and cardiovascular mortality also changed — and in the appropriate direction; at the same time, there was no differential change in non-cardiovascular mortality (16). Between 1950 and 1960, the water became harder in five towns and softer in six. During this period, there was a general increase in cardiovascular mortality, but its magnitude was a function of water hardness. Towns where water had become softer had an increase of 20% which was almost twice the average increase, and towns where water had become harder had an increase of only 8.5% which was somewhat less than the average increase. At the same time, the non-cardiovascular mortality fell 11 to 13% for all 83 towns regardless of the change, or lack of it, in water quantity (Table 2). Lacey and Shaper reexamined these data of Crawford et al., using newer and more refined statistical techniques. The effect remained unchanged, but the statistical significance decreased, with the p changing from its original reported value of 0.02 to 0.06 (17).

Table 2 Mean percentage change in death rate from 1951 to 1961 as function of change in water hardness

Cause of death	Hardness of drinking water		
	Increased (5 towns)	No change (72 towns)	Decreased (6 towns)
Cardiovascular	8.5	11.2	20.2
Other	−10.8	−13.0	−12.4

In search of underlying mechanisms, Crawford and Crawford compared hearts from Glasgow, a soft-water area, with hearts from London, a hard-water area (18). From 1960 to 1962, the mortality rate for ischemic heart disease for men from 45 to 65 years old was 613 per 100,000 in Glasgow versus only 398 in London. The authors considered two series of subjects, each approximately evenly divided between Glasgow and London: 121 men who died sudden accidental deaths and 196 men who died of ischemic heart disease. They examined: (1) the myocardium for fibrosis, as a guide to the amount of actual infarction which a subject had sustained; (2) the coronary arteries for "confluent atheroma" and "lumen stenosis", as an index of the anatomic lesion which they felt was most often associated with myocardial infarction; and (3) the coronary arteries for their content of calcium and magnesium, since these elements are primarily responsible for hardness in water. Their findings were complex, but they can be simplified and summarized as follows:

(1) Old healed myocardial infarcts were more common in Glasgow than in London for both accident victims and subjects dying of ischemic heart disease.

(2) Coronary artery lesions in accident victims were less severe in London than in Glasgow.

(3) Among those dying of ischemic heart disease, Englishmen had more severe lesions (both atheromata and stenosis) than Scots, suggesting that the English environment decreased vascular changes as well as raising the tolerance to those that did occur. Thus, the two effects apparently reinforced each other.

(4) Concentrations of calcium and magnesium were much lower in the relatively normal coronary arteries of both groups from Glasgow, where the water had low concentrations of these elements.

Since Scots developed fatal myocardial infarction with less anatomic disease of the coronary arteries than the English, the authors speculated that soft water might be associated with an increased tendency toward more severe arteriosclerotic lesions. These investigators also found that Scots had low concentrations of bone magnesium more often than Englishmen (19), suggesting that a low content of magnesium in the water depleted total body magnesium stores and not just coronary artery magnesium.

Extending Crawford and Crawford's impression that something more than just anatomic difference was involved in the high mortality rates of ischemic heart disease in soft water areas, Anderson and his coworkers have suggested that the major relationship between water hardness and ischemic heart disease might involve rapidly fatal arrhythmias. Using 1967 data for subjects 35 to 75 years old in the province of Ontario, they divided the deaths from ischemic heart disease into "coroner" (sudden, unexpected death) and "non-coroner" groups. The two groups happened to be of similar size. When correlations were sought, the coroner group showed the characteristic marked inverse correlation between death rate from ischemic heart disease and hardness of water, and the non-coroner group showed no such inverse correlation (20).

More recently Anderson et al. (21) matched autopsy subjects from areas high in water magnesium with those from areas low in water magnesium. These investigators found lowered levels of magnesium in heart and other muscles from male residents of soft water areas dying from either myocardial infarction or accident. These findings are consistent with those of Crawford and Crawford (18) and with the hypothesis that the magnesium found in hard water is protective. In contrast, when Chipperfield et al. compared non-cardiovascular deaths in a soft and a hard water town, they found 25% more magnesium in heart muscle of subjects from the former. The towns, however, were characterized as having hard or soft water on the basis of the calcium in their water supply, while magnesium levels were not specified. Moreover, the authors interpreted their findings as compatible with a protective effect of magnesium since they considered the decedents from the soft water town as having a decrease in magnesium relative to potassium (22).

In a major effort to understand mechanism, the British Regional Heart Study was designed to seek factors responsible for the marked regional variations in stroke and coronary artery disease in Great Britain. Examination of 253 towns with populations exceeding 50,000 in 1971 reaffirmed the negative correlation between water hardness and cardiovascular mortality (23). Although considerable scatter in standardized mortality rates (SMR's) was observed at any given hardness, all but one of the towns with SMR's over 120 had soft water (less than 1 mmol per liter = calcium carbonate equivalent of 100 mg/liter), and 95% of the towns with water hardness over 2 mmol/liter had SMR's less than 100. In a multiple regression model using the SMR during the period in 1969–1973 for all cardiovascular disease in men and women aged 35 to 75, there were five variables that collectively had a highly significant effect on the SMR: water hardness, percentage of days with rain, mean daily maximum temperature, percentage of manual workers, and car ownership (Table 3). Each of these variables made a separate and significant contribution to explaining regional variations in cardiovascular mortality. The influence of climate was considered to be of

Table 3 Major factors related to cardiovascular mortality
(From ref. 23)

Variable	Standardized regression effect
Water hardness:	
Up to 1–7 mmol/l	−7.8
Over 1–7 mmol/l	−0.8
% Manual workers	+5.1
Rain	+4.1
Maximum temperature	−3.0
Car ownership	−2.9

particular importance since high rainfall and areas with soft water tend to coincide. Total hardness was not the only water parameter associated with cardiovascular mortality; not unexpectedly, high correlation coefficients with cardiovascular mortality were observed for carbonate hardness ($r = -0.65$) and for calcium ($r = -0.67$). Magnesium ($r = -0.13$) and sodium ($r = -$ -0.16), on the other hand, did not appear to be associated with cardiovascular mortality.

The report of the British Regional Heart Study presents the geometric means of the SMR's for cardiovascular disease for towns grouped according to water hardness; Fig. 1 presents the curves which best fit these means, both with and without adjustments for the effects of the other four variables

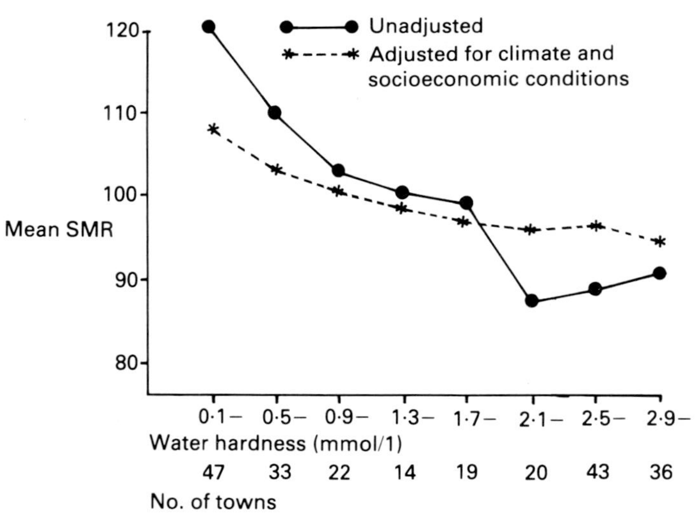

Fig. 1 Geometric means of SMR (for all men and women aged 35–74 with cardiovascular diseases) for towns grouped according to hardness of water

Water hardness: 1 mmol/liter = calcium carbonate equivalent of 100 mg/liter

(From ref. 1. Reproduced, with permission, from the Annual Review of Nutrition, Vol. 1. © 1981 by Annual Reviews Inc.)

(23). Adjusting for the two climatic and the two socioeconomic variables considerably reduces, but certainly does not eliminate, the hard water effect. This effect of water hardness is non–linear, being significant in the range of very soft to medium-hard water, but negligible in the range of medium to very hard water. The effects of hardness on SMR were therefore considered separately for the intervals above and below 1.7 mmol/liter. In the lower range, an increase in total hardness of 1 mmol/liter (i.e. from 0.5 to 1.5 mmol/liter) while keeping the other variables constant should result in a 7% decrease in cardiovascular mortality; however, there is no evidence of an equivalent decrease in the higher range. Thus, these data suggest a 10 to 15% difference in cardiovascular mortality between medium hard and very soft water areas. Moreover, there is no effect between non-cardiovascular mortality and water hardness in any range.

POSSIBLE SUBSTANCES INVOLVED IN THE HARD WATER EFFECT

General Considerations: As indicated, the mechanism of the "hard water effect" and the possible substance(s) responsible for it have been the subject of extensive speculation. Hardness is not a specific constituent of water, but rather a complex characteristic which is usually measured by titration with a chelating agent and is often expressed as the calcium carbonate equivalent of the total calcium and magnesium present (24). It seems likely that the adverse effect of soft water is due to the presence of a "toxic" substance or to the absence of a protective substance which is found in hard water.

When considering the effects of a water-borne substance, its concentration in the critical target region would seem to be the important datum. To obtain this concentration, however, requires quantitative information which is rarely available, necessitating the use of various approximations, some of which are dubious resulting in uncertainties about the significance of the candidate substances. First, the concentration in the water supply—and not just the concentration in the resevoir—but rather the concentration as it is drunk. Many things can change the concentration of one or another of the candidate substances between the reservoir and the mouth, e.g., water softeners and galvanized or lead pipes. Second, an individual's daily consumption of water from the supply in question. A recent New Zealand study indicates a more than ten-fold range of water intake from individual to individual from just above a quarter liter to almost three liters a day (25); presumably there is also an intraindividual variation. Third, how much of the substance which enters the alimentary tract in water actually crosses the gut wall and gets into the blood stream. Fourth, what fraction of the total intake of the substance comes from the water supply in question. Fifth, how much of the fluid intake comes from boiled or otherwise processed water, (e.g., tea or coffee). It is generally assumed that considerable amounts of calcium and magnesium carbonates are precipitated on the vessel walls during boiling, thus resulting in significant softening. Finally, it is also necessary to know how much water comes from an entirely different supply (e.g. beer or soft drinks). Comparable information regarding estimates of intake from the different water supplies, from food, and from other sources (i.e., ambient air) require similar consideration. In addition, the question of availability becomes important because some substances differ greatly in their availability for absorption across the gut, depending on chemical form, the presence of binding compounds, and the like.

Overall body burden, or even burden in the particular compartment of the body responsible for the critical effect, may not be the most critical parameter. It may be a ratio between the concentrations of two or more substances. For instance, in the case of cadmium it seems likely that the ratio of zinc to cadmium rather than the absolute amount of cadmium is crucial to cadmium toxicity. Moreover, in attempting to arrive at acceptable intake levels, we ordinarily deal with the average exposure for a population. Perhaps we should be attempting to identify the 10 or 20% of the population with a somewhat higher than usual intake, or perhaps a smaller percentage with an unusually high exposure or unusual susceptibility. These considerations are summarized in Table 4.

Possible Substances: As indicated in Table 5, the current candidate substances for the cause of the "hard water effect" are: (1) calcium and/or magnesium, the major contributors to water hardness; (2) sodium or potassium, the other major metallic electrolytes in living systems; (3) trace substances which would be effective in much lower concentrations. Calcium and magnesium have been obvious candidates for a protective substance in hard water.

Table 4 Considerations in estimating importance of intake from water

I. Concentration of substance in water
   A. In local water supply
      Changes in water itself prior to ingestion (softeners, pipes, etc.)
      Additional changes in converting to other beverages (i.e. boiling for tea or coffee) and fraction taken as such beverages
   B. In non-local water converted to beer, soft drinks, etc. and fraction of intake from this source
   C. Absorbtion across gut wall
   D. Excretion and inactive storage

II. Intake from food
   A. Fraction ingested and availability from food versus water

III. Body burden
   A. Concentration in critical compartment
   B. Ratio of its concentration to that of regulating substances (e.g. Zn:Cd)

IV. Fraction of population above critical level
   A. Particularly high-risk groups
   B. Particularly high-exposure groups

Table 5 Contributions from water

	Possible effect	Typical concentrations in water	Typical intake from water	Maximum intake from water
Ca	Protective	26 ppm	5–10%	60%
Mg	Protective	6 ppm	2–5%	50%
Na	Adverse	28 ppm	1–3%	25%
Cd	Adverse	<10 ppb	<5 %	65%
Pb	Adverse	13 ppb	<10%	40%

Both sodium and potassium have also been mentioned, although neither contributes directly to hardness. Sodium, as a toxic substance, would have to be associated with soft water; whereas, potassium, as a protective substance, would have to be associated with hard water. There is a considerable literature relating excess sodium to hypertension which, as indicated previously, is directly related to heart attacks and strokes. However, soft water tends to have a low sodium content except when water has been artificially softened by ion exchange. Potassium has attracted less attention as a potential participant in the "hard water effect", although high concentrations often accompany high concentrations of calcium and magnesium. Potassium, a dearth of which has long been recognized as potentiating dangerous arrhythmias, has recently come to be regarded as weakly antihypertensive.

Finally, several trace metals have also been considered as potential toxic substances, particularly lead and cadmium. To be involved in the "hard water effect", a trace metal would have to be more concentrated in, or possibly more available from, soft water. There is no evidence that, at the concentrations involved, either cadmium or lead has any biologic effect in man; however, there is no contrary evidence, and they are present in widely varying but sometimes quite high concentrations in human tissue, apparently as a result of widely varying environmental exposure (26). Moreover, in animals both cadmium and lead can induce hypertension (27, 28); this hypertension is characteristically mild and resembles human essential hypertension, which if present in man, would produce major health effects, e.g., doubling of cardiovascular mortality (29). Very early in this investigation of the "hard water effect", Schroeder suggested that drinking water composition and cardiovascular disease mortality could be indirectly related through high blood pressure which is a major risk factor for apoplectic stroke, myocardial infarction and cardiovascular arrhythmia (10). Currently hypertension has been invoked as a possible mechanism for all of the candidate substances discussed below except magnesium.

Calcium and Magnesium: In both the United States and Canada, the concentrations of these alkaline earths in drinking water have negative correlations of approximately equal strength with cardiovascular mortality. In contrast, in England, strong negative correlations are found between calcium and cardiovascular mortality, but magnesium generally appears to be unrelated (24). Using the American data, attempts have been made to evaluate the possible independent effects of calcium and magnesium by statistical means, with neither element having a marked effect in the absence of the other (24). Despite the apparent lack of relationship with the British data, magnesium is generally considered to be a strong candidate for the causal substance. The previously cited data of Crawford and Crawford on the tissue concentrations of both calcium and magnesium, i.e. low in the soft water areas, are from Great Britain and support the involvement of magnesium as much as calcium (19). Some data which, on the surface at least, seem to separate the effects of these two substances are available. McCarron and co-workers have cited evidence tending to demonstrate the protective effect of calcium (30). Adults between 35 and 74 years without cardiovascular disease or diet modification from the American National Health and Nutrition Examination Survey (NHANES) were compared with respect to blood pressure after controlling for age and sex. Hypertensives, regardless of age, reported significantly less calcium consumption than did normal subjects (17 % versus 22 %) (31). This group has also reported that calcium exposure is inversely related to blood pressure in SHR rats (32). As part of their argument, they have also proposed that low sodium can be associated with elevated blood pressure, and this concept has met with considerable resistence and has reduced enthusiasm for the rest of their thesis. The data from Great Britain of Stitt et al. also demonstrated an inverse relationship between calcium exposure from water sources and both systolic and diastolic blood pressures (33) and so are consistent with a protective role for calcium.

The evidence favoring magnesium as the cause is less consistent and more difficult to summarize. The findings of decreased levels of magnesium in coronary artery and bone from "low magnesium areas" by Crawford et al. (18), and the apparently contrary findings of increased levels in heart muscle by Chipperfield (22) have already been noted. Other magnesium data are complex and subject to more than one interpretation; for instance, a Finnish study found that levels of both calcium and magnesium in water were inversely related to mortality from coronary heart diesease (34). In areas with high mortality, however, tap water of coronary decedents had significantly less magnesium than the water of study subjects who were free of coronary disease. The results, however, were not consistent, since subjects less than 60 years old who had died of coronary disease had higher tap water magnesium than controls.

Moderate and severe magnesium deficiency has also been reported to produce graded degrees of hypomagnesemia and graded elevation of blood pressure in rats (35).

Sodium and Potassium: Although sodium concentration in water may have significant health-related effects, its concentration is not usually inversely correlated with the concentration of calcium or magnesium, rather it tends to travel with potassium and chloride; hence it seems unlikely that it is the toxic factor in soft water. Folsom and Prineas list nine epidemiologic studies seeking a relationship between blood pressure and sodium content of drinking water, in seven of these there was a direct relationship, although some of the differences seemed trivial (6). In more general terms, Freis lists four principal lines of evidence indicating that, under some circumstances, blood pressure is directly related to dietary sodium intake: (1) epidemiological studies in unacculturated populations indicating that the prevalence of hypertension is inversely correlated with salt intake; (2) hemodynamic studies suggesting that chronic experimental hypertension is a homeostatic response to a long-term increase in extracellular fluid volume (ECF); evidence that the ECF of "salt eaters" is expanded in comparison to that of those limiting their salt intake; and (4) investigations in hypertensive patients receiving either diets greatly restricted in salt or continuous diuretic therapy which relate the fall in blood pressure with a reduction in ECF (36). Finally, there is a recent suggestion that much of the "sodium data" are really related to chloride rather than sodium.

Kempner's successful treatment of severe human hypertension in the 1940's with a diet maximally restricted in sodium (10 mEq/day) (37) can be contrasted with Meneely's maximally high sodium diets (up to 20 % of diet by weight) which markedly raised blood pressure and shortened survival in rats (38). These studies amply demonstrate that extremes of sodium intake can influence both blood pressure and survival. The pertinent question involves the effect of smaller and more practical modifications of sodium intake in the range of acceptable human diet. One well controlled trial has claimed an antihypertensive effect from moderate as opposed to severe sodium restriction (39). The study was relatively short and the fall in blood pressure minimal. Apparently a reduction of salt intake to about 1 gm (17 mEq of sodium per day) is required to produce more than a minimal reduction of blood pressure.

Potassium is not often mentioned in relation to the "hard water effect", although it is generally considered to be beneficial. The first of my three major points is that potassium may cause such an effect and that some recent data from the "MRFIT" Study are consistent with this hypothesis. These data raise the question of whether thiazide-induced hypokalemia could be related to unanticipated excess deaths of hypertensive subjects with baseline electrocardiograph abnormalities. In the group of more than 1,200 hypertensives with such baseline abnormalities who may have received intensive thiazide therapy, the mortality rate was increased by two-thirds over comparable subjects who probably received less thiazide (40). These data have caused a great deal of concern; however, because of the study design which included no control group, they are subject to different interpretation, and as yet there are no confirmatory data. The suggestion that hypokalemia might induce potentially fatal arrhythmias and sudden unexpected deaths recalls the excess mortality reported by Anderson in soft water areas of Ontario (20). It cannot be too strongly emphasized that there is no real evidence that chronic thiazide usage is a significant hazard. Nonetheless, the worry persists, particularly when one thinks of decades of treatment for very large numbers of asymptomatic hypertensive patients, the great majority of whom would survive many years without treatment and without any complications of their hypertension. Finally, it should also be noted that thiazides induce hypomagnesemia as well as hypokalemia, thus once again a magnesium-mediated effect could be invoked.

It has also been suggested that excess potassium may lower blood pressure and that a dearth of potassium may be hypertensive, but that effect is probably small, the data are very limited, and no strong case can be made at the present time. It is certainly true that Kempner's ''rice-fruit'' diet was not only very low in sodium but also high in potassium (37), and that Meneely's rats were protected by added potassium (38).

Trace Metals: Among the candidates suggested as causing the ''hard water effect'' are a group of trace metals which are seldom discussed in any detail because the definitive data are limited. Tissue concentrations of trace metals can vary a great deal, perhaps ten- or a hundred-fold. Such variation is obviously not possible for major tissue components. If hard water contains a ''beneficial'' trace element, vanadium, lithium, zinc, selenium, and possibly chromium are candidates. If soft water contains harmful metals, cadmium and lead are likely candidates, with copper and barium as additional possibilities.

My second major point is that cadmium and lead are valid candidate substances as causes for the ''hard water effect''. These metals, along with barium, have been reported to elevate blood pressure in animals at the same low concentrations in drinking water to which many Americans are continuosly exposed (28, 41, 2). Although there is no evidence that any of these metals is involved in human hypertension, there is no evidence that they are not, and some of the available data are consistent with a pressor effect in man. In rats the long-term ingestion of these metals has caused elevations of between 15 and 25 mm Hg in average systolic pressure, without affecting growth rates or seeming to induce any toxic manifestations (Fig. 2). These average increases in pressure are consistently present and are statistically significant. Although the basis of the metal-induced pressor effect remains obscure, all three metals produce similar changes in the pattern of energy-related, phosphate-containing compounds in the perfused rat heart, as determined by nuclear magnetic resonance spectroscopy. The high energy phosphate bonds in ATP and phosphocreatinine are decreased by a quarter, while ADP and inorganic phosphate are comparably increased, thus significantly decreasing the ''phosphorylation potential'' (Fig. 2) (43).

Cadmium: Rats chronically exposed to cadmium at levels of 0.1 to 5 ppm

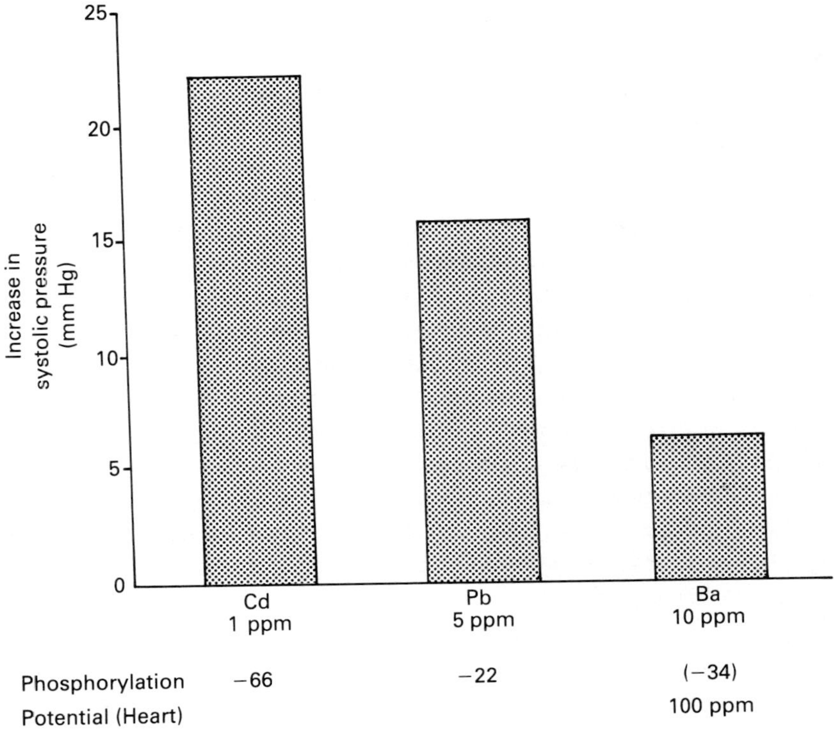

Fig. 2 Average increase in systolic pressure of unanesthetized female Long-Evans rats exposed for about a year to the indicated metal concentrations

Average decreases in cardiac phosphorylation potential are on similar rats with similar exposures except for the parenthetic value which was for rats exposed to 100 ppm barium for 16 months. All six indicated changes are statistically significant

in drinking water from the time of weaning are not sick and show a normal growth pattern (44). Their average systolic pressure is increased about 20 mm Hg (Table 6), and some of the exposed animals develop much larger increases in pressure, with a sixth of the rats in one report having increases of at least 50 mm Hg (41). In addition to the pressor effect, there are marked

Table 6 Cadmium-induced hypertension and cadmium balance after 18 months of exposure

Mean values for female Long-Evans rats exposed for 18 months from the time of weaning to the indicated amounts of cadmium

	Increase in systolic pressure (mm Hg)	Ingested cadmium/animal (mg)	Total body cadmium (mg)	Cadmium retained (%)	Kidney cadmium (γ/gm)
Control	0	0.20	0.0005	0.15	0.06
0.1 ppm	18	1.5	0.010	0.67	0.99
1 ppm	20	14.8	0.14	0.95	11.7
5 ppm	22	74.0	0.70	0.94	44.3

biochemical and physiological changes in the heart: not only "high energy phosphate", but both cardiac contractility and conductivity are also decreased. Finally, there are very significant increases in tissue cadmium levels, and, if these changes are large, there is a concomitant increase in tissue zinc (43).

A total of 10 laboratories have reported attempts to induce hypertension by chronically exposing rats to cadmium in drinking water (41); seven succeeded (45–54) (Table 7), thus demonstrating the reality of the pressor effect. The pressor doses of cadmium in the drinking water ranged from 0.1 ppm to 17 ppm. In general, there are two possible explanations for failure to induce hypertension with cadmium in drinking water that deserve emphasis. The first is that too large a dose of cadmium was used, i.e. a toxic rather than a pressor dose. The mechanism of cadmium-induced hypertension in rats appears to be different from the renal dysfunction induced in man by heavy toxic exposure. The hypertensive dose for a rat is small and not associated with proteinuria or glucosuria. Larger doses do not induce more severe hypertension; in fact they do not induce any hypertension at all. Instead they are depressor and produce other toxic symptoms. The second is that control animals may be exposed to enough cadmium in the food or the environment that they, as well as the cadmium-fed animals, have cadmium-induced hypertension. Because of the relatively flat dose-response curve, even a low control exposure might induce a near maximum pressor response. Figure 3 provides an example of this. The difference in systolic pressure between control and cadmium-fed rats gradually declined when the food was Purina Chow; whereas when our usual low cadmium diet with only

Table 7 Reported attempts to induce hypertension in rats by adding cadmium to drinking water

The first seven groups of investigators found a statistically significant increase in systolic pressure following cadmium exposure; the other groups found no significant difference. All cited pressures are averages

Number in exposed group	Rats: Sex, age & strain[a]	Cadmium in water (ppm)	Cadmium exposure (Months)	Systolic pressure		Reference
				Control (mm Hg)	Cadmium (mm Hg)	
22	F, weanling, LE	5	10	84	127	Schroeder (45)
20	F, weanling, LE	0.1	15	101	123	Perry (46)
8	M, weanling, SD	17	9	121	136	Petering (47)
8	M, adult, SD	10	5	106	135	Boscolo (48)
10	F, weanling, Dahl S	1	4	148	170	Ohanian (49)
6	M, 200–300 gm, SD	3	2	control < Cd-exposed by 25 mm Hg		Revis (50)
5	F, 4 mos, SD	10	8	96	155	Walker (51)
10	F, weanling, SD	5	11		NS[a]	Doyle (52)
10	M, weanling, OSU Brown	10	24	142	142	Eakin (53)
	F, weanling, Wistar	5	16	NS[a]		Lener (54)

[a] LE = Long Evans, SD = Sprague Dawley, Dahl S = Dahl Sensitive, OSU Brown = Oregon State University Brown, and NS = no significant difference

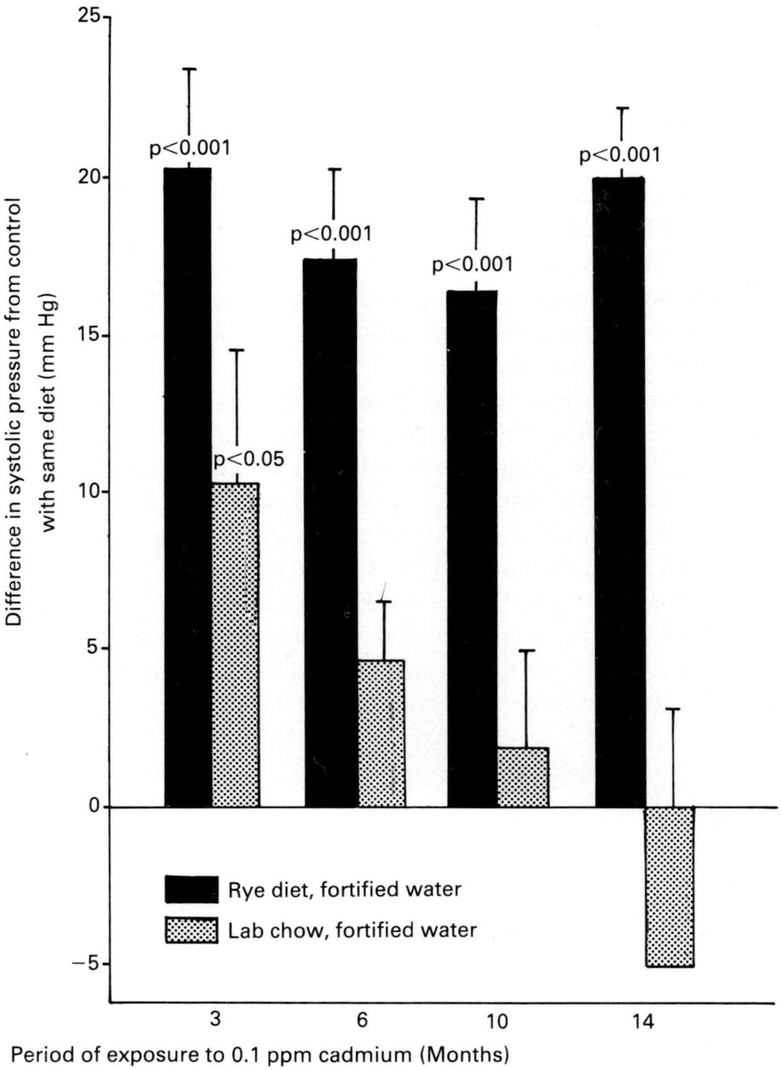

Fig. 3 Bars indicate average pressure difference between control and cadmium-fed animal; lines extending from bars indicate SEM

The solid bar in each time period represents rats fed rye-based diet plus fortified water and the stippled bar, rats fed stock chow plus fortified water. P-value indicates the significance of the pressure difference between control and cadmium-fed animals, by using Student's t-test

1/10 as much cadmium was used, the difference between control and cadmium-fed rats persisted (41). Finally, it should be noted that in four unsuccessful experiments, cadmium was added to the food where it may well be less available than in water (41).

Table 6 gives cadmium balance data after 18 months of exposure, including cadmium concentration in the kidney where cadmium is most concentrated. Under our conditions, 0.1 ppm of cadmium is the minimum consistently pressor dose and 5 ppm is the highest consistently pressor dose. The minimum pressor dose induced total body cadmium and renal cadmium concentration of about 20 times the values found in control rats and about 1/50 of the values found with the maximum pressor dose.

Cadmium-induced hypertension in rats can be influenced by the presence of several other metals added to drinking water. Small amounts of selenium, moderate amounts of copper, and large amounts of zinc can lessen the cadmium-induced increases in pressure by 50 % to 90 % (55). Dissolving the cadmium in hard water has a similar effect (56). In contrast, lead in concentrations equal to the concentration of cadmium can increase the pressor effect of cadmium (28).

There is no convincing evidence that chronic environmental exposure to the small doses of cadmium considered here has any effect in man; on the other hand, there is no indication that it does not. Nine relatively small studies have compared the renal cadmium concentration in normotensive and hypertensive individuals (Table 8). All normotensive groups had average renal cadmium concentrations of 15 to 32 μg per gm of whole kidney. In five of the nine studies, the hypertensive groups had from 32 to 51 μg of cadmium per gram of kidney. In these five, the hypertensive subjects had significantly higher renal cadmium concentrations than their normotensive counterparts (57–60). In three of the nine studies, there was no significant

Table 8 Human studies comparing renal cadmium in hypertensives and normotensives

Data from nine small series that have compared renal cadmium concentration in hypertensive and "matched" normotensive subjects. Six of the nine comparisons found statistically significant differences, with five showing more renal cadmium in hypertensive subjects than in normotensive subjects and one showing the reverse

Total number in study	Normotensive mean (γ/gm kidney)	Hypertensive mean (γ/gm kidney)	Author/Country
134	29	42	Schroeder–US[a] (57)
40	32	51	Schroeder–non-US[a] (57)
18	15	32	Karlicek–Czechoslovakia[a] (58)
22	27	36	Lener–Czechoslovakia[a] (59)
22	26	40	Perry–US[a] (60)
37	25	25	Morgan–US (61)
58	27	20	Syversen–Norway[b] (62)
136	15	16	Indraprasit–US[b] (63)
82	21	12	Ostergaard–Denmark[a] (64)
Range	15–32	32–51 (in 5 of 9)	

[a] Difference between normotensive and hypertensive were statistically significant, with $p < 0.05$

[b] These two studies were apparently designed for other purposes, with incidental division of population into hypertensive and normotensive cohorts.

difference in the mean concentrations of the two groups (61–63); however, two of these three studies were designed for other purposes and division into hypertensive and normotensive groups was done retrospectively. The last study is the most puzzling. It was performed very carefully, and the normotensive mean was close to those of the other studies. The hypertensive mean, however, was not only well below the other hypertensive means but was also below any of the normotensive means of the other studies (64).

Lead: Like cadmium, lead seems to be a possible candidate for involvement in the "hard water effect". The available data suggest that lead has two different mechanisms for inducing hypertension: In animals, at least, long-term, low-dose lead exposure induces a relatively mild hypertension which resembles essential human hypertension, and there are data suggesting that the same effect may occur in man. Considerably more intense exposure, e.g., industrial exposure, induces renal damage which may in turn result in hypertension. Any relationship to the "hard water effect" would involve the essential type of hypertension associated with low lead exposure. Only three epidemiologic studies have been reported in which blood pressure, itself, has been examined in relation to lead in drinking water (65, 66). Cerebrovascular deaths have been reported to be associated with occupational lead exposure (67), and there are reports failing to find such an association.

In a case-comparison study of 135 hypertensives and 135 age- and sex-matched normotensives, Beevers et al. (65) found that on average hypertensives' drinking water contained more lead than did that of controls and mean blood lead levels were correspondingly higher in hypertensives than in normotensives. A study in Finland, however, found this relationship in only one geographic area (68). If any relationship does exist, it may be only in areas with uncommonly high lead levels.

Preliminary studies by Crawford and her associates found higher concentrations of both lead and cadmium in the bones of subjects from hard water areas than in those from soft water areas (19). A direct association between blood lead and blood pressure has recently been reported in the British Regional Heart Study. In addition, a chelate challenge in hypertensive patients evoked more lead excretion in those with renal failure as compared to those with normal function suggesting that an unsuspected increase in the body burden of lead had induced renal damage and perhaps associated hypertension (69). Such hypertension would seem to be renal in origin and to result from a large unrecognized lead exposure.

Finally, like cadmium, chronic low-level, long-term exposure to lead leads to hypertension in rats. This hypertension, like that induced by low dose cadmium, is characteristically not the marked increase in blood pressure which has come to typify experimental hypertension and which seems to be neccessary to arouse interest in hypertension. Instead lead induces hypertension which is usually mild and only occasionally severe. This pattern resembles human essential hypertension which also is usually mild and has no obvious associated abnormalities, yet which markedly increases the risk of myocardial infarction. The required doses of lead to induce such hypertension resemble those of cadmium in both intensity and duration. Moreover the physiologic and biochemical changes in the heart are similar for lead and cadmium. Since exposure to low dosages of both cadmium and lead must occur frequently, it should be noted that the initial response to the combination is relatively marked hypertension (Fig. 4) (28).

Hydralazine, a Metal Binding Antihypertensive Agent: My third major point involves some observations on patients who received long-term high dose hydralazine. These observations are consistent with binding, and presumably removal, by hydralazine of a metal associated with human hypertension. This is entirely speculative; however, the data, which are seldom considered in this context, are sufficiently striking to warrant mention. Hydralazine is a direct peripheral vasodilator which strongly binds

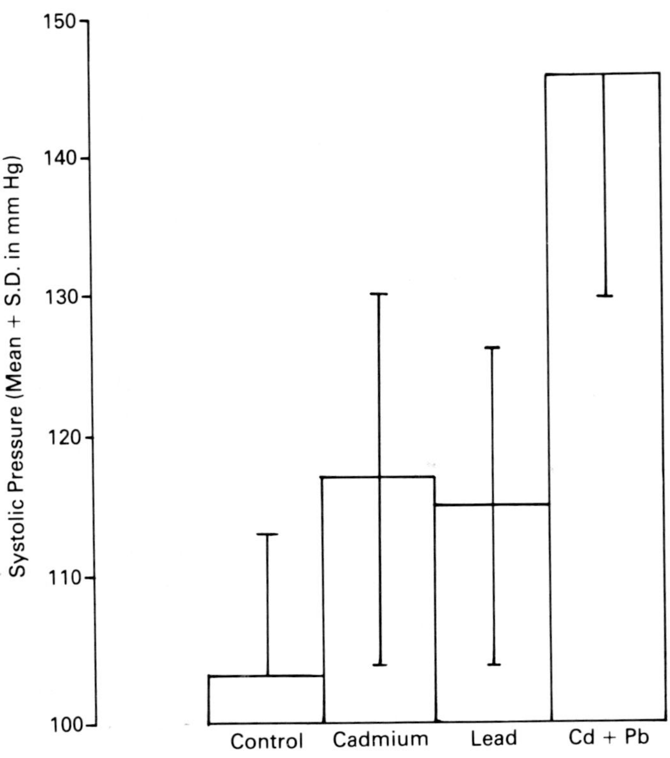

Fig. 4 Early synergistic hypertensive effects of lead and cadmium

Average systolic pressures ± standard deviations are presented for 45 control rats and for groups of 15 rats fed 1 ppm cadmium and/or lead for three months

many metals. In addition to its antihypertensive effect it has unique effects in man. It can induce an autoimmune reaction that stimulates idiopathic systemic lupus erythematosus, but only in subjects who are slow metabolizers of the hepatic enzyme acetyl transferase which degrades hydralazine. Hydralazine lupus (HL) is characterized by normotension even in patients who originally had severe or malignant underlying hypertension; in fact, the only recognized prodrome of HL is normotension. Some data documenting the reciprocal relationship between HL and blood pressure are briefly presented in Table 9. Forty-two of 308 similarly and simultaneously treated white patients developed HL after an average daily intake of just over 0.5 gm hydralazine for an average of 17 months. The 42 HL were compared both to the entire 266 non-HL patients and to 42 of them who were matched with respect to sex, age, and the presence of accelerated hypertension (70). Before treatment, their diastolic pressures were higher while during and after treatment, their diastolic pressures were lower than the controls without HL. Moreover, when their symptoms were most intense, HL patients were normotensive. Of more importance, 10 years after all HL symptoms had disappeared, the normotension often persisted *without any treatment in patients who felt well and led normal lives*. The clinical picture often is consistent with a depletion phenomenon. The permanent normotension in some instances suggests that a permanent change has been induced. Myocardial infarction and stroke which are usually incapacitating are the only other circumstances known to occasionally restore severe hypertension to normotension.

In addition to changes cited with HL, there was a gradual decrease in average drug requirement for *all controlled patients* on a single regimen of hydralazine in combination with ganglioplegic agent (71). After three years of treatment, the average reduction for those with a sitting diastolic pressure less than 100 mm Hg was 50% for each of the two drugs. In contrast, the "partially controlled" group was taking nearly 100% of its initial doses at

Table 9 Average diastolic pressure (mm Hg) as measured on the seated patient at home several times daily

Data in the third and fourth columns of figures are averages at 18 and 30 months after treatment began. "Most Recent" pressure is averaged only for patients who survived at least 10 years after beginning treatment; in this group there were 26 HL and 183 non-HL patients, of whom 17 were "matched" non-HL patients

	Before therapy	After one month of therapy at home	One month before first HL symptom	At time of maximum HL symptoms	Most recent
42 HL patients	130	93	88	80	89
42 matched non-HL patients	126	99*	97**	98**	101**
All 266 non-HL patients	120*	99*	98**	99**	101**

* and ** indicate averages which differed significantly from the average for the HL patients, with $p < 0.05$ and < 0.001, respectively.

Table 10 Decrease in severity of treated hypertension with time as manifested by decreasing drug requirement in controlled patients

The tabulated numbers indicate the percentages of the originally effective drug dosages still required after one and three years. The subjects are 114 consecutive patients, with varyingly severe pretreatment hypertension, who are divided here solely on basis of whether home diastolic pressures averaged < 100 or > 100 mm Hg (22)

	One year		Three years	
	Percent hexa-methonium	Percent hydrala-zine	Percent hexa-methonium	Percent hydrala-zine
79 patients controlled by treatment	74	89	42	55
35 patients uncontrolled on treatment	97	99	84	77

the end of one year and was still taking 80% at the end of three years, when their mean diastolic pressure was somewhat higher than when therapy had been initiated. These observations could provide a clue to a cause of the inverse relationship of hard water and cardiovascular disease if a trace metal or several trace metals are contributing factors to that negative correlation.

CONCLUSION

The "hard water" effect is real. The cause or causes for the negative correlation with mortality are not delineated. Further investigation is needed to elucidate the mechanism.

From the Medical Service, Veterans Administration Medical Center and the Hypertension Division, Department of Internal Medicine, Washington University School of Medicine, St. Louis, Missouri.

REFERENCES

1. MASIRONI, R. & SHAPER, A. G. (1981). Epidemiological studies of health effects of water from different sources. *Ann. Rev. Nutr.* 1, 375.
2. COMSTOCK, G. W. (1980). The epidemiologic perspective: Water hardness and cardiovascular disease. *J. Environ. Pathol. Toxicol.* 4, 9.
3. HEYDEN, S. (1976). The hard facts behind the hard water theory and ischemic heart disease. *J. chron. Dis.* 29, 149.
4. NERI, L. C. & JOHANSEN, H. L. (1978). Water hardness and cardiovascular mortality. *Ann. N.Y. Acad. Sci.* 304, 203.
5. SHARRETT, A. R. (1981). Water hardness and cardiovascular disease. *Circulation* 63, 247A.
6. FOLSOM, A. R. & PRINEAS, R. J. (1982). Drinking water composition and blood pressure: A review of the epidemiology. *Amer. J. Epidem.* 115, 818.
7. *U.S. National Committee for Geochemistry* (1979). *Geochemistry of Water in Relation to Cardiovascular Diseases.* National Academy of Sciences, Washington, D.C.
8. KOBAYASHI, J. (1957). On geographical relationship between the chemical nature of river water and death-rate from apoplexy. *Ber. Ohara Inst. Landwirtsch. Biol.* 11, 12.
9. SCHROEDER, H. A. (1960). Relationship between mortality from cardiovascular disease and treated water supplies. Variations in states and 163 largest municipalities of the United States. *J. Amer. Med. Ass.* 172, 1902.
10. SCHROEDER, H. A. (1960). Relations between hardness of water and death rates from certain chronic and degenerative diseases in the United States. *J. chron. Dis.* 12, 586.
11. MORRIS, J. N., CRAWFORD, M. D. & HEADY, J. A. (1961). Hardness of local water supplies and mortality from cardiovascular disease. *Lancet* 1, 860.
12. MASIRONI, R., PISA, A. & CLAYTON, D. (1979). Myocardial infarction and water hardness in the WHO Myocardial Infarction Registry Netword. *Bull. World Health Org.* 57, 291.
13. GREATHOUSE, D. G. & OSBORNE, R. H. (1980). Preliminary report on nationwide study of drinking water and cardiovascular diseases. *J. Environ. Pathol. Toxicol.* 4, 65.
14. MASIRONI, R., MIESCH, A. T., CRAWFORD, M. D. & HAMILTON, E. I. (1972). Geochemical environments, trace elements, and cardiovascular diseases. *Bull. World Health Org.* 47, 139.
15. MARIER, J. R., NERI, L. C. & ANDERSON, T. W. (1978). *Water Hardness, Human Health, and the Importance of Magnesium,* p. 119. Rep. ISSN 0316-0114 NRCC No. 17581 Natl. Res. Counc., Canada, Ottawa.
16. CRAWFORD, M. D., GARDNER, M. J. & MORRIS, J. N. (1971). Changes in water hardness and local death-rates. *Lancet* 2, 327.
17. LACEY, R. F. & SHAPER, A. G. (1984). Changes in water hardness and cardiovascular death rates. *Int. J. Epidem.* 13, 18.
18. CRAWFORD, T. & CRAWFORD, M. D. (1967). Prevalence and pathological changes of ischemic heart disease in a hard water and in a soft water area. *Lancet* 1, 299.
19. CRAWFORD, M. & CRAWFORD, T. (1969). Lead content of bones in a soft and a hard water area. *Lancet* 1, 699.
20. ANDERSON, T. W. & LERICHE, W. H. (1971). Sudden death from ischemic heart disease in Ontario and its correlation with water hardness and other factors. *Can. Med. Ass. J.* 105, 1551.

21. ANDERSON, T. W., NERI, L. C., SCHREIBER, G. B., TALBOT, F. D. F. & ZDROJEWSKI, A. (1975). Ischemic heart disease, water hardness and myocardial magnesium. *Can. Med. Ass. J.* 113, 199.
22. CHIPPERFIELD, B., CHIPPERFIELD, J. R., BEHR, G. & BURTON, P. (1976). Magnesium and potassium content of normal heart muscle in areas of hard and soft water. *Lancet* 1, 121.
23. POCOCK, S. J., SHAPER, A. G., COOK, D. G., PACKHAM, R. F., LACEY, R. F., POWELL, P. & RUSSELL, P. F. (1980). British regional heart study: Geographic variation in cardiovascular mortality, and the role of water quality. *Brit. med. J.* 280, 1243.
24. SHARRETT, A. R. (1979). The role of chemical constituents of drinking water in cardiovascular diseases. *Amer. J. Epidem.* 110, 401.
25. GILLIES, M. W. & PAULIN, H. V. (1983). Variability of mineral intakes from drinking water: A possible explanation for the controversy over the relationship of water quality to cardiovascular disease. *Int. J. Epidem.* 12, 45.
26. PERRY, H. M., JR., TIPTON, I. H., SCHROEDER, H. A., STEINER, R. L. & COOK, M. J. (1961). Variation in the concentrations of cadmium in human kidneys as a function of age and geographic origin. *J. chron. Dis.* 14, 259.
27. PERRY, H. M., JR., ERLANGER, M. W. & PERRY, E. F. (1979). Increase in the systolic pressure of rats chronically fed cadmium. *Environ. Hlth Perspect.* 28, 251.
28. PERRY, H. M., JR., ERLANGER, M. W. & PERRY, E. F. (1983). Effect of a second metal on cadmium-induced hypertension. *Arch. environ. Hlth* 38, 80.
29. KANNEL, W. B. & SORLIE, P. (1975). Hypertension in Framingham. In *Epidemiology and Control of Hypertension,* p. 553. Ed. by O. Paul.
30. MCCARRON, D. A., MORRIS, C. D. & COLE, C. (1982). Dietary calcium in human hypertension. *Science* 217, 267.
31. MCCARRON, D. A. (1983). Calcium and magnesium nutrition in human hypertension. *Ann. intern. Med.* 98, 800.
32. MCCARRON, D. A. (1982). Calcium, magnesium, and phosphorus balance in human and experimental hypertension. *Hypertension* Suppl. III, 27.
33. STITT, F. A., CRAWFORD, M. D., CLAYTON, D. G. & MORRIS, J. N. (1973). Clinical and biochemical indicators of cardiovascular disease among men living in hard and soft water areas. *Lancet* 1, 122.
34. PUNSAR, S., ERAMETSA, O., KAWONEN, M. J., et al. (1975). Coronary heart disease and drinking water. *J. chron. Dis.* 28, 259.
35. *Magnesium Deficiency and Hypertension. Nutr. Rev.* 1984: 42, 235.
36. FREIS, E. D. (1976). Salt, volume and the prevention of hypertension. *Circulation* 53, 589.
37. KEMPNER, W. (1948). Treatment of hypertensive vascular disease with rice diet. *Amer. J. Med.* 4, 545.
38. MENEELY, G. R. & BALL, C. O. (1957). Chronic sodium chloride toxicity and the protective effect of potassium chloride, Proc. Council for High Blood Pressure Research. *AHA* 6, 65.
39. PARIJS, J., JOOSENS, J. V., DER LINDEN, L. V. et al. (1973). Moderate sodium restriction and diuretics in the treatment of hypertension. *Amer. Heart J.* 85, 22.
40. *Multiple Risk Factor Intervention Trial Research Group.* (1982). Multiple risk factor intervention trial: Risk factor changes and mortality results. *JAMA* 248, 1465.
41. PERRY, H. M., JR & ERLANGER, M. (1982). Cadmium and hypertension: The effect of diet. *Trace Subst. environ. Hlth* 16, 280.

42. PERRY, H. M., JR., KOPP, S. J., ERLANGER, M. W. & PERRY, E. F. (1983). Cardiovascular effects of chronic barium ingestion. *Trace Subst. environ. Hlth* 17, 155.

43. KOPP, S. J., PERRY, H. M., JR., PERRY, E. F. & ERLANGER, M. (1983). Cardiac physiologic and tissue metabolic changes following chronic low-level cadmium and cadmium plus lead ingestion in the rat. *Toxicol. appl. Pharmacol.* 69, 149.

44. PERRY, H. M., JR., ERLANGER, M. & PERRY, E. F. (1977). Elevated systolic pressures following chronic low level cadmium feeding. *Amer. J. Physiol.* 232, H114.

45. SCHROEDER, H. A. (1964). Cadmium hypertension in rats. *Amer. J. Physiol.* 207, 62.

46. PERRY, H. M., JR. & ERLANGER, M. W. (1982). Effect of diet on increases in systolic pressure induced in rats by chronic cadmium feeding. *J. Nutr.* 112, 1983.

47. PETERING, H. G., MURTHY, L., SORENSEN, J. R., LEVIN, L. & STEMMER, K. L. (1979). Effect of sex on oral cadmium dose responses in rats: Blood pressure and pharmacodynamics. *Environ. Res.* 20, 289.

48. BOSCOLO, P., PROCELLI, G., CARMIONANI, M. & FINELLI, V. N. (1981). Urinary kallikrein and hypertension in cadmium-exposed rats. *Toxicol. Letters* 7, 189.

49. OHANIAN, E. V. & IWAI, J. (1979). Effects of cadmium ingestion in rats with opposite genetic predisposition to hypertension. *Environ. Hlth Perspect.* 38, 261.

50. REVIS, N. (1978). Possible mechanism for cadmium-induced hypertension in rats. *Life Sci.* 22, 479.

51. WALKER, H. L. & MOSES, H. A. (1979). Cadmium: Hypertension induction and lead mobilization. *J. Nat. Med. Ass.* 71, 1187.

52. DOYLE, J. J., BERNHOFT, R. A. & SANSTEAD, H. H. (1975). The effects of a low level of dietary cadmium and blood pressure, 24Na, 42K, and water retention in growing rats. *J. Lab clin. Med.* 86, 57.

53. EAKIN, D. J., WHANGER, P. D. & WESWIG, P. H. (1980). Cadmium and nickel influence on blood pressure, plasma renin, and tissue metal concentrations. *Amer. J. Physiol.* 238, 353.

54. LENER, J. & BIBR, B. (1970). Cadmium content in some food stuffs in respect of its biological effects. *Int. J. Vital Zivilisation* 14, 125.

55. PERRY, H. M., JR., ERLANGER, M. W. & PERRY, E. F. (1980). Inhibition of cadmium-induced hypertension in rats. *Sci. Total Environ.* 14, 153.

56. SCHROEDER, H. A. (1965). Cadmium as a factor in hypertension. *J. chron. Dis.* 18, 647.

57. PERRY, H. M., JR., PERRY, E. F. & ERLANGER, M. W. (1974). Reversal of cadmium-induced hypertension by selenium or hard water. *Trace Subst. environ. Hlth* 8, 51.

58. KARLICEK, B., TOPOLCAN, O., BILKOVA, L., KOTT, J. & SOVA, J. (1971). Stopove proky v. ledvinarch hypertoniku, stanovene metodou neutronve aktivacni analyzy. *Čas. Lék. čes.* 110, 756.

59. LENER, J. & BIBR, B. (1971). Cadmium and hypertension. *Lancet* 1, 970.

60. PERRY, H. M., JR. A preliminary examination of renal and hepatic cadmium and zinc in normotensive and hypertensive men from St. Louis (In preparation).

61. MORGAN, J. M. (1969). Tissue concentration in man. *Arch. intern. Med.* 123, 405.

62. SYVERSEN, T. L. M., STRAY, T. K., SYVERSEN, G. B. & OFSTAD, J. (1976). Cadmium and zinc in human liver and kidney. *Scand. J. clin. Lab. Invest.* 36. 251.
63. INDRAPRASIT, S., ALEXANDER, G. V. & GONIC, H. C. (1974). Tissue composition of major and trace elements in uremia and hypertension. *J. chron. Dis.* 27, 135.
64. OSTERGAARD, K. (1977). Cadmium and hypertension. *Lancet* 1, 677.
65. BEEVERS, D. G., ERSKINE, E., ROBERTSON, M. et al. (1976). Blood-lead and hypertension. *Lancet* 2, 1.
66. CALABRESE, E. J. & TUTHILL, R. W. (1978). Elevated blood pressure levels and community drinking water characteristics. *J. environ. Sci. Hlth* A13, 781.
67. DINGWALL-FORDYCE, I. & LANE, R. E. (1963). A followup study of lead workers. *Brit. J. ind. Med.* 20, 313.
68. PUNSAR, S., ERAMETSA, O., KARVONEN, M. J. et al. (1975). Coronary heart disease and drinking water: A search in two Finnish male cohorts for epidemiologic evidence of a water factor. *J. Chron. Dis.* 28, 259.
69. BATUMAN, V., LANDY, E., MAESAKA, J. K. & WEDEEN, R. P. (1983). Contribution of lead to hypertension with renal impairment. *New Engl. J. Med.* 309, 17.
70. PERRY, H. M., JR. (1981). Possible mechanisms of the hydralazine-related lupus-like syndrome. *Arthr. and Rheum.* 24, 1093.
71. PERRY, H. M., JR. & SCHROEDER, H. A. (1956). Studies on the control of hypertension. VI. Some evidence for reversal of the process during hexamethonium and hydralazine therapy. *Circulation* 13, 528.

Discussion (the paper by Perry)

Chairman: WESTER

CHRISTOPHERSEN: I would like to make a comment on the calcium and magnesium. We did a study in Norway where we compared areas with the same total hardness but with different calcium/magnesium ratios in the water, because we thought perhaps there should be less mortality with more magnesium. We found the opposite, that the mortality was lower where the calcium/magnesium ratio was higher. So we thought it might be explained best by assuming that it was due to a technical effect of calcium in preventing corrosion.

If you compare studies in Great Britain and in the United States, the United States has mostly a similar correlation coefficient for calcium and for magnesium when you study both elements, but in Great Britain there is a difference with better correlation for calcium and with magnesium insignificant. Obviously, the composition of the water in the United States must be correlated with the composition of the soil when you consider a large geographical area. Calcium in the drinking water has usually been correlated with calcium in the soil which, again, will be correlated with soil pH which in turn will influence the uptake of various nutrients and toxic elements in the plants. So there must be a false correlation. This food correlation will probably show better when you compare larger geographical areas and this is what we find in the United States. When you compare states, there is a better correlation between cardiovascular mortality and water hardness than if you only compare cities. But in Great Britain you find good correlation with cities and what I believe this means is that you have a toxic factor in water in Great Britain and that calcium might be a protecting factor. In the United States this factor is much less important than it is in Great Britain. If we ask what is different in the United States and Great Britain, the most plausible answer would be lead because of the utilization of lead pipes in the drinking water supply system in Great Britain. But, drinking water is only one of the environmental sources of lead, and what is the effect of the total lead intake?

PERRY: It is disturbing that questions regarding the correlation between hardness of water and cardiovascular mortality remain unresolved more that 20 years after a relationship was first proposed. This suggests to me either the involvement of some generally unsuspected factor(s), that the analytic methodology is inadequate to quantitate the culprit(s), or that the relationship is more complex than we have supposed. I do believe that the relationship is real, but the literature fails to provide me with a convincing candidate. Among the trace metals I would place lead as the most likely and cadmium as the next in line.

ANDERSON: I have a question regarding ion-exchange water softeners. These are certainly very popular in many regions of the United States. First of all, have there been any studies where they have looked at death rates in households where people used water softeners as opposed to non-water softener users? Second, what is your opinion of ion-exchange water softeners?

PERRY: There have been attempts to address the problem of water softeners—does water softened in this way have the same deleterious effect ascribed to normally occurring soft water? These attempts are not convincing. For one thing, many home water softeners in the United States are often installed to soften only the hot water and hence bypass drinking water. For another, the "soft water effect" was certainly present long before water softeners were widely used.

ANDERSON: I do use a water softener. Should I continue to use it or should I throw it out?

HURLEY: Get a hard water tap put on it.

ANDERSON: Would you agree with that?

PERRY: At the present time, I would have some hesitancy about using a water softener on my drinking water line.

HURLEY: You can use a water softener for your washing and have a hard water tap which is a very simple plumbing job and use that for your drinking water. That's what we've done.

ANDERSON: Yes, but if your drinking water has iron in it, it turns all your glasses orange.

HURLEY: Well, you take your choice—heart disease or orange glasses.

SALONEN: I'm a big believer in human studies, because I don't think humans are rats. You mentioned that the comparisons between hypertensives and normals have no value. Is that because you think hypertension effects renal cadmium concentration or what's the reason for your statement?

PERRY: First let me say that I am suggesting there are two kinds of toxicity associated with ingested cadmium. They differ in extent of exposure and in toxic manifestations. The first is the commonly accepted human industrial cadmium toxicity and involves long high exposure, with the toxic manifestations primarily involving the kidney which has accumulated a great deal of cadmium. The second effect is an entirely different one. It certainly can occur in rats but is unproven in man. It too involves prolonged exposure but at a much lower level; again the kidney is the organ with the highest accumulation but it is far less than occurs in industrial exposure. The manifestation is hypertension. It is worth emphasizing that hypertension is a major manifestation of human industrial exposure and it is not seen in animals after high exposures; and exposures make rats sick but not hypertensive.

Now, let me answer your specific question as to why I said that the available studies comparing renal cadmium concentrations in hypertensives and normotensives were of limited value. In simplest terms, our sampling technique is flawed, and we are not examining the material we should be examining. It is difficult to get autopsy samples, and that is what we need to examine tissue cadmium levels. The studies that have been done, therefore, involved very small numbers of subjects but the larger problem has to do with the appropriateness of the population sample. Only rarely do the hypertensives have early uncomplicated hypertension without other disease. Early uncomplicated hypertension is normally not fatal. Matching normotensives without disease are equally hard to find for the same reasons. Automobile accidents would seem to provide a possible source, but the most available of them are related to a distinct life style of drinking, drugs and fast driving. It should be emphasized that those who die of their hypertension or who have severe or malignant hypertension have end stage—disease or at least late—kidney disease, with much of the parenchyma, where the cadmium was located, having been replaced by fibrous tissue.

WESTER: When you are talking about the one factor, adverse or beneficial, I think we also have to consider the pathophysiology. You have made some points on hypertension, you have made some points on arrhythmias. If we consider the MRFIT study, there were more deaths than expected in the thiazide-treated group. You mentioned the hypokalemia. You said, also, that perhaps we should consider magnesium, because thiazides cause urinary losses of magnesium. That's true. What I would like to point out is that magnesium is essential for the potassium balance which is important for the development of arrhythmias. The membrane potential is built up by the relation between extra- and intracellular potassium and magnesium is necessary for the sodium potassium pump. So magnesium is an important factor for the relationship between extra- and intracellular potassium. If you get a magnesium deficiency you will change the ratio between the extra- and intracellular potassium, so you have in lack of magnesium a pathophysiological factor for developing arrhythmias. Another thing is also that magnesium is a calcium antagonist and it lowers blood pressure. So there are, indeed, pathophysiological reasons to point at magnesium as a possible factor.

PERRY: There is considerable evidence that magnesium may be involved in the "soft water effect". It is worth noting that I mentioned MRFIT because its results are causing considerable concern and because they could give us a lead to the etiology of the soft water effect which has not been emphasized before. Although there is concern, there is no evidence that the excess mortality was related to hypokalemia or to hypomagnesemia *or* that it was preceded by arrhythmias. There was one particular group that was responsible for the excess MRFIT deaths: These were the hypertensives who had pretreatment electrocardiographic abnormalities. That is really all we know at this time.

SHAMBERGER: In the United States we have at least a modest amount of lead and cadmium in our drinking water. A small amount of cadmium is in the air due to air pollution. We have some lead in our food because of the leaded gasoline we burn. Can you speculate, possibly, how these amounts that we take in compare to the amounts of lead and cadmium you gave your rats in the drinking water?

PERRY: On a "per kilogram" basis, the lowest intake of cadmium which regularly causes hypertension in our rats is higher than the average cadmium intake which is consumed in the United States or Europe, but it is equivalent to the intake which some 10 or 20% of Americans ingest—and here I am talking about general environmental exposure, not specific industrial exposure to cadmium. Probably somewhat more than 20% of Americans ingest the equivalent of what would be a pressor dose of lead for a rat. To extrapolate from a rat to a human being on the basis of intake per kg body weight, however, seems to be a very large assumption.

NORRMAN: The selenium content in the water was not measured. We could assume that in an area where you had hard water, the selenium content in the water and in the native crops would be higher than in other areas. Couldn't selenium perhaps add something to your answer because of the well-known interaction between selenium and cadmium?

PERRY: Yes, it is entirely possible that such an interaction occurs and has a significant effect. A WHO study looking at, among other things, selenium and cadmium in tissues of hypertensive and normotensive human beings has observed a significantly higher selenium level in the kidneys of normotensive subjects than in the kidneys of hypertensive subjects. In rat experiments, selenium can block the pressor effect of cadmium. The data, as you indicated, are too limited to go much further at the present time. Moreover, the WHO experiments I am citing here have the same flaws I mentioned above, i.e. the samples were very small and probably not "representative".

CHRISTOPHERSEN: I would like to ask, if you are aware of any studies on the effects of cadmium and lead, each of them alone and together, on the metabolism of heme and myoglobin levels in the heart, and the importance this might have for myocardial infarction because it is, of course, well known that lead inhibits the heme biosynthesis. It is also known that various toxic metals can induce heme oxygenase in the liver. I don't think this has ever been studied in the heart. Myoglobin is obviously very important for the oxygen supply in the heart, so that if you get an inhibition of the heme synthesis in the heart together with accelerated heme degradation, you get a change in the myoglobin concentration as a result of this. This would have the same effect on the oxygen supply as constriction on the coronary arteries. All together they will probably work synergistically with respect to each other.

PERRY: No, I am not aware of any such studies. When considering the mechanism of the soft water effect, a major problem is that we are talking about an event rate—and they are "all-or-none" events—that involves a few individuals in a large population. At present it is simply not practical to measure a parameter like heme synthesis in the large population at risk, and it might be difficult to interpret in the involved individuals after a catastrophe has occurred.

AGGETT: I would just like to invite Dr Perry, if he can, to say if there is any information at all on the differential effects of cadmium and lead on diastolic and systolic blood pressure and, also, if it has any effect on the blood pressure response to stress?

PERRY: There are no such data on human beings that I know about, and I know of no differential effect on systolic versus diastolic pressure in animals. In our experience diastolic pressure follows systolic pressure. Of course, stress that results in catechol release might be expected to induce a temporary dissociation beween systolic and diastolic pressures. If one is seeking a real and persistent differential effect in man, however, the most likely mechanism would seem to involve an increased (or decreased) rate of progression of arteriosclerosis with its loss of arterial elasticity and resultant increase in systolic pressure relative to diastolic pressure.

BERLIN: Dr Perry, are you aware of any data concerning the hard water effect on smokers and non-smokers? There is a two-fold difference in cadmium intake in these two groups. It would be very interesting to learn if there are any studies on these two different groups.

PERRY: I know of no such data. Obviously smokers have a higher intake and a higher body burden of cadmium. There is of course the question of whether the precise intracellular location of cadmium is the same for inhaled cadmium. In addition there is the peculiar maximum at about age 50 for the body burden of cadmium. Why does it occur and does it occur earlier in smokers with their higher body burdens? Does it occur because those with the highest values die, because the aging process leads to a reduction in renal parenchyma which binds the cadmium, or is cadmium excreted without the loss of renal parenchyma? Answers to these questions would improve our understanding.

DANIELSON: Dr Perry, in the United States chelation therapy is used, for instance, in order to reduce the risk of cardiovascular disease, for example hypertension, by binding heavy metals. Have you any comment on whether that method is effective or not?

PERRY: The potent chelator EDTA certainly has some effect when injected into man. The calcium chelate of EDTA temporarily lowers circulating cholesterol more dramatically than anything else I know of. It will also produce fever if given in high enough doses! Its toxic effect may result from scavenging any available metals in the body and releasing them in the kidney as a result of a pH change. It is not, however, very effective in lowering blood pressure acutely, and of course it is impractical to use daily injections over a long period of time to determine its chronic effect. When given orally, 0.5 to 1% is absorbed. This can be enough to lower elevated levels of cholesterol and to cause xanthomata to regress; we have not tested the antihypertensive effect of chronic oral EDTA.

You are correct, there are those who advocate weekly injections of EDTA to prevent heart attacks. I am afraid that some of our early work is responsible for some of what is being done in the United States; however, we do not use EDTA in this manner, and I know of no evidence that it is beneficial.

Zinc Metabolism in Alcoholic Cirrhosis

By Kaare Weismann

Liver cirrhosis is the first human disease in which alteration in Zn metabolism has been documented. Vikbladh (44) in 1951, using the dithizone method for analysis, reported lowered serum Zn levels in cirrhotic patients. A few years later Vallee at al. (42, 43) performed more extensive Zn studies on alcoholic liver cirrhosis. They found low serum Zn levels associated with hyperzincuria and decreased Zn content in the liver. The changes in Zn metabolism have been corroborated by several later reports (37). The degree of aberrant Zn metabolism seems to reflect the severity of liver disease, but is useless in differentiating the various forms of cirrhosis.

So far it remains unknown whether the abnormal Zn metabolism is involved in the pathogenesis of the disease, or it is a harmless secondary phenomenon. It is also unknown if alcoholic cirrhosis benefits from additional Zn and if the patients should be treated with Zn supplementation.

In the following, characteristic abnormalities observed in the Zn metabolism of cirrhotic patients, their causes and significance will be discussed (Table I).

Table I Some pathogenic factors involved in the altered Zn metabolism of alcoholic cirrhosis

Possible causes	Observation
Inadequate nutrition Ethanol Hypoalbuminæmia Dysproteinaemia	Hypozincaemia
Increased tubular secretion of Zn Increased Zn absorption	Hyperzincuria
Defective metallothionein synthesis Decreased Zn uptake in liver cells	Low hepatic Zn

NUTRITIONAL FACTORS

There is a continuous loss of Zn with urine, faeces, sweat, desquamated cells from hair, skin and mucous membranes, accounting for 1 to 2 mg Zn per day. This calls for a net supply of the same magnitude to maintain Zn equilibrium in the body. Under normal conditions a nutritional supply of 15 mg Zn daily in adults is considered safe. If the absorption is blocked, the loss increased or the need for Zn is augmented due to weight gain or repletion of preexisting Zn deficiency, considerably larger amounts will have to be supplied. The most important Zn source in the diet is protein-rich products of animal origin. Red meat contains on average 37 mg Zn/kg (wet weight), and cheese about 57 mg Zn/kg (30). Extremely high Zn concentrations are found in shellfish, oysters containing up to 1,000 mg Zn/kg. Legumes, nuts, whole grain and leafy vegetables are additional important Zn sources, but due to the variable presence of fibers and phytate, Zn is generally less available than from animal protein. A daily Zn supply of 15 mg is supplied with about 100 g animal protein, the nitrogen : zinc ratio being about 1,000 : 1. Beverages, tea, coffee and fruits are poor Zn sources. Very low Zn concentrations are found in wine, spirits and beer. Danish beer contains 10 to 50 μg Zn/l. This means that a person living on 18 to 20 bottles of beer per day receives less than 2% of the recommended Zn allowance. To cover this would demand an intake of about 300 l beer daily. Addiction to beer, wine and spirits leads to an insufficient Zn supply in consequence of the low Zn content and the poor appetite and eating associated with the abuse. The most unfortunate in this respect would be an alcoholic vegetarian if such a combination is likely to exist. In a clinical study comprising 36 alcoholics attending an out-patients' clinic for alcoholics, all patients had normal serum Zn levels. All were well-nourished and had at least one hot meal daily (29). Other studies have shown hypozincaemia to be present in about 50% of alcoholics without cirrhosis, probably reflecting severe addiction and poor general condition of the patients (319).

HYPOZINCAEMIA AND ALTERED SERUM PROTEINS IN LIVER CIRRHOSIS

Low serum Zn levels in liver cirrhosis have been reported by several investigators (37, 42–44). Hypozincaemia can be found in approximately 70% of alcoholic cirrhotics but the frequency much depends on the general condition of the patients and the stage of disease. Zn circulates in serum bound to proteins and to a minor degree ultrafiltrable amino acid complexes and low-molecular ligands. About 70 to 80% of total serum Zn is albumin-Zn, and roughly estimated 18 to 28% is firmly bound to circulating α_2-macroglobulin. The albumin level is physiologically decreased in old age and is associated with a moderately lowered serum Zn level. The two parameters have been found to be positively correlated (53). In liver cirrhosis, plasma albumin is decreased, which partly explains the hypozincaemia frequently associated with the disease. In a clinical study on Zn therapy in stable alcoholic cirrhosis 60% of the patients had subnormal plasma albumin levels (49). Of these, the majority, 70% had normal serum Zn values. There were 10 cases of hypozincaemia, all of them associated with hypoalbuminaemia (Fig. 1). No case of low serum Zn concentration associated with a normal plasma albumin level was found. The moderately lowered serum Zn level was partly explicable by the cirrhotic dysproteinaemia although a defective Zn metabolism and other mechanisms may have been involved.

A normal serum Zn level despite a low plasma albumin concentration may reflect an increase in other Zn binding proteins and compunds in serum, or a raised albumin-Zn fraction. Albumin contains 16 imidazol groups per mole, to which Zn, copper, cadmium, and lead can compete to bind in a 1:1 molar ratio (14). Under normal conditions about 10 µmol/l of a total serum Zn level

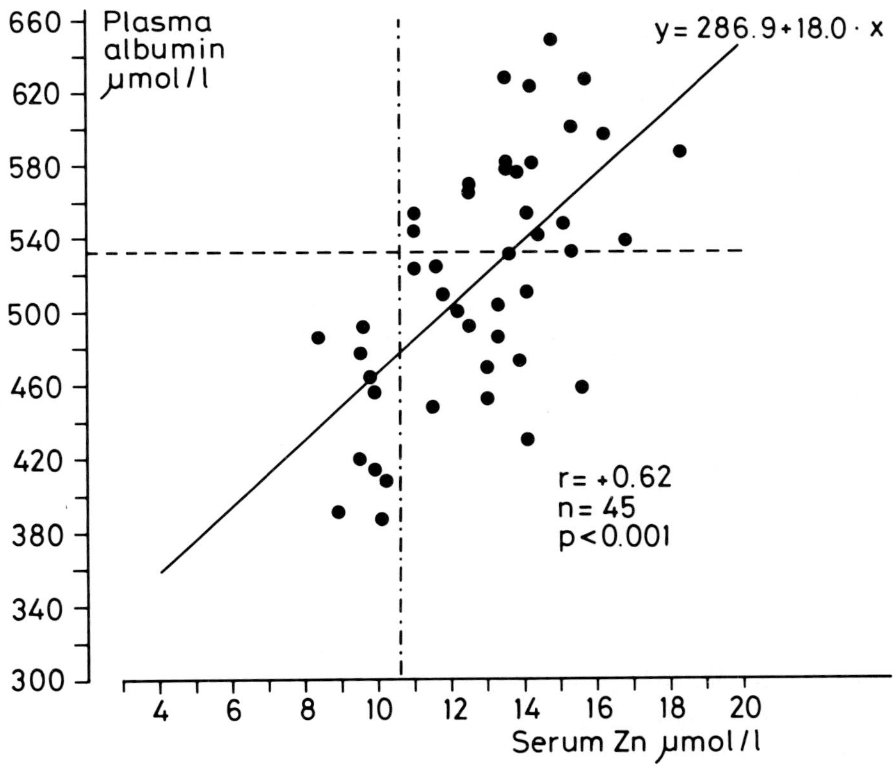

Fig. 1 Positive correlation between plasma albumin and serum Zn levels in alcoholic cirrhosis

Dashed line denotes lower normal limit for plasma albumin (normal range 532 to 813 µmol/1). Dotted-dashed line indicates the lower normal limit for serum Zn (normal range 10.6 to 18.9 µmol/l)

of 13 μmol/l is albumin-Zn. If plasma albumin is 600 μmol/l the theoretical maximum binding of Zn is 9,600 μmol, or about a thousand times more than under normal conditions. If albumin is reduced to 300 μmol/l, a value often seen in cirrhosis, an unchanged total serum Zn concentration would be maintained by involving an extra 0.2% of the albumin binding for Zn. The relation between Zn and albumin, however, is more complicated than considered here. Other divalent cations compete with Zn for identical binding sites and there is reduced affinity of albumin for Zn in cirrhosis (12). The change in binding properties of albumin is believed to be related to increased concentrations of free fatty acids and bilirubin which also bind to the albumin, but a full explanation for the findings remains to be established.

In cirrhosis there are often increased levels of serum IgG. Boyett and Sullivan (5) found significant amounts of Zn bound to the IgG, about three times more than in normals. They also demonstrated Zn binding to transferrin in cirrhotic samples which in one case exceeded the α_2-macroglobulin-Zn level. It was concluded that the bulk of serum Zn in cirrhosis is bound to albumin and a reduction in albumin concentration is associated with a reduction in the serum Zn level, specifically Zn bound to albumin. There was a positive correlation between albumin-bound Zn and total serum Zn ($r = +0.89$) (5).

HYPERZINCURIA IN CIRRHOSIS

Vallee et al. (42, 43) demonstrated increased urinary Zn excretion, about twice the amount of normals in their original reports on alcoholic liver cirrhosis. A loss of this magnitude is significant in patients whose Zn nutrition may be suffering due to nutritional factors and advanced liver disease. The cause of the hypozincuria is not clear. Some have tried to explain it by an increased fraction of diffusible Zn in serum, but as yet such a fraction has not been identified. Studies on the amino acid excretion with urine of cirrhotics have shown decreased levels of taurine, aspargine/glutamine, histidine and 3-methyl-histidine (37). Thus, an increased Zn loss related to an augmented amino acid excretion is not the explanation. Other studies have revealed a positive correlation between urinary creatin and Zn levels, so possibly the urinary Zn loss is a consequence of protein catabolism under conditions of an inadequate protein nutrition (9). It remains to be defined to which extent diuretic therapy interferes with the hyperzincuria in cirrhosis (see further on p. 230). A role of ethanol is also to be considered. Earlier studies failed to show consistant changes in the urinary excretion of Zn after administration of ethanol to normal adults and alcoholics with or without cirrhosis (36, 39). Later studies reported a significant increase in urinary Zn and lowered serum Zn levels after ingestion of ethanol (13). In five alcoholic subjects admitted to the ward for one month, ethanol was supplied to maintain a blood level of 100 mg/100 ml (31). The urinary Zn excretion was increased about twofold during the ethanol ingestion as compared with the ethanol-free period. Serum Zn decreased, only to bounce back to normal values after ethanol had been discontinued. In Zn-deficient rats ethanol adds to the Zn depletion by increasing urinary Zn as demonstrated by Ahmed and Russell (2). Concurrent with the urinary loss, or triggered off by it, there is a significant reduction in Zn of testes, liver, spleen, kidneys and hair, and a higher faecal Zn loss than in the Zn-deficient control animals not receiving ethanol. The mechanism of action of ethanol is not known. Ethanol impairs the Zn absorption (2) and may act on the renal tubular handling of filtered Zn. It may also have an effect on the release of hepatic Zn and storage of Zn in the liver.

ABSORPTION OF ZINC

Normals. In a human study on normal humans, Matseshe et al. (20) demonstrated that the amount of Zn in the intestinal lumen passing the ligament of Treitz was greater than the quantity ingested with the meal. The step-up in Zn concentration of the chyme is propably mainly due to delivery of pancreatic juice and bile into the intestinal lumen. The amount of Zn reaching the distal ileum is only slightly less than supplied with the meal itself. This indicates that Zn is reabsorbed in the distal small intestine. It was estimated (20) that about 7.5 to 14.4 mg endogenous Zn is exposed to the chyme each day. A similar quantity is ingested with the food, so the intestine receives two equivalent meals of Zn, one exogenous from the diet and one endogenous from duodenal secretions. Because of the selective concentration of Zn by the pancreas and the role of Zn in pancreatic enzymes such as carboxypeptidases, it is assumed that the pancreatic secretion rather than the bile contributes to the majority of endogenous Zn secretion (8). By the use of whole-body counting technique and ^{65}Zn as radionuclide, Zn absorption has been studied repeatedly in man (for reveiw see 35). After an oral ^{65}Zn dose the radioactivity is measured by intervals until the elimination of retained ^{65}Zn becomes stable. By extrapolation back to the time of ^{65}Zn administration an estimate of the absorbed fraction can be obtained (so-called net absorption). In some studies the values are corrected for the endogenous loss by a factor obtained by intravenously administered ^{65}Zn (so-called fractional absorption) (1). This yields absorption values which are about 20% higher. The mean absorption of ^{65}Zn in various studies has ranged from 38% to 69% (1, 35). The fractional absorption values of the study by Aamodt et al. (1) ranged from 40 to 86%, with a mean of 65%, following a Gaussian distribution. In an additional study net absorption of ^{65}Zn ranged from 27 to 65%, mean 43% (50). The variance in the absorption values of Zn is explained by different methods of calculation, experimental conditions, fasting or non-fasting of the patients and the vehicle used for ^{65}Zn.

Cirrhosis. ^{65}Zn absorption was studied in 10 ambulatory patients with compensated liver cirrhosis by means of whole-body counting technique (22). The net absorption ranged from 27 to 90% with a mean value of 69%. The results are significantly increased as compared to the normal mean value of 42% and a range of 27 to 65% (50). This indicates an intact Zn absorption and rules out Zn malabsorption as the cause of the low serum Zn values in these patients. The cause of the increased absorption of Zn is unclear. It could be due to a primary defect in the absorption mechanisms, or a secondary phenomenon related to increased urinary loss of Zn or a reduced pool size (reduced hepatic Zn?). The ^{65}Zn half-life was increased significantly, 156 versus 103 days in normal controls. Previous studies on the kinetics of intravenously administered ^{65}Zn have indicated a diminished Zn pool size in cirrhosis and a slower elimination of retained ^{65}Zn (38).

Oral Zn tolerance tests performed in cirrhotic patients have shown a significant reduction in the serum Zn increase, determined as the time-concentration integral of the curve, as compared to normal controls (4). The results are apparently at variance with those obtained by whole-body counting, but the methods are not comparable. By the oral Zn test the change in the serum Zn levels occurring within a few hours after administration can only be taken as a semiquantitative measure of Zn absorption. A rapid turnover of absorbed Zn (redistribution within the body, increased rate of urinary excretion and endogenous intestinal secretion) will lead to low serum Zn levels just as well as malabsorption of the element will do. Furthermore, Zn binding to serum proteins in cirrhosis differs substantially from normal conditions. The Zn salt also plays a role. In cirrhosis, oral Zn sulphate was found equivalent to Zn dipicolinate, whereas in case of pancreatic insufficiency the picolinate was superior to the sulphate (4).

METHALLOTHIONEIN AND ZINC IN THE LIVER

The liver plays a central role in the metabolism of Zn. Human and animal studies have indicated that a major part of absorbed Zn is temporarily stored in the liver (7, 50). When the liver Zn concentration exceeds a level of about 30 μg/g, extra Zn is bound to *de novo* synthesized metallothionein (7). Actinomycin D, cordycepin and cycloheximide block the formation of metallothionein whereby the hepatic accumulation of Zn can be stopped. Metallothionein has a short half-life of 18 to 20 hrs and concomitantly with proteolysis the tightly bound metal is set free. Glucocorticoids cause a marked rise in hepatic Zn accumulation after a lag of about 4 hrs. The accumulation can be suppressed by actinomycin D and cycloheximide. It appears that the hepatic metallothionein and mRNA synthesis induced by glucocorticoids is indirectly caused by an enhancing effect on the hepatocellular Zn uptake (7). Glucagon has a synergistic effect on the glucocorticoid stimulation of the Zn accumulation, but the facilitation is not dependant on mRNA synthesis and cannot be blocked by cytostatics.

Whether these complicated mechanisms remain intact in cirrhosis is not known. It is possible that the equilibrium is disturbed in advanced cases of cirrhosis and that the liver storage for Zn decreases as the active hepatocytes are replaced with metabollically inactive collagen.

ZINC CONTENT IN THE CIRRHOTIC LIVER

Several reports have documented a significantly reduced Zn concentration in the cirrhotic liver (6, 19, 42). It is only partly explicable by increased amounts of collagen which has a low Zn content compared with the liver cells. Boyett and Sullivan (6) determined the Zn concentration in autopsied livers and found a 50% reduction in the content of 43 specimens. A decrease in Zn concentration was verified in 1980 by Kiilerich et al. (19). They performed analyses of liver biopsies performed *in vivo* and corrected the Zn concentration to the mass of the liver cells. In 24 patients with alcoholic liver disease (9 with fatty liver and 15 with cirrhosis) the liver Zn concentration was reduced by about 30%. It is believed that the low liver Zn content indicates a depletion of body Zn, although there is no definite proof of this notion. The question arises whether the low Zn content is primary or secondary to the cirrhosis and whether the hepatic Zn depletion bears any relation to the well-known changed biochemical functions of the organ. Experimental studies have shown that Zn supplementation ameliorates the CCl_4-induced liver damage. It has long been generally accepted that the effect is due to interference of Zn ions with lipid peroxidation of the cell membrane and, additionally, an inhibition of the macrophage function. A recent experimental study shows that Zn probably also has a direct effect on the CCl_4-induced collagen formation by inhibiting proline hydroxylase which mediates a crucial step in the collagen synthesis (3).

Leucocyte Zn has been found reduced in cirrhotics (18) which indicates that other nucleated tissues apart from the liver are depleted of Zn in cirrhosis. Jackson et al. (17) have evaluated which organs and tissues show the lowest Zn levels during dietary deprivation of Zn. Using experimental rats receiving a Zn-depleted diet, a 30% decrease in total body Zn was demonstrated. There were no consistent changes in the Zn content of skeletal muscles, hair, skin or heart, whereas a significant reduction was found in liver, plasma, bone and testes. Analysis of human tissues have indicated that man reacts to Zn deficiency in a similar way as rats. The finding in cirrhosis of a low liver Zn concentration together with decreased serum Zn and leucocyte levels may therefore point to a general Zn deficiency associated with the disease rather than a selective Zn depletion of the liver.

ZINC ENZYMES AND THE LIVER

A large number of mammalian enzymes contain Zn or depend on the presence of Zn. So far about 70 different Zn enzymes have been identified in various species and tissues. Examples are alcohol dehydrogenase, aldolase, δ-aminolaevulinic acid dehydratase (δ-ALAD), NADH diaphorase and carbonic anhydrase. Zn is involved in both DNA and RNA synthesis as originally demonstrated on liver cells by Fujioka and Lieberman (11). In cirrhosis, lack of Zn or redistribution of Zn to other binding sites might cause alterations in the biochemistry of the liver. At present little is known about such possible changes of the activity of Zn enzymes related to a decreased Zn content in the liver. Such studies would be of great interest to enlighten the question about the significance of Zn depletion and the need for Zn supplementation in cirrhosis.

ZINC AND VITAMIN A

In the Zn-deficient, rat serum Zn and serum vitamin A are depressed. Vitamin A supplementation fails to restore the vitamin A levels to normal, whereas Zn therapy has such an effect (32–34). Zn is believed to stimulate the synthesis of retinol-binding protein which is essential for hepatic release of vitamin A and for the serum transport of the vitamin (about 95% of total serum vitamin A circulates with retinol-binding protein, forming complexes with prealbumin in a 1: 1 molar ratio).

Patients with alcoholic cirrhosis may suffer from night blindness usually attributable to hypovitaminosis A (26). But not all patients are curable by vitamin A. This may be due to a concomitant Zn deficiency as recently shown by Morrison et al. (23). They reported five patients with alcoholic liver cirrhosis and night blindness, who all showed reversal to normal dark adaptation thresholds with Zn replacement. Two of the patients initially had received vitamin A 10,000 IU per day for 2 to 4 weeks without any beneficial effect. When oral Zn sulphate 220 mg per day was added for 1 to 2 weeks, their dark adaptation was restored to normal. In a similar study (21) six night-blind patients with alcoholic cirrhosis and depressed serum Zn levels failed to improve by vitamin A therapy, whereas 660 mg of Zn sulphate daily restored the dark adaptation to normal in all patients. Russell et al. (32) performed a study on cirrhosis aimed at evaluating whether the increase in vitamin A concentrations after oral supplementation of the vitamin was due to release of hepatic vitamin A (retinol) or to an increased absorption of retinyl esters. It was demonstrated that the primary defect in cirrhosis was that of the hepatic vitamin A release. In two patients, vitamin A therapy failed to normalize the dark adaptation. Both had subnormal serum Zn concentrations below 65 g per 100 ml (10 μmol/l). The dark adaptation became normal after one week's therapy with 220 mg Zn sulphate daily.

Table II Some drugs interfering with normal Zn absorption

Drug	Effect	Studied on	Citation	
Phenytoin	increase	rats	Weismann et al.	1978 (52)
D-penicillamine	increase	rats	Weismann & Knudsen	1978 (48)
Iodochlorohydroxyquin (Vioform)	increase	rats	Weismann & Knudsen	1978 (48)
Tetracycline hydrochloride	decrease	rats	Weismann et al.	1978 (51)
Diethyldithiocarbamate	increase	rats	this study	

Another area of a possible Zn–vitamin A interaction in cirrhosis is the interconversion of vitamin A (retinol) to retinal in the retina. The reaction involves catalysis by NAD and a specific alcohol dehydrogenase, denounced retinal reductase or retinol dehydrogenase. Several mammalian alcohol dehydrogenases have been identified to be Zn metalloenzymes. Huber and Gershoff (16) studied the effects of Zn deficiency on retinol dehydrogenase activity in the adult male rat. The conversion of retinol to retinal, which is crucial for the formation of rhodopsin, was significantly reduced. The activity of the enzyme was depressed in the testes, but not in the liver. Another enzyme involved in vitamin A metabolism, retinol oxidase, also displayed a reduced activity. Zn deficiency causes marked morphological changes of the testes. Cirrhosis is often associated with gonadal dysfunction and testicular atrophy which might bear relation to a combined deficiency of Zn and vitamin A.

ZINC METABOLISM AND DRUGS

It is important to consider the current medication when evaluating a patient's Zn metabolism, because drugs may change serum Zn, urinary Zn levels and the absorption of Zn (Tables II and III). Many cirrhotics receive diuretic therapy to control oedema and ascites. Often the medication con-

Table III Some drugs affecting the serum Zn level

Drug	Effect	Studied on	Citation	
Glucocortiocoids	decrease	humans	Flynn et al.	1971 (10)
Thiazides	increase	humans	Wester	1975 (54)
Loop-diuretics	increase	humans	Wester	1980 (55)
Disulfiram (Antabuse)	increase	humans	Rasmussen & Tønnesen	1984 (29)
Diiodohydroxyquin (Diiodoquin)	increase	humans	Neldner & Hambidge	1975 (24)
Clofibrate	decrease	rats	Powanda et al.	1978 (27)
Birth control pill	(decrease)	humans	Prasad et al.	1975 (27)
Spironolactone	nil	humans	Szadkowski et al.	1969 (41)

sists of aldosterone antagonists, thiazides and loop-diuretics. Neither aldosterone nor spironolactone cause any significant changes in the Zn metabolism (41). Furosemide, thiazides and chlorthalidone cause a slight increase in the serum Zn concentration of normal subjects (54). The urinary Zn excretion is increased 60 to 65% by bendroflumethiazide, chlorthalidone and hydrochlorthiazide, an effect that persists during prolonged treatment. Half of the extra excretion is attributable to a rise in Zn concentration, the other half to an increased urine volume (55). Loop-diuretics cause a diminished urinary Zn concentration, but the amount of excreted Zn is augmented due to the large urine volume produced. The mode of action is believed to be an enhanced Zn absorption or tissue release of Zn, first of all in the liver. Wester (54) found evidence in favour of this explanation by showing a decreased Zn concentration in livers from patients who had been treated with diuretics.

Antabuse® (disulfiram) possesses heretofore neglected effects on divalent metals such as nickel and Zn. In an open study, six normal volunteers and 16 alcoholic patients were given oral disulfiram 400 mg daily for four weeks (29). All had normal pretreatment serum Zn values. There was a significant increase, averaging 20% (range −5 to +50%), in the serum Zn level equally present in patients and controls. The results indicate an enhancing effect on Zn absorption in accordance with ^{65}Zn absorption studies performed on rats receiving 100 mg dithiocarbamate by mouth daily (Table IV). Dithiocarbamate is chemically related to disulfiram, and has strong chelating effects on divalent heavy metal ions (Fig. 2). The ^{65}Zn retention curves show a significantly increased net absorption of 45.3 ± 7.1% (mean ± S.D.), range 34 to 56%, as compared with the normal values of 37.0 ± 6.9% (Fig. 3). The findings indicate that disulfiram and dithiocarbamate chelate Zn ions in the intestinal lumen or in the mucosal cells and hereby enhance the absorption of Zn. The effect seems to be similar to that of halogenated 8-hydroxyquinolines and D-penicillamine as studied in rats (48). 8-hydroxyquinolines were formerly used in the treatment of acrodermatitis enteropathica and probably act by enhancing Zn absorption. Neldner and Hambidge (24) showed a 50% increase in the serum Zn level of a patient suffering from acrodermatitis enteropathica who was started on a daily oral dose of 2.6 g diiodoquin.

Table IV Effect of oral dithiocarbamate (Dithiocarb) on ^{65}Zn absorption in experimental rats

	Dithiocarbamate 100 mg/day (n=6)		Controls (n=8)
Net absorption, percent (mean ± S.D.)	45.3 ± 7.1		37.0 ± 6.9
Biological half-life, days (mean ± S.D.)	16.2 ± 2.2		19.2 ± 2.7
		$p < 0.05$	

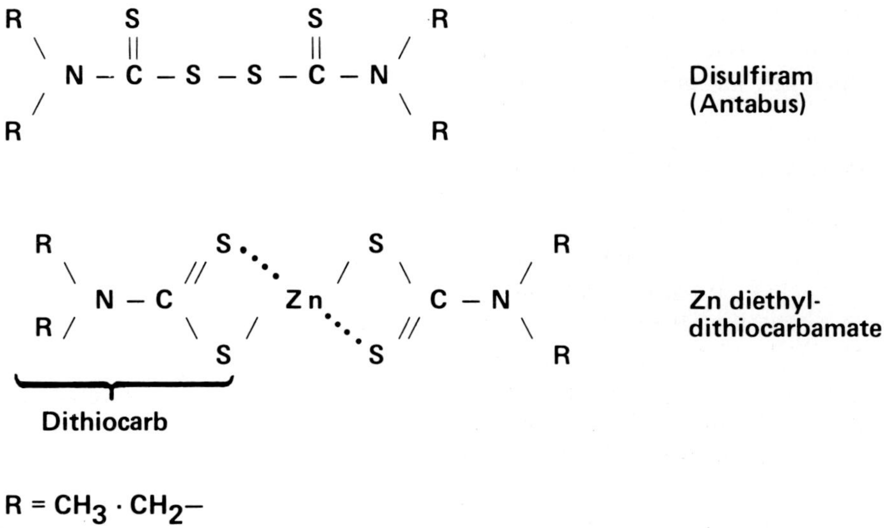

Fig. 2 After absorption disulfiram is believed to undergo chemical reactions which lead to its reduction to the parent thiol diethyldithiocarbamate

Chelation of Zn by diethyldithiocarbamate in a 2:1 molar ratio is indicated

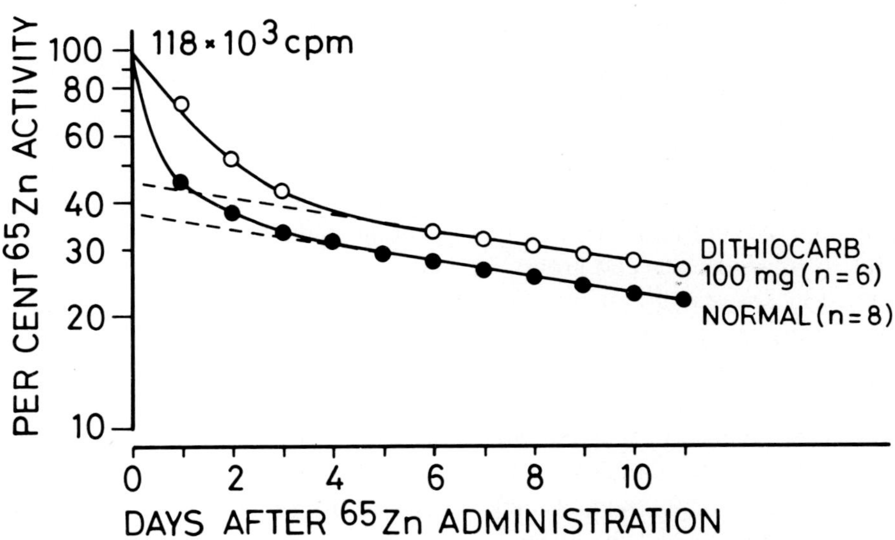

Fig. 3 Whole-body retention of orally administered ^{65}Zn (0.7 μCi $^{65}ZnCl_2$ with a specific activity of 1 mCi per mg Zn) in diethyldithiocarbamate-treated rats (100 mg orally per day) and in untreated normal rats

Mean values are indicated. Net absorption and biological half-life of ^{65}Zn are seen in Table IV

Whether disulfiram and dithiocarbamate have similar effects on Zn absorption in acrodermatitis entereopathica would be interesting to know but apparently has never been studied.

ORAL ZINC SUPPLEMENTATION IN LIVER CIRRHOSIS

In the investigations by Vallee et al. (42, 43) it was noted that the bromsulphalein test improved in six patients with alcoholic cirrhosis who were given 20 mg oral Zn daily. There were no controls and the subjects were benefiting from hospital care and abstinence from alcohol. Hammond et al. (15) treated 15 ambulatory patients with alcoholic cirrhosis or post-necrotic cirrhosis with 90 mg oral Zn daily for three months. In ten of the patients the bromsulphalein retention was studied during Zn therapy and placebo supplementation. No effect of Zn apart from a rise in serum Zn was detected.

Sullivan et al. (40) investigated the effect of 50 mg oral Zn daily to 16 hospitalized patients with advanced decompensated liver cirrhosis treated in the hospital ward. The mean serum Zn increased from about 9 μmol/l to 13 μmol/l after one week. Urinary Zn rose from an elevated pretreatment mean value of 2,000 μg Zn to 3,200 μg Zn per 24 hrs. Routine serum liver enzymes, bilirubin, cholesterol and ammonia levels declined during the hospitalization. The authors did not consider the improvement to be mediated by the Zn supplementation. Their aim was primarily to study the effect of Zn on serum and urinary Zn levels in cases of severe cirrhosis.

In a randomized double-blind clinical trial (49), 16 patients with biopsy-verified alcoholic cirrhosis received 600 mg Zn sulphate and 14 patients placebo for six weeks. All were in a stable phase and had been controlled regularly in the out-patients clinic. Only 22% of the patients showed subnormal serum Zn levels, in all cases associated with a decreased plasma albumin concentration (Fig. 1). Except for an unexplained fall in the plasma IgG level in the placebo group, statistically significant changes were only noted in Zn-treated patients (Fig. 4). As expected, there was a significant rise in the mean serum Zn level from 13.3 to 17.4 μmol/l. Plasma prothrombin increased from 0.85 to 0.94 arbitrary units, and serum bilirubin showed a decrease from a mean value of 12.9 to 10.1 μmol/l. As seen from Fig. 4, the mean serum alkaline activity rose from 270 to 304 U/l, but the change only reached statistical significance after two weeks. Serum vitamin A remained unaltered whereas serum carotene decreased from 1.11 to 0.91 μmol/l. The taste function, which has been suggested as a functional measure of Zn deficiency, was studied by a semiquantitative test by which the patients recognize increasing concentrations of sucrose, sodium chloride, citric acid and quinine chloride. The overall taste acuity improved significantly in the Zn-supplemented group. Three patients on Zn sulphate declared that their well-being had improved during the trial. These patients displayed a marked

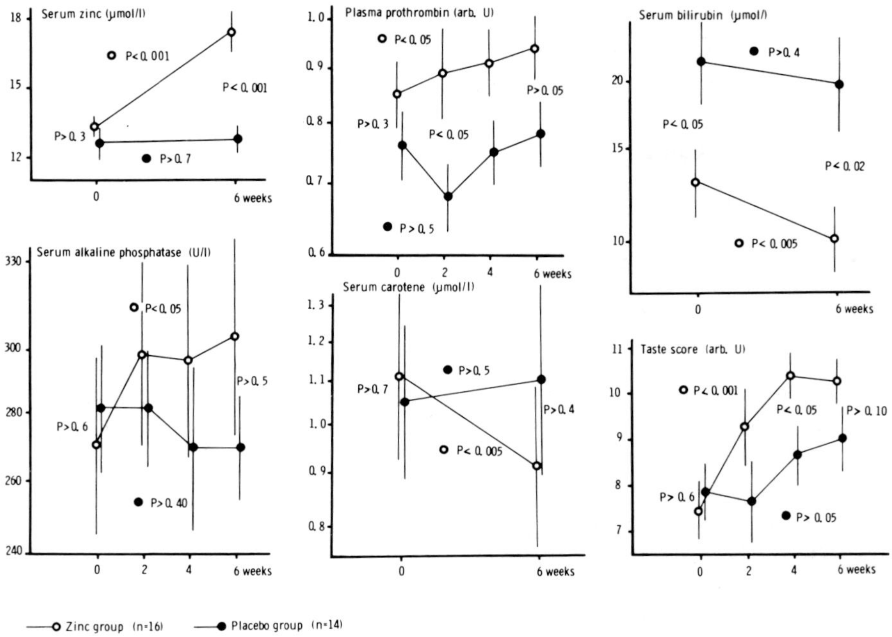

Fig. 4 Results of Zn sulphate supplementation 0.6 g daily and placebo in alcoholic liver cirrhosis

Sixteen patients received Zn and 14 patients the placebo for six weeks. Single open and closed circles indicate p-values as calculated by paired t-test of values before and after six weeks. Otherwise the p-value is calculated by unpaired t-test, comparing the results of the two groups. Vertical lines denote S.E.M. Prothrombin, bilirubin, alkaline phosphatase and carotene levels are not normally distributed. The ordinates are logarithmic and the mean is calculated as the antilog of the mean of logarithmic values. Likewise, the S.E.M. in these cases is based on the logarithmic values. (49)

increase in the taste and smell acuity. They had essentially normal serum Zn, vitamin A and carotene levels.

The dark adaptation was evaluated by a Goldmann–Weeker adaptometer, and the colour vision by Ishikara's test and pseudoisochromatic plates. The investigations failed to disclose significant changes by Zn therapy (Table V). In view of the low prevalence and the overall moderately disturbed Zn metabolism of the group combined with a relatively low incidence of night blindness in cirrhosis, the results are perhaps not unexpected.

The fall in serum carotene concentration might reflect an increased conversion of carotene to retinaldehyde, retinol and retinyl esters, processes which take place in the mucosal epithelial cells (31). An effect of Zn is a possibility, but remains to be studied further.

It is conceivable that the beneficial effects of Zn supplementation in cirrhosis is due to restoration of a marginal Zn deficiency. The rise in serum

Table V Dark adaptation threshold values in alcoholic cirrhotics before and after oral Zn sulphate and placebo (49)

	Zn sulphate group (n=16)		Placebo group (n=14)	
	Before	After 6 weeks	Before	After 6 weeks
Normal	4	5	5	4
Border-line	11	7	9	6
Abnormal	1	4	0	4
		$p>0.05$		

alkaline phosphatase activity in the Zn group supports this notion. Alkaline phosphatase is a metalloenzyme containing 4 Zn atoms per molecule enzyme. In Zn deficiency in acrodermatitis enteropathica and in prolonged total parenteral nutrition, serum alkaline phosphatase activity is depressed but returns to normal with Zn supplementation (45). The activity runs a parallel course with the serum Zn level, and the correlation coefficient has been found statistically significant. In a recent study, it was demonstrated that serum alkaline phosphatase activity does not increase in normozincaemic patients receiving oral Zn sulphate supplementation (47).

In *biliary cirrhosis*, the liver copper is increased. Penicillamine, a copper chelating agent, has been shown to improve the survival time of the patients. Zn competes with the binding sites of copper and increases the faecal copper output, which might be of therapeutic use. A trial with oral Zn sulphate 600 to 900 mg daily for 12 months in four patients with biliary cirrhosis failed to show any effect on the routine liver tests or on the liver copper concentration (25). But the lack of rise in the serum Zn levels, which is an unexpected event, could explain the negative results.

ZINC DEFICIENCY DERMATOSIS IN ALCOHOLIC CIRRHOSIS

Liver cirrhosis is one of the diseases in which clinical Zn deficiency may be observed. The conditional factors triggering the depletion of Zn include, apart from the cirrhosis, severe pancreatitis, gastric and intestinal resections, prolonged diarrhoea associated with malabsorption, chronic gastritis and malnutrition. Zn deficiency dermatosis was reported in two 52-year-old alcoholics, one of them in a miserable condition with pneumonia and renal insufficiency, the other receiving high doses of bumetamid (46). Both had skin and hair changes, low serum Zn levels and responded promptly to oral Zn sulphate (Fig. 5).

None of the cases reported have displayed the severe acute type of Zn deficiency with oozing vesicular and bullous lesions on acral parts of the extremities and periorificial lesions as seen in acrodermatitis enteropathica or during prolonged parenteral nutrition. Patients with liver cirrhosis and

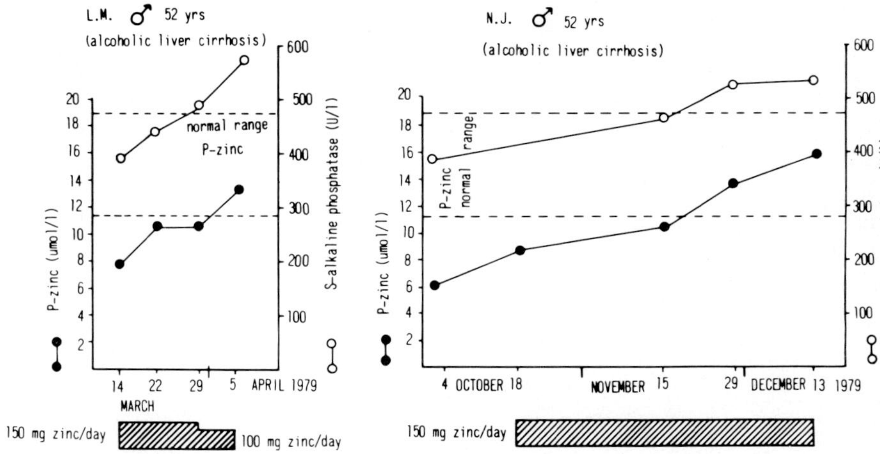

Fig. 5 Response to oral Zn sulphate in two alcoholic cirrhotics with clinical Zn deficiency

Both displayed a concomitant rise in serum Zn and serum alkaline phosphatase levels during therapy. Filled circles indicate Zn values and open circles alkaline phosphatase activity in serum. (46)

chronic Zn deficiency have shown a type of widespread eczematous skin changes known as eczema craquelé, hair loss and transverse depressions (Beau's lines) on the finger nails appearing after supplementation with oral Zn (Fig. 6a–d).

SUMMARY

Alcoholic liver cirrhosis is associated with a high frequency of low serum Zn levels, hyperzincuria and a low hepatic Zn concentration. The decreased serum Zn level is partly explicable by hypoalbuminaemia, but a poor nutritional status, ingestion of alcohol and a decreased affinity for Zn of circulating plasma proteins are also operating. Whole-body counting studies have shown a significant increase in the ^{65}Zn absorption, so malabsorption of Zn is probably not involved. The hyperzincuria may be related to a disturbed protein metabolism, but the renal mechanism involved is unknown. The low hepatic Zn concentration in alcoholic cirrhosis may be related to a distorted storage function of the liver, a defective transport of Zn into the hepatic cells or a decrease in the metallothionein synthesis. Certain drugs are capable of changing the Zn absorption, serum Zn and urinary Zn levels. Disulfiram (Antabuse) and its split-product dithiocarbamate have been found to increase serum Zn and Zn absorption, respectively. Diuretics and

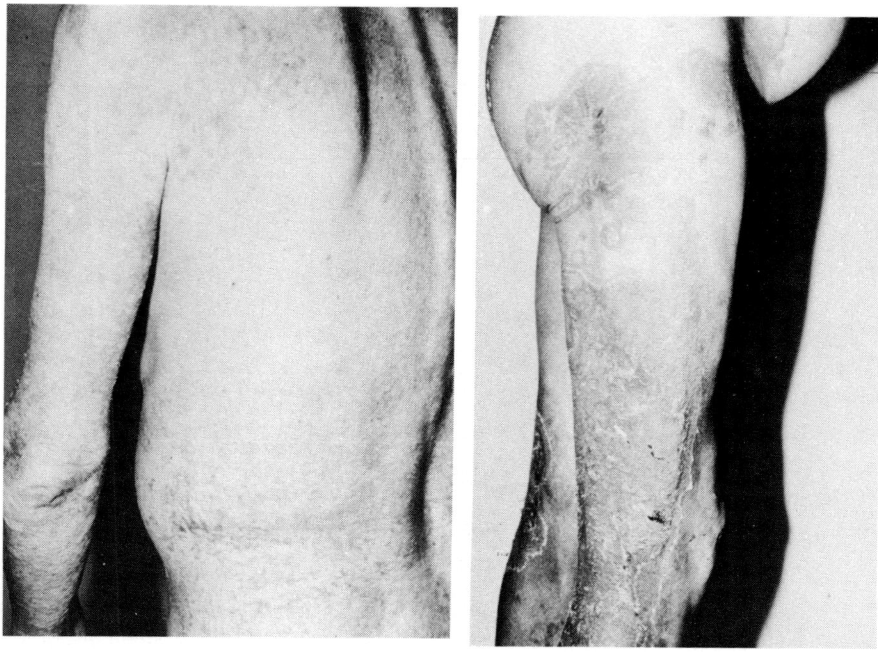

6 a 6 b

Fig. 6 Extensive Zn deficiency dermatitis

A 53-year-old male suffering from decompensated alcoholic cirrhosis, chronic pancreatitis, malabsorption and malnutrition. There is widespread eczema craquelé on the trunk (a) and sharply marginated psoriasiform lesions with a broad erythematous border on the lower extremities (b). Hair loss is seen in chronic Zn deficiency (c), often progressing further after the Zn supplementation is started. The appearance of Beau's lines on finger nails, appearing 2–3 weeks after Zn therapy is initiated (d), is a retrospective sign of severe Zn deficiency. The patient was a 52-year-old malnourished alcoholic male with decompensated, advanced liver cirrhosis, pneumonia and renal insufficiency

6 c

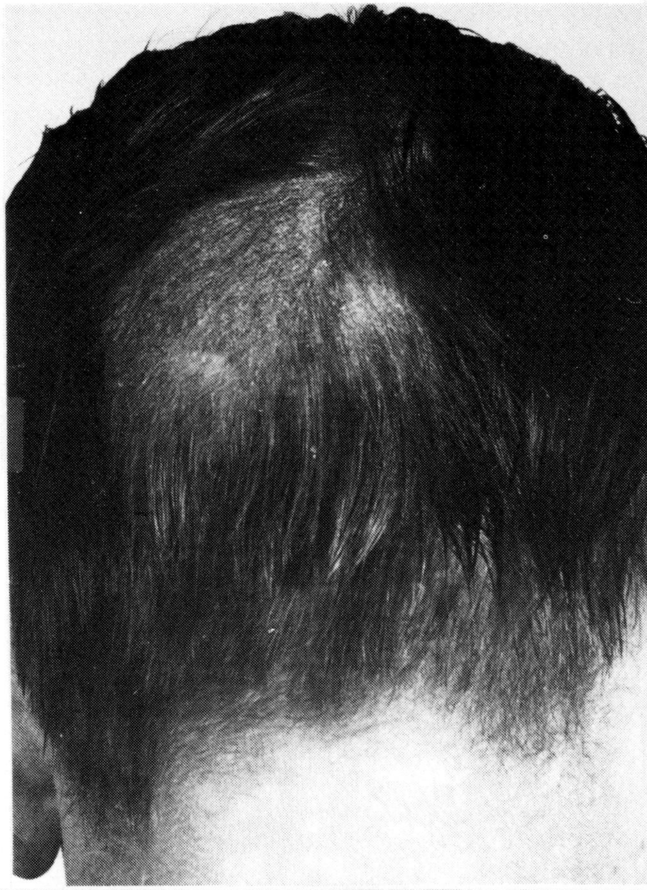

6 d

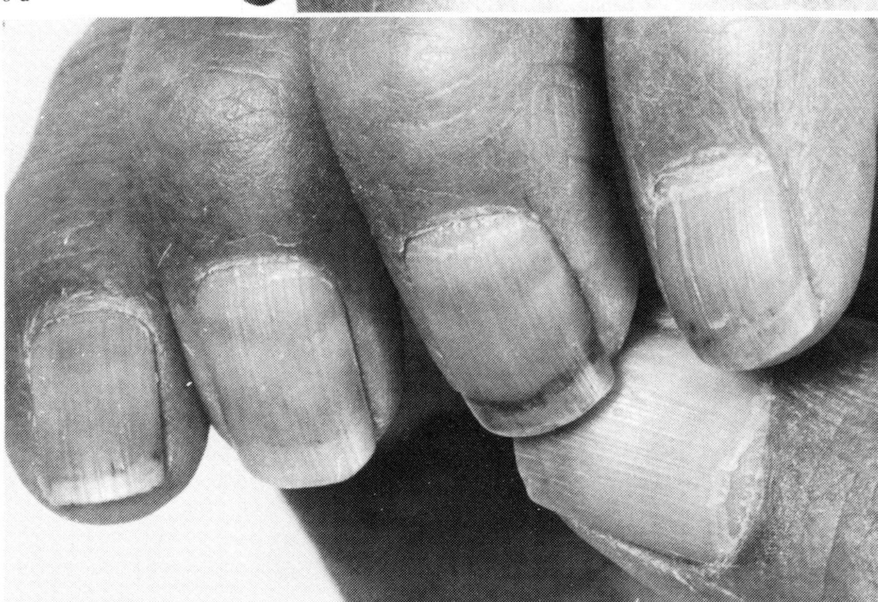

steroids influence serum Zn and urinary Zn levels, so the current medication of the patients should always be taken into consideration when efforts are made to evaluate the Zn metabolism. A relationship between Zn and vitamin A plays a role in alcoholic cirrhosis with vitamin A-resistant night blindness. Positive effects with Zn therapy were recorded in a clinical double-blind trial. The taste function improved, serum bilirubin decreased and prothrombin levels increased. A rise in serum alkaline phosphatase activity with Zn supplementation adds to the accumulating evidence of border-line Zn deficiency being present in cirrhosis. Generally, cirrhotics do not show clinical signs of the deficiency, but a few cases of manifest Zn deficiency dermatitis in cirrhosis have been reported. The patients showed widespread dry eczematous changes, hair loss and nail changes. Conditioning factors in the form of pancreatitis, prolonged diarrhoea, gastrointestinal resections or severe alcohol abuse with malnutrition and malabsorption are operating to produce the Zn depletion.

REFERENCES

1. AAMODT, R.L., RUMBLE, W.F., JOHNSTON, G.S., MARKLEY, E.J. & HENKIN, R.I. (1981). Absorption of orally administered ^{65}Zn by normal human subjects. *Amer. J. clin. Nutr.* 34, 2648.
2. AHMED, S.B. & RUSSELL, R.M. (1982). The effect of ethanol feeding on zinc balance and tissue zinc levels in rats maintained on zinc deficient diets. *J. Lab. clin. Med.* 100, 211.
3. ANTTINEN, H., RYHÄNEN, L., PUISTOLA, U., ARRANTO, A. & OIKARINEN, A. (1984). Decrease in liver collagen accumulation in carbonic tetrachloride-injured and normal growing rats upon administration of zinc. *Gastroenterology* 86, 532.
4. BOOSALIS, M.G., EVANS, G.W. & MCCLAIN, C.J. (1983). Impaired handling of orally administered zinc in pancreatic insufficiency. *Amer. J. clin. Nutr.* 37, 268.
5. BOYETT, J.D. & SULLIVAN, J.F. (1970). Distribution of protein-bound zinc in normal and cirrhotic serum. *Metabolism* 19, 148.
6. BOYETT, J.D. & SULLIVAN, J.F. (1970). Zinc and collagen content of cirrhotic liver. *Digest. Dis.* 15, 797.
7. COUSINS, R.J. (1979). Regulatory aspects of zinc metabolism in liver and intestine. *Nutr. Rev.* 37, 97.
8. *Editorial.* On the entero-pancreatic circulation of endogenous zinc (1981).*Nutr. Rev.* 39, 162.
9. FELL, G.S., CUTHBERTSON, D.P., MORRISON, C., FLECK, A., QUEEN, K., BESSENT, R.G. & HUSAIN, S.L. (1973). Urinary zinc levels as an indication of muscle catabolism. *Lancet* I, 280.
10. FLYNN, A., PORIES, W.J., STRAIN, W.H., HILL, O.A. et al. (1971). Rapid serum zinc depletion associated with corticosteroid therapy. *Lancet* II, 1169.
11. FUJIOKA, M. & LIEBERMAN, I. (1964). A Zn^{++} requirement for synthesis of deoxyribonucleic acid by rat liver. *J. biol. Chem.* 239, 1164.
12. GIROUX, E., SCHECHTER, P.J., SCHOUN, J. & SJOERDSMA, A. (1977). Reduced binding of added zinc in serum of patients with decompensated liver cirrhosis. *Europ. J. clin. Invest.* 7, 71.

13. GUDBJARNASON, S. & PRASAD, A.S. (1969). Cardiac metabolism in experimental alcoholism. In *Biochemical and clinical Aspects of Alcohol Metabolism*, p. 266. Ed. by V.M. Sardesai. Charles C. Thomas Publisher, Springfield.
14. GURD, F.R.N. & GOODMAN, D.S. (1952). Preparation and properties of serum and plasma proteins. XXXII. The interaction of human serum albumin with zinc ions. *J. Amer. Chem. Soc.* 74, 670.
15. HAMMOND, J.B., BLACK, H.R. & CULLISON, J.L. (1960). Effect of oral zinc therapy in cirrhosis. *Amer. J. dig. Dis.* 5, 923.
16. HUBER, A.M. & GERSHOFF, S.N. (1975). Effects of zinc deficiency on the oxidation of retinol and ethanol in rats. *J. Nutr.* 105, 1486.
17. JACKSON, M.J., JONES, D.A. & EDWARDS, R.H.T. (1982). Tissue zinc levels as an index of body zinc status. *Clin. Physiol.* 2, 333.
18. KEELING, P.W.N., JONES, R.B., HILTON, P.J. & THOMPSON, R.P.H. (1980). Reduced leukocyte zinc in liver disease. *Gut* 21, 561.
19. KIILERICH, S., DIETRICHSON, O., LOUD, F.B., NÆSTOFT, J., CHRISTOFFERSEN, P., JUHL, E., KJEMS, G. & CHRISTIANSEN, C. (1980). Zinc depletion in alcoholic liver disease. *Scand. J. Gastroent.* 15, 363.
20. MATSESHE, J.W., PHILLIPS, S.F., MALAGELADA, J.R. & McCALL, J.T. (1980). Recovery of dietary iron and zinc from the proximal intestine of healthy man. *Amer. J. clin. Nutr.* 33, 1946.
21. McCLAIN, C.J., THIEL, D.H. VAN, PARKER, S., BADZIN, L.K. & GILBERT, H. (1979). Alterations in zinc, vitamin A, and retinol-binding protein in chronic alcoholics: a possible mechanism for night blindness and hypogonadism. *Alcohol. clin. exp. Res.* 3, 135.
22. MILMAN, N., HVID-JACOBSEN, K., HEGNHØJ, J. & SØLVSTEN SØRENSEN, S. (1983). Zinc absorption in patients with compensated alcoholic cirrhosis. *Scand. J. Gastroenterol.* 18, 871.
23. MORRISON, S.A., RUSSELL, R.M., CARNEY, E.A. & OAKS, E.V. (1978). Zinc deficiency: a cause of abnormal dark adaptation in cirrhotics. *Amer. J. clin. Nutr.* 31, 276.
24. NELDNER, K.H. & HAMBIDGE, K.M. (1975). Zinc therapy of acrodermatitis enteropathica. *New Engl. J. Med.* 292, 879.
25. OLSSON, R. (1982). Oral zinc treatment in primary biliary cirrhosis. *Acta med. scand.* 212, 191.
26. PATEK, A.J. & HAIG, C. (1939). The occurrence of abnormal dark adaptation and its relation to vitamin A metabolism in patients with cirrhosis of the liver. *J. clin. Invest.* 18, 609.
27. POWANDA, M.C., BLACKBURN, B.S., BOSTIAN, K.A., FOWLER, J.P. et al. (1978). Clofibrete-induced alterations in zinc, iron and copper metabolism. *Biochem. Pharmacol.* 27, 125.
28. PRASAD, A.S., OBERLEAS, D., LEI, K.Y., MOGHISSI, K.S. et al. (1975). Effect of oral contraceptive agents on nutrients. I. Minerals. *Amer. J. clin. Nutr.* 28, 377.
29. RASMUSSEN, E.B. & TØNNESEN, H. (1984). Zink-niveau hos alkoholmisbrugere i deisulfirambehandling. *Ugeskr. Læg.* 146, 3034.
30. REITH, J.F., ENGELSMA, J.V. & DITMARSCH, J. (1974). Lead and zinc contents of food and diets in the Netherlands. *Z. Lebensm. Unters. Forsch.* 156, 271.
31. RUSSELL, R.M. (1980). Vitamin A and zinc metabolism in alcoholism. *Amer. J. clin. Nutr.* 33, 2741.
32. RUSSELL, R.M., MORRISON, S.A., SMITH, F.R., OAKS, E.V. & CARNEY, E.A. (1968). Vitamin A reversal of abnormal dark adaptation in cirrhosis. Study of effects on the retinal transport system. *Ann. internal Med.* 88, 622.

33. SMITH, J.C., MCDANIEL, E.G., FAN, F.F. & HALSTED, J.A. (1973). Zinc: a trace element essential in vitamin A metabolism. *Science* 181, 954.
34. SMITH, J.E., BROWN, E.D. & SMITH, J.C. (1974). The effect of zinc deficiency on the metabolism of retinol-binding protein in the rat. *J. Lab. clin. Med.* 84, 692.
35. SOLOMONS, N.W. (1982). Biological availability of zinc in humans. *Amer. J. clin. Nutr.* 35, 1048.
36. SULLIVAN, J.F. (1962). Effect of alcohol on urinary zinc excretion. *Quart. J. Stud. Alc.* 23, 216.
37. SULLIVAN, J.F. & BURCH, R.E. (1976). Potential role of zinc in liver disease. In *Trace Elements in Human Health and Disease*, I, p. 67. Ed. by A.S. Prasad and D. Oberleas. Academic Press, New York.
38. SULLIVAN, J.F. & HEANEY, R.P. (1970). Zinc metabolism in alcoholic liver disease. *Amer. J. clin. Nutr.* 23, 170.
39. SULLIVAN, J.F. & LANKFORD, H.G. (1962). Urinary excretion of zinc in alcoholism and post-alcoholic cirrhosis. *Amer. J. clin. Nutr.* 10, 153.
40. SULLIVAN, J.F., WILLIAMS, R.V. & BURCH, R.E. (1979). The metabolism of zinc and selenium in cirrhotic patients during six weeks of zinc ingestion. *Alcoholism: Clin. exp. Res.* 3, 235.
41. SZADKOWSKI, D., WEIMERSHAUS, E., LINDNER, K., SCHALLER, K.H. & LEHNERT, G. (1969). Einfluss von Aldosteron auf den Interflux und Efflux arbeitsmedizinisch relevanter Mineralien und Spurenelement des menschlichen Organismus. *Int. Z. angew. Physiol.* 27, 99.
42. VALLEE, B.L., WACKER, W.E.C., BARTHOLOMAY, A.F. & ROBIN, E.D. (1956). Zinc metabolism in hepatic dysfunction. I. *New Engl. J. Med.* 255, 403.
43. VALLEE, B.L., WACKER, W.E.C., BARTHOLOMAY, A.F. & HOCH, F.L. (1957). Zinc metabolism in hepatic dysfunction. II. *New Engl. J. Med.* 257, 1055.
44. VIKBLADH, I. (1951). Studies on zinc in blood. *Scand. J. clin. Lab. Invest.* 3, Suppl. 2.
45. WEISMANN, K. & HØYER, H. (1979). Serum alkaline phosphatase activity in acrodermatitis enteropathica: an index of the serum zinc level. *Acta derm-venereol. (Stockh.)* 59, 89.
46. WEISMANN, K. & HØYER, H. (1980). Acquired zinc deficiency in alcoholic liver cirrhosis: report of two cases. *Acta derm-venereol. (Stockh.)* 60, 447.
47. WEISMANN, K. & HØYER, H. (1984). Serum alkaline phosphatase and serum zinc levels in the diagnosis of zinc deficiency. *Amer. J. clin. Nutr.* (in press).
48. WEISMANN, K. & KNUDSEN, L. (1978). Effects of penicillamine and dihydroxyquinoline on absorption of orally ingested ^{65}zinc in the rat. *J. invest. Derm.* 71, 242.
49. WEISMANN, K., CHRISTENSEN, E. & DREYER, V. (1979). Zinc supplementation in alcoholic cirrhosis. A double-blind clinical trial. *Acta med. scand.* 205, 361.
50. WEISMANN, K., HOE, S., KNUDSEN, L. & SØLVSTEN SØRENSEN, S. (1979). ^{65}Zn absorption in patients suffering from acrodermatitis enteropathica and in normal adults assessed by whole-body counting technique. *Brit. J. Derm.* 101, 573.
51. WEISMANN, K., KNUDSEN, L. & HØYER, H. (1978). Effects of tetracycline on the absorption of ^{65}zinc in rats. *Arch. Derm. Res.* 263, 135.
52. WEISMANN, K., KNUDSEN, L. & HØYER, H. (1978). Phenytoin increases ^{65}zinc absorption in the rat. *J. invest. Derm.* 71. 396.
53. WEISMANN, K., WANSCHER, B. & KRAKAUER, R. (1978). Oral zinc therapy in geriatric patients with selected skin manifestations and a low plasma zinc level. *Acta derm.-venereol. (Stockh.)* 58, 157.

54. WESTER, P.O. (1975). Zinc during diuretic treatment. *Lancet* I, 578.
55. WESTER, P.O. (1980). Urinary zinc excretion during treatment with different diuretics. *Acta. med. scand.* 208, 209.

Trace Element Metabolism in Coeliac Disease

By Sten Jameson

Trace elements are absorbed in the proximal part of the gut, mainly in the duodenum and jejunum. The uptake is an active, controlled process, but the homeostatic regulation system is not fully understood (26). The bioavailability of trace elements from daily diets varies according to the amounts of different foods and their quality, the cooking and eating habits, and the ingestion of drugs, especially antacids, and chelating substances. Marked differences can thus exist between different countries and ethnic groups, which further accentuates the difficulties in understanding the complex system of trace element homeostasis.

Diseases affecting the proximal gut interfere with the digestion of food and the availability and uptake of essential nutrients. Examples of conditions which may adversely influence the absorptive function and reduce the mucosal surface area are atrophic gastritis and achylia, villous atrophy of varying degree, hepatic and pancreatic diseases, parasitic infestations, bacterial overgrowth, inflammatory bowel diseases, and surgical procedures such as gastric resection, enteroanastomosis, and jejuno-ileal shunts.

Knowledge of the aetiology and pathogenesis of coeliac disease is incomplete. Many attempts have been made to give the disease a strict definition. The diagnosis requires the presence of pretreatment signs of mucosal damage, a demonstration of improvement in the mucosal lesions upon gluten restriction, and evidence of deterioration when gluten is reintroduced (6, 25). It is generally accepted that coeliac disease in children and that in adults is the same disorder. Follow-up studies of children with coeliac disease suggest that it is a life-long illness (31).

The clinical picture of coeliac disease is changing (1, 7). The classical pattern of a patient with weight loss, bowel complaints, diarrhoea and severe anaemia is not often seen today. Many patients are now diagnosed on the basis of rather vague symptoms in the presence of a family history of coeliac disease and mild haematological abnormalities. A number of diseases associated with coeliac disease are also identified, as diabetes mellitus, primary biliary cirrhosis (PBC), idiopathic pulmonary haemosiderosis, fibrosing alveolitis, polymyositis, dermatitis herpetiformis (DH) (25), and depressive syndromes with alterations in the cerebral monoamine metabolism (17).

In the untreated typical case of advanced coeliac disease the jejunal mucosa is flat, with signs of severe inflammation and cellular hyperplasia in the crypts. Less severe lesions are referred to as subtotal villous atrophy, and minor lesions as partial villous atrophy (35). The lesions may be patchy (34), which will make the evaluation of biopsy results more difficult.

The demonstration of malabsorption has mostly relied upon the finding of steatorrhoea, folate deficiency, abnormally decreased urinary D-xylose excretion after an oral loading test, or a defective lactose absorption test. These factors are claimed to be insensitive indicators (7, 15). In a comparison of absorption assays with morphometric data on the proximal jejunal biopsy specimen, no distinct correlations were found (9). However, all diseases affecting the proximal intestinal mucosa can induce some malabsorption, which can be detected if a sufficiently specific and sensitive technique is used. A cellobiose and mannitol absorption test has given favourable results in this respect (10). Early mucosal lesions, such as the presence of an increased number of intraepithelial lymphocytes, can be detected with special techniques. A positive correlation between the degree of pathological mucosal changes, on the one hand, and malabsorption of D-xylose and the occurrence of circulating antibodies against reticulin and gluten, on the other, has been demonstrated (28).

The knowledge of trace element metabolism in humans with proximal intestinal disease is incomplete and little reference to this matter is to be found in the literature (33). The clinical and biochemical effects of trace element aberrations would seem to be an important field of investigation and treatment. As recently as 1983 a comprehensive review article concerning new clinical aspects of coeliac disease did not give any information about trace elements (25).

The essential trace elements iron, zinc, copper, manganese and selenium seem to be of specific interest, as they are also components of metalloenzymes, which together with the fat-soluble vitamins A and E and the water-soluble vitamin C are involved in the free radical defence system of the tissues (12).

The aims of the present study were to collect clinical and biochemical data concerning the metabolism of trace elements, especially iron, zinc and copper, from patients referred routinely to our gastro-enterological unit, and to establish working routines for the investigation and treatment of deficiencies and overload.

PATIENTS AND METHODS

Adult patients referred to our unit with suspected proximal gastrointestinal disease were investigated according to a basic scheme. Those with diagnosed intestinal blood losses, tumours and ulcers, hepatic and pancreatic diseases without proximal intestinal mucosal damage, or inflammatory bowel disease such as Crohn's disease and ulcerative colitis, were excluded. The remaining group consisted of 174 adults, 90 females and 84 males, with proven or suspected proximal gastrointestinal disease: 85 with coeliac disease, 24 with both coeliac disease and DH, 22 with probable coeliac disease who did not accept a gluten-free diet, 5 with PBC and proximal intestinal mucosal lesions, 10 with chronic inflammatory cell infiltrates in duodenal mucosal biopsies, 5 with primary lactose intolerance, and 23 with chronic diarrhoeas of unknown origin.

All patients underwent oesophago-gastro-duodenoscopy, recto-sigmoidoscopy or colonoscopy, with biopsies. The mucosal biopsy specimens were obtained from the postpapillary area of the duodenum with a gastroscope or from the duodeno-jejunal junction by means of a biopsy capsule under fluoroscopic control. Villous atrophy was classified as "total" (no villi, elongated crypts and an extensive inflammatory reaction of the chronic type in the lamina propria), "subtotal" (no or almost no villi, which were shortened, elongated crypts and an extensive inflammatory reaction of the chronic type in the lamina propria), or "partial" (broad, sometimes shortened villi, with slight crypt hyperplasia and slight or moderate inflammation). A finding of no villous changes but an increased lymphocyte count, more than 40/100 epithelial cells, was regarded as "inflammation" by the Department of Clinical Pathology.

Haematological and biochemical screening was undertaken in all patients, using standard laboratory techniques as part of the diagnostic routine at the Department of Clinical Chemistry.

All laboratory data refer to investigations performed at the same time as the biopsy procedure. All blood samples were drawn in the morning after an overnight fast.

For D-xylose absorption tests, 25 g of D-xylose dissolved in 500 ml of water was administered orally in the morning after an overnight fast. Xylose concentrations in serum were determined after 30 and 60 minutes. Based on a local control material, a serum xylose concentration after 60 minutes of more than 2.3 mmol/l was considered normal.

The faecal fat content was determined in stools collected over a period of three days while the patients were on a standard hospital diet giving about 70 g of fat per day. Elimination of more than 8 mmol lipids per day was considered abnormal.

Serum zinc and copper concentrations were determined by atomic absorption spectrophotometry (Perkin–Elmer 203). Serum selenium and manganese concentrations were assayed by energy dispersive x-ray fluorescence (Kevex-Ultratrace) at Scandlab, Sollentuna. Red cell glutathione-peroxidase activity (GSH-Px) was measured at the Department of Experimental Medicine, Pharmacia AB, Uppsala.

All biochemical methods were not used on all patients, some samples were lost, some patients were acutely ill and some analytical methods were not available for daily routine use or without delay. Some patients were studied on different occasions and therefore the number of patients in the tables differs from the total patient population. Data from patients receiving iron, zinc, folate or vitamin B_{12} supplementation at the time of investigation were excluded from the calculations of these mean values.

RESULTS

The reported results refer to the results of the pathologico-anatomical grouping of the duodenal biopsies and simultaneously obtained haematological and biochemical values.

The patients with the most pronounced mucosal lesions showed the most extensive aberrations in values obtained and the highest frequencies of abnormal values (Tables 1–4).

Table 1 *Mean haemoglobin g/l (Hb), normal range females 113–139, males 134–166; mean red cell volume fl (MCV), normal range 76–96; serum folate nmol/l (S-folate), normal range 7–34; vitamin B_{12} pmol/l (S-B_{12}), normal range 105–600; plus standard deviation (SD) and number of observations (n)*

The significance of difference between means was tested with double-sided Student's t-test. * $p < 0.05$, ** $p < 0.01$, *** $p < 0.001$. Mucosal biopsies graded according to patients and methods

Mucosal biopsy	Hb	(SD) (n)	MCV	(SD) (n)	S-folate	(SD) (n)	S-B_{12}	(SD) (n)
A. Total atrophy	120	(18.2) (60)	91	(9.7) (43)	8.0	(6.3) (47)	218	(116) (47)
	**							
B. Subtotal atrophy	129	(17.1) (57)	90	(8.5) (38)	9.9	(5.4) (37)	239	(91) (41)
	*				**			
C. Partial atrophy	137	(15.3) (55)	90	(6.9) (37)	14.9	(8.8) (32)	224	(115) (31)
							*	
D. Inflammation	134	(16.5) (22)	87	(9.7) (19)	19.1	(9.5) (25)	303	(120) (18)
							*	
E. Diarrhoea, no changes	140	(16.8) (17)	91	(6.6) (14)	14.0	(5.6) (13)	396	(106) (12)
F. Gluten-free, no changes	143	(14.6) (16)	91	(4.0) (10)	17.0	(5.1) (10)	422	(120) (7)

Table 2 *Mean serum levels of albumin g/l (S-alb), normal range 38–55; transferrin µmol/l (S-transf), normal range 45–72; D-xylose 60 min µmol/l (D-xyl 60), normal level > 2.3*

Faecal lipid elimination per 24 hours mmol (F-lip), normal amount < 8 mmol. See Table 1 for details

Mucosal biopsy	S-alb	(SD) (n)	S-transf	(SD) (n)	D-xyl 60	(SD) (n)	F-lip	(SD) (n)
A. Total atrophy	37	(7.3) (51)	54	(14.6) (53)	1.35	(0.6) (36)	28	(31) (46)
B. Subtotal atrophy	39	(6.6) (46)	55	(13.2) (44)	1.46	(0.6) (23)	18	(20) (29)
C. Partial atrophy	41	(5.6) (44)	53	(11.9) (43)	* 2.09	(1.0) (20)	14	(24) (21)
D. Inflammation	41	(5.1) (28)	54	(17.9) (25)	2.49	(0.7) (14)	13	(16) (11)
E. Diarrhoea, no changes	* 44	(3.7) (16)	53	(8.9) (15)	2.20	(0.5) (12)	7	(4) (14)
F. Gluten-free, no changes	45	(4.3) (10)	61	(19.7) (11)	2.87	(0.9) (7)	5	(3) (3)

Table 3 *Mean serum levels of iron µmol/l (S-Fe), normal range 11–35; zinc µmol/l (S-Zn), normal range 11–20; copper µmol/l (S-Cu), normal range 13–21; selenium µmol/l (S-Se), normal range 0.7–2.1*

See Table 1 for more details

Mucosal biopsy	S-Fe	(SD) (n)	S-Zn	(SD) (n)	S-Cu	(SD) (n)	S-Se	(SD) (n)
A. Total atrophy	12.2	(8.1) (57)	7.5	(2.3) (53)	16.2	(5.3) (13)	—	
B. Subtotal atrophy	15.0	(9.3) (44)	** 9.1	(2.3) (44)	18.1	(4.8) (9)	1.0	(0.4) (7)
C. Partial atrophy	** 21.4	(9.0) (43)	*** 10.8	(1.7) (42)	21.3	(5.1) (9)	—	
D. Inflammation	16.4	(8.2) (25)	11.6	(2.0) (27)	18.1	(2.0) (5)	1.1	– (1)
E. Diarrhoea, no changes	21.8	(10.7) (15)	12.7	(1.1) (15)	—		—	
F. Gluten-free, no changes	17.1	(3.8) (11)	12.2	(1.1) (12)	20.8	(1.7) (2)	—	

Table 4 Percentage frequencies of abnormal values, see normal ranges Tables 1–3

Transferrin-(Tf)-saturation with iron <16% is considered abnormal

Mucosal biopsy	Laboratory parameter												
	Hb <125	MCV >96	MCV <76	S-fol <7	S-B12 <105	S-alb <38	F-lip >8	D-xyl <2.3	S-Fe <11	Tf-sat <16	Tf <45	S-Zn <11	S-Cu <13
A. Total atrophy	55	33	9	60	15	47	83	89	51	43	26	92	46
B. Subtotal atrophy	32	18	3	30	0	30	55	87	41	30	18	80	22
C. Partial atrophy	22	11	3	22	10	23	33	50	9	5	30	60	11
D. Inflam-mation	36	5	16	0	6	21	36	43	24	20	24	63	0
E. Diarrhoea, no changes	18	0	7	0	0	0	36	67	20	20	20	0	—
F. Gluten-free, no changes	6	10	0	0	0	0	33	14	0	0	9	8	0

The mean serum levels of the essential vitamins B_{12} and folate decreased and the frequencies of deficiency of these vitamins increased with advancing degrees of mucosal damage. Similar observations were made for the essential trace elements iron, zinc, and copper.

Anabolic function and protein synthesis, as judged from the levels of albumin, transferrin and haemoglobin decreased with increasing degrees of mucosal impairment. Malabsorption, measured as loss of faecal lipids and reduction of D-xylose uptake, was more pronounced the greater the degree of mucosal damage.

Eight blood samples were analysed for serum selenium and for red cell GSH-Px activity. The mean serum selenium concentration, 1.0 μmol/l, was lower than that of the laboratory, 1.4 μmol (range 0.7–2.1). Two patients had serum selenium levels of only 0.6 μmol/1, both had subtotal villous atrophy. The mean GSH-Px value, 1.0 μkat/g Hb, was significantly lower than the mean in 100 healthy blood donors, 1.33 μkat/g Hb ($p < 0.01$).

Serum samples from four patients were analysed for manganese. One of these patients, who also had a low serum zinc value, had a very low manganese level, 13 nmol/1 (normal range of the laboratory 20–150), but did not have hypoalbuminaemia. A biopsy revealed subtotal villous atrophy.

One patient who originally was found to have hypothyroidism displayd a very low intestinal isotope uptake in a I^{131} test, which, in turn, led to a gastrointestinal investigation, disclosing total villous atrophy.

Serum zinc assay and measurement of D-xylose uptake were the most sensitive tests for revealing proximal mucosal damage, although the D-xylose test had a low specificity. The most specific indicator of villous damage was serum folate, although this was less sensitive than serum zinc, the D-xylose test and faecal lipid elimination (Table 4).

The tests gave no information about the possibility of increased intestinal losses of proteins or basic raw materials such as trace elements. Serum zinc, copper, and iron were negatively correlated with the faecal lipid content (r −0.46, n 113, $p < 0.001$; r −0.37, n 21, $p < 0.1$; r −0.33, n 124, $p < 0.001$). Serum zinc was positively correlated with serum albumin (r 0.66, n 188, $p < 0.001$).

DISCUSSION

Most patients with mucosal disorders in the proximal intestine in our part of the world have coeliac disease. It has been difficult to define this disease, and as there is no specific sign or symptom that is diagnostic, it has been necessary to rely upon the histological demonstration of mucosal changes and the clinical and biochemical effects of a gluten-free diet and gluten challenge, which is a troublesome and inconvenient method. However, clinicians are becoming more aware of the possibility of proximal intestinal disease, which, consequently, is more often diagnosed today (1).

Iron uptake has been found to be reduced in patients with untreated coeliac disease and normalized on administration of a gluten-free diet; the uptake of haemoglobin iron was not reduced, however (2). Decreased serum albumin, pre-albumin, and transferrin levels have been found in severe zinc deficiency (4), but may also be secondary to intestinal leakage or an inflammatory reaction.

Low serum or plasma zinc levels in patients with villous atrophy and malabsorption have been observed by several research groups (19, 32, 33). A reduced zinc uptake from an oral test dose has also been reported (11, 21). In addition, we have observed that patients with villous atrophy and folate deficiency absorb zinc better if the folate deficiency is corrected. The uptake was not restored to normal until a gluten-free diet was given (21). Moreover, serum zinc values increase towards a normal level both in coeliac patients on a gluten-free diet (22, 32), and in patients with DH on this diet (22). The low serum zinc values cannot be entirely explained by reduced serum albumin in coeliac disease in adults (19) or in children (32). Zinc deficiency may affect the capacity of albumin synthesis. Low zinc levels can be secondary to combined effects of a reduced uptake, increased loss, and redistribution of circulating zinc, although a true deficiency seems most probable in coeliac disease.

Lowered serum copper levels in coeliac disease and a reduced copper uptake from an oral isotope dose have been noted by other authors (36). The first report on reduced copper uptake from an oral copper sulphate test dose in patients with proximal intestinal mucosal damage, and signs of copper deficiency in the form of severe neutropenia, which were normalized by a gluten-free diet, is in press (23). These results are further supported by the finding of a low serum copper level in about one-half of the patients with total villous atrophy, although the number of observations is still fairly small.

GSH-Px is a selenium-containing enzyme. Reduced activity of this enzyme is considered to be a feature of selenium defiency (29). Patients with DH, which is correlated with coeliac disease, have been shown to have reduced red cell GSH-Px-activity (24). Although our observations are few, the finding of significantly low GSH-Px-activities and low serum selenium levels indicates the presence of a disturbed selenium balance in patients with proximal intestinal disease.

Manganese in serum was only assayed in four patients. One of them, with subtotal villous atrophy and a low serum zinc value, had a serum manganese level below the lowest normal limit. This, although a single finding, merits further investigation, as there is a connection between coeliac disease and epilepsy (8), and neurological disorders and manganese inbalance (5).

Our results show that patients with advanced mucosal damage in the proximal intestine have a common decrease in circulating levels of iron, zinc, copper and probably selenium. This reduction is more pronounced the more advanced the mucosal lesion, as demonstrated both histologically and in conventional malabsorption tests, with increased faecal lipid losses and a decreased uptake of D-xylose. In a previous study we found that patients with coeliac disease had a low serum zinc level, low urinary zinc excretion, low serum copper and in some cases also no stainable bone marrow iron. The women in that study suffered from infertility of long standing, two of them secondarily after giving birth to infants with foetal malformations (19). Infertility with sperm abnormalities, elevated levels of serum-luteinising hormone, and lowered dihydrotestosterone values, have been found in untreated male coeliac patients (13). Similar observations have been made in patients treated with haemodialysis having low serum zinc levels, who showed a positive effect of zinc therapy (3).

Zinc deficiency profoundly affects pregnancy. Abortions, foetal malformations, slow foetal growth, and abnormal parturitions have been described (20). A high frequency of abortions and small-for-gestational-age (SGA) infants has been found among women with coeliac disease who have not kept to a gluten-free diet (7, 14). Women with a jejuno-ileal shunt performed for obesity have also shown a high frequency of SGA gestations (18). SGA infants and their mothers have been found to have a low granulocyte zinc level (30). It has been reported that rhesus monkeys on a zinc-deficient diet from conception gave birth to growth-retarded offspring at abnormal parturitions (16).

Our results confirm the earlier finding by our group of a correlation between the degree of mucosal changes and malabsorption of D-xylose (28).

It has been claimed that conventional malabsorption tests are relatively insensitive (7, 15). However, if all patients referred for investigation, and not only those who fit into the narrow definition of coeliac disease and/or DH, are considered, the conventional tests are not only relatively insensitive, but also unspecific. Newly introduced tests measuring trace element levels seem to give better results, discriminating patients with proximal mucosal damage from those without. We suggest that a combination of serum folate, albumin, zinc and copper assays, and a one-hour D-xylose uptake test will give the best chance of detecting a disease with proximal intestinal mucosal damage.

Our results also indicate that the observed abnormalities in haematological and biochemical parameters develop stepwise. A fall in the circulating zinc level seems to be the first event, followed by reductions in serum folate, albumin and transferrin levels. Pronounced steatorrhoea appears to be a late phenomenon. Zinc deficiency correlates with defective synthesis of transport proteins (4), which might accentuate the metabolic aberrations. It has also been suggested that folate conjugase, the enzyme that cleaves complex folates into monofolates in the gut, is a zinc enzyme, the activity of which decreases in man on induction of zinc deficiency (38).

Zinc, copper, manganese and selenium are essential for the development of an effective immunological response (5) and for the free radical tissue defence system (12). Low selenium levels in the blood have been associated with later development of cardiovascular disease and malignancy (39). Patients with coeliac disease and DH run an increased risk of developing malignant disease, expecially lymphomas (27, 37). Disturbed metabolism of essential trace elements might be an important factor in this respect.

SUMMARY

Proximal intestinal mucosal damage, mainly coeliac disease, interferes with the metabolism of essential trace elements. Abnormally low uptake of iron, but not of haemiron, zinc, and copper, has been demonstrated. The more pronounced the mucosal lesion, as judged from duodenal biopsy specimens, the lower the circulating levels of iron, zinc and copper. Some few data indicate that selenium and manganese levels might also be affected. Our data suggest the presence of multiple essential trace element deficiencies, and/or defects in their transport, in patients with proximal intestinal mucosal damage. These changes could have secondary effects, as these trace elements are basic raw materials in the free radical tissue defence system and in the immunological response. Patients with coeliac disease and dermititis herpetiformis run an increased risk of developing malignant diseases.

REFERENCES

1. *Anonymous*. (1984). Coeliac disease in the elderly. *Lancet* i, 775–776.
2. ANAND, B.S., CALLENDER, S.T. & WARNER, G.T. (1977). Absorption of inorganic and haemoglobin iron in coeliac disease. *Brit. J. Haematol.* 37, 409–414.
3. ANTONIOU, L.D., SHALHOUB, R.J., SUDHAKAR, T. & SMITH, J.C. (1977). Reversal of uraemic impotence by zinc. *Lancet ii,* 895–898.
4. BATES, J. & MCCLAIN, C.J. (1981). The effect of severe zinc deficiency on serum levels of albumin, transferrin, and prealbumin in man. *Amer. J. clin. Nutr.* 34, 1655–1660.
5. BEACH, R.S., GERSHWIN, M.E. & HURLEY, L.S. (1982). Zinc, copper, and manganese in immune function and experimental oncogenesis. *Nutr. and Cancer* 3, 172–191.
6. BOOTH, C.C. (1974). Definition of coeliac disease. In *Coeliac Disease,* pp. 17–22. Ed. by W.T.J.M. Hekkens and A.S. Pena. Stenfert Kroese, Leiden.
7. CAMPBELL, B.C., ROBERTS, R.K. & COWEN, A.E. (1977). The changing clinical presentation of coeliac disease in adults. *Med. J. Aust.* i, 89–93.
8. CHAPMAN, R.W.G., LAIDLOW, J.M. & COLIN-JONES, D. (1978). Increased prevalence of epilepsy in coeliac disease. *B.M.J.* 2, 250–251.
9. CLUYSENAER, O.J.J., SCHILLINGS, P.H.M. & VAN TONGEREN, J.H.M. (1982). Mucosal lesions and malabsorption in celiac sprue. *J. clin Gastroenterol.* 4, 425–429.
10. COBDEN, I., ROTHWELL, J. & AXON, A.T.R. (1980). Intestinal permeability and screening tests for coeliac disease. *Gut* 21, 512–518.
11. CROFTON, R.W., GLOVER, S.C., EWEN, S.W.B., AGGETT, P.J., MOWAT, N.A.G. & MILLS, C. (1983). Zinc absorption in coeliac disease and dermatitis herpetiformis: a test of small intestinal function. *Amer. J. clin. Nutr.* 38, 706–712.
12. DELMAESTRO, R.F. (1980). An approach to free radicals in medicine and biology. *Acta physiol. scand.* Suppl. 492, 153–168.
13. FARTHING, M.J.G., REES, L.H., EDWARDS, C.R.W. & DAWSON, A.M. (1983). Male gonadal function in coeliac disease. *Gut* 24, 127–135.
14. FERGUSON, R., HOLMES, G.K.T., & COOKE, G.T. (1982). Coeliac disease, fertility, and pregnancy. *Scand. J. Gastroenterol.* 17, 65–68.
15. GILLBERG, R., DOTEVALL, G., KASTRUP, W., LINDSTEDT, G., MOBACKEN, H. & SWOLIN, B. (1984). Conventional malabsorption tests: do they detect the adult patient with villous atrophy? *Scand. J. clin. Lab. Invest.* 44, 91–98.
16. GOLUB, M.S., GERSHWIN, M.E., HURLEY, L.S., BALY, D.L, & HENDRICKX, A.G. (1984). Studies of marginal zinc deprivation in rhesus monkeys: II. Pregnancy outcome. *Amer. J. clin. Nutr.* 39, 879–887.
17. HALLERT, C., ÅSTRÖM, J. & SEDVALL, G. (1982). Psychic disturbances in adult coeliac disease. III. Reduced central monoamine metabolism and signs of depression. *Scand. J. Gastroenterol.* 17, 25–28.
18. INGARDIA, C.J. & FISCHER, J.R. (1978). Pregnancy after jejuno-ileal bypass and the SGA-infant. *Obstet. Gynec.* 52, 215–218.
19. JAMESON, S. (1976). Zinc deficiency in malabsorption states: a cause of infertility? *Acta med. scand.* Suppl. 593, 38–49.
20. JAMESON, S. (1982). Zinc status and pregnancy outcome in humans. In *Clinical Applications of Recent Advances in Zinc Metabolism,* pp. 39–52. Ed. by A.S. Prasad, I.E. Dreosti and B.S. Hetzel. Alan R. Liss, New York.
21. JAMESON, S., BJÖRKLUND, O., LÖÖF, L. & ULFBERG, J. (1981). Zinc and folate malabsorption in coeliac disease. In *Trace Element Metabolism in Man and Animals,* pp. 495–497. Ed. by J. McC. Howell, J.M. Gawthorne and C.L. White. Australian Academy of Science, Canberra.

22. JAMESON, S., JÄRNEROT, G., MOI, H. & JAMESON, M. (1979). Zinc deficiency in coeliac disease and dermatitis herpetiformis. *Opusc. med.* 24, 14–15.

23. JAMESON, S., HELLSING, K. & MAGNUSSON, S. (1984). *Copper Malabsorption in Coeliac Disease*. Elsevier Science Publishers, in press.

24. JUHLIN, L., EDQVIST, L.-E., EKMAN, L.G., LJUNGHALL, K. & OLSSON, M. (1982). Blood glutathione-peroxidase levels in skin diseases: effect of selenium and vitamin E treatment. *Acta dermato-vener. (Stockh.)* 62, 211–214.

25. KLUGE, F., KOCH, H.K., KÖTTGEN, E. & GEROK, W. (1983). Glutensensitive Enteropathie im Lichte neuer klinischer und patogenetischer Aspekte. *Klin. Wschr.* 61, 669–679.

26. LAURIE, S.H. (1983). Transport and storage of metals. *J. inher. metab. Dis.* 6, Suppl. 1, 9–14.

27. LEONARD, J.N., TUCKER, W.F.G., FRY, J.S., COULTER, C.A.E., BOYLSTON, A.W., MCMINN, H.M., HAFFENDEN, G.P., SWAIN, A.F. & FRY, L. (1983). Increased incidence of malignancy in dermatitis herpetiformis. *B.M.J.* 286: 1, 16–18.

28. LJUNGHALL, K., LÖÖF, L., GRIMELIUS, L., FORSUM, U., JONSSON, J., SCHEYNIUS, A. & SCHILLING, W. (1983). Dermatitis herpetiformis: relation between circulating antibodies against reticulin and gluten, small-intestinal mucosal status and absorptive capacity. *Acta dermato-vener. (Stockh.)* 63, 27–34.

29. MCKENZIE, R.L., REA, H.M., THOMSON, C.D. & ROBINSON, M.F. (1978). Selenium concentration and glutathione-peroxidase activity in blood of New Zealand infants and children. *Amer. J. clin. Nutr.* 31, 1413–1418.

30. MEADOWS, N.J., RUSE, W., SMITH, M.F., DAY, J., KEELING, P.W.N., SCOPES, J.W. & THOMPSON, R.P. (1981). Zinc and small babies. *Lancet* i, 1135–1136.

31. MORTIMER, P.E., STEWART, J.S., NORMAN, A.P. & BOOTH, C.C. (1968). Follow-up study of coeliac disease. *Brit. med. J.* 3, 7–9.

32. NAVEH, Y., LIGHTMAN, A. & ZINCER, O. (1983). A prospective study of serum zinc concentration in children with celiac disease. *J. Pediatr.* 102, 734–736.

33. PRASAD, A.S. (1983). The role of zinc in gastrointestinal and liver disease. *Clin. Gastroenterol.* 12, 713–741.

34. SCOTT, B.B. & LOSOWSKY, M.S. (1976). Patchiness and duodenal-jejunal variation of the mucosal abnormality in coeliac disease and dermatitis herpetiformis. *Gut* 17, 984–992.

35. SHINER, M. & DONIACH, I. (1960). Histopathologic studies in steatorrhoea. *Gastroenterology* 38, 419–440.

36. STERNLIEB, I. & JANOWITZ, H.D. (1964). Absorption of copper in malabsorption syndromes. *J.clin. Invest.* 43, 1049–1055.

37. SWINSON, C.M., COLES, E.C., SLAVIN, G. & BOOTH, C.C. (1983). Coeliac disease and malignancy. *Lancet* i, 111–115.

38. TAMURA, T., SHANE, B., BAER, M.T., KING, J.C., MARGEN, S. & STOKSTAD, E.L.R. (1978). Absorption of mono- and polyglutamyl folates in zinc-depleted man. *Amer. J. clin. Nutr.* 31, 1984–1987.

39. WILLETT, W.C., MORRIS, J.S., PRESSEL, S., TAYLOR, J.O., POLK, B.F., STAMPFER, M.J., ROSNER, B., SCHNEIDER, K. & HAMES, C.G. (1983). Prediagnostic serum selenium and risk of cancer. *Lancet* ii, 130–134.

Discussion (the papers by Weismann and Jameson)

Chairman: BOSTRÖM

ABDULLA: I have one question to Dr Jameson and one to Dr Weismann. The first one to Dr Jameson is about the coeliac patients with very low copper levels. I would like to know whether you have looked at the plasma electrophoresis and if so, was there any inflammatory reaction? Was ceruloplasmin very low in these patients?

The other question, to Dr Weismann, is about your patients with alcoholic liver cirrhosis and encephalopathy. I wonder if you had treated them with zinc and got any positive results, because there was a report in Lancet a few weeks ago that a group of cirrhotic patients who had encephalopathy had very positive effect with oral zinc treatment.

JAMESON: We have described our patients in a paper that will appear from the meeting in Amsterdam this May (1984). I'm sorry but we have not measured ceruloplasmin levels. The patients did not have inflammatory reactions of severe degree. I'm quite convinced that these low copper levels we found are difficult to understand, unless you try to analyse plasma proteins. We hadn't the ability at that time to look into the problem. But there is a possibility, which is suggested by Danks, to measure the ceruloplasmin levels at start and then again after a few days, when giving copper supplementation. If there is a significant increase, it would indicate a true copper deficiency and that's what we are going to do the next time we have the possibility.

WEISMANN: In response to your question, Dr Abdulla, about encephalopathia, there were no patients with encephalopathia in our group. They were all out-patients and I have not been involved in the treatment of such patients. Of course, it would be very interesting to see if this can be true.

JAMESON: We have tried, but did not see any dramatic changes in Swedish patients with liver insufficiency.

AGGETT: I would like to ask Dr Weismann to comment on the question of leucocyte zincs. This is an area I brought up yesterday and it goes back to what we were talking about on the first day—that we really should know what we are measuring. I think we should bear in mind that considerable changes in the white cell population occur during hepatic cirrhosis and with various other conditions associated with the liver. We should remember that in measuring the entire leucocyte population we may well be distorting the zinc concentration and as a consequence we should look at subsets which I don't think have as yet been published.

The other thing I'd like to comment on is the idea of a reduced zinc pool. There is, in fact, a paper from a Glasgow group, Mills et al., which has shown that the total body zinc in a group of patients with alcoholic cirrhosis is in fact increased, it's much higher than normal. But this just makes it even more fascinating; that no doubt many of these patients truly do have zinc-responsive symptoms. Our own studies suggest that the zinc, in fact, is going to the skeleton; there's decreased uptake by the liver, increased retention of the zinc the liver does take up and it appears in the skeleton much more rapidly than it does in normal individuals. So it really just points to fatty-cirrhosis not just being a zinc deficiency state but a totally aberrant zinc metabolism.

WEISMANN: I agree with you about the question of the leucocyte zinc. I've not worked with this myself and I have cited Dr Keeling and co-workers for the information.

It's very probable that leucocyte zinc actually reflects an inflammatory response or some other reaction in the body, but the study has shown that if you have a decreased zinc pool in the body, there is a low leucocyte zinc level that could be used as a parameter for zinc deficiency. But, I agree with you, it's not quite clear.

About the other point you raised on the group that has been able to show an increased zinc contained in the whole body of the patient, I'm not quite aware of this study. Do we know how they measured this?

AGGETT: This was the radio-isotopic dilution of zinc 65. They gave zinc 65 to measure zinc absorption and confirmed the other study, also finding that zinc absorption as measured by this technique was increased. They also showed, in fact, the whole-body retention was marginally increased, if I remember correctly. Even though urinary loss, again, was marginally increased. At 24–32 weeks, by determining the dilution of zinc 65 in the body pool, they calculated the total-body zinc, which was increased by about 50%. But this doesn't get over the problem that there's no doubt that these patients, as in the many studies you cited, can have zinc-responsive features.

ANDERSON: I have a question to Dr Weismann in that when you're supplementing your patients with ten times the RDA as far as for zinc, I have a little trouble thinking that's a nutritional effect rather than a pharmacological effect. I'm sure you would disagree with that and I think I would say in this case that you're right. But have you considered doing a study where you treat the group with, for example, a multivitamin plus minerals plus and minus zinc and do it that way? Then, hopefully, you wouldn't have to put in 150 mg of zinc but you could put in the remainder of the vitamins and minerals and then one or two times the RDA of zinc because if, indeed, it is a zinc deficiency, it should respond in that way just as well or better.

WEISMANN: I agree that the doses we used were pharmacological but if you remember the response in serum zinc, it was not very impressive. You can give a rather high amount of zinc without producing toxic effects. We gave the high dose because we, of course, wanted enough zinc to be absorbed, also because at that time it was believed that the patient had a decreased zinc absorption. So, clearly, if I were to do the study again today, I would give a much smaller amount, 20 mg for example.

In regard to your question about multivitamin, multimetal supplementation, yes, of course this would be very interesting, but I think it would be very difficult to interpret the results.

ANDERSON: No, you would just give one of those, plus or minus zinc. I wouldn't just shotgun approach it.

WEISMANN: Oh yes, then that would be a very good idea. I have no plans at the time but it clearly would be very interesting to do that.

BOSTRÖM: Can I also ask you two questions? The first one is, how is zinc bound in plasma? You mentioned albumin but is there a certain amount of free or ionised zinc so we have the same situation as with calcium, for instance? If so, would the ionised zinc be the active, important part? If it is, I think you can compensate even if you have hypoalbuminia with an increased ionisation of the zinc. So perhaps you shouldn't have too drastic effects just because of a decreased total zinc. Can you say something about this?

WEISMANN: Yes, I think zinc is quite different from calcium. I don't think anyone has been able to demonstrate ionised zinc in serum. If there are zinc ions, they at once react with circulating proteins or complexes. But your question is an interesting one, because there's a small portion of the total serum zinc which is bound to amino acids and this small fraction is very likely to be very active in terms of carrying zinc to the tissues. But only one or two per cent of serum zinc is bound to such ultra-filtrable complexes. Dr Kiilerich, you have worked with this, can you comment on it?

KIILERICH: We can't measure the ionised zinc fraction, but the theory is that the zinc that is bound to albumin equiliberates the ionised zinc fraction, which is about one per cent of the total serum zinc. So if you take the albumin into account it should be enough in clinical purposes, I think.

BOSTRÖM: I would also ask another question. Would there be any relationship between zinc deficiency and the foetal alcoholic syndrome, which we know about one child in one thousand is suffering from in varying degrees? I think there might be some studies on this.

JAMESON: There is a paper by Flynn in the Lancet 1981 which showed that alcoholic mothers had lower circulating zinc levels than the controls. This study has been criticised since then, because the control group had a high frequency of abnormal children too. So I guess that the question isn't settled yet. There are many similarities and, as far as I know, there are at least two studies going on looking into this question but I haven't heard any answers.

HURLEY: I just wanted to add to the comment on the foetal alcohol syndrome and the possible relationship with zinc. As Dr Jameson said, there is work going on currently. There is also some work from animal experiments that suggest that zinc may be a factor. From what we know, not only about zinc, but also about other nutrients that may be deficient in alcoholics, such as folate and magnesium, deficiencies of all three of these nutrients do produce congenital malformations in experimental animals and there is some evidence for effects in human reproduction as well. So I think that it is entirely possible that zinc deficiency may be one of the factors involved in the foetal alcohol syndrome. All cases of FAS are also not necessarily exactly the same in their aetiology. There is currently a certain amount of controversy about this. Some people believe that the effects of alcohol on the foetus are purely toxic, that is, the toxic effects of the alcohol itself, and that there is no nutritional component, but I think that is very far from having been proved. I think that in the end we're going to find that there is a nutritional component as well.

WENGLE: I have a question to put to Dr Jameson about his coeliac disease material. I wonder how the diagnosis was confirmed, was it by biopsies taken from the duodenum or from the jejunum?

JAMESON: Most of the cases are biopsied several times via endoscope, that is, postpapillary biopsies. Some early cases in the series were biopsied by capsule. The diagnosis is according to the Booth idea that you need to see an improvement when a gluten-free diet is introduced and, then, damage again on a gluten diet.

AASETH: I have a question to Dr Jameson. Have you tried the zinc treatment on any of these patients?

JAMESON: Yes, we have, certainly. I think the first publication about that was by Elmes in Cardiff eight years ago. We have the same impression, that coeliacs recover faster when given extra zinc, but there is no need for it if they keep to a true gluten-free diet, because they will normalise spontaneously then. And then we have the increase in serum zinc as a good parameter that they keep to a gluten-free diet. If they do, they normalise. If there is a hurry, or if they have septic fever or are in a very bad state, there's obviously a need for trace elements, not only zinc, and that ought to be given in high doses, intravenously sometimes.

AASETH: In Oslo we had almost the same findings, but we had one patient, a non-responder, with ulcers in jejunum, a complication which we treated with a combination of zinc and prednisone with a dramatic effect on improvement.

JAMESON: I quite agree. This is a very dangerous syndrome and it has been reported from several groups. The combination of zinc and steroids is possibly effective, but it's very difficult to gather patient material enough to prove that this is an effective treatment.

HURLEY: I'd like to ask Dr Jameson two questions. The first is, how did you measure the copper uptake? The second is that you mentioned a patient who apparently had a copper deficiency without folate deficiency or other deficiencies. Presumably the copper deficiency arose from the lesion in the intestinal absorption. How do you explain such a specific effect that only copper was not absorbed?

JAMESON: The copper uptake is measured as the area under the plasma curve, measuring serum copper after giving an oral dose. It's, of course, a crude measurement, but it probably gives some idea of the copper uptake. Of course, the distribution could be very rapid so we instead measure a severe copper deficiency.

The other thing is that, as I think, there is a sequence of events in coeliac disease. As the lesions increase, there is a stepwise decrease in uptake of basic nutrients to the circulation. To me it's obvious that one of the first steps in this event is falling zinc levels. Then iron and copper levels decrease in step two. As step three, there is a decrease in circulating folate levels. It seems to me that this is a regular finding. The enzyme, called folate conjugate for some reason, which divides complex folates into mono-folates, is probably a zinc-dependent enzyme in man. The activity of this enzyme is decreasing when a zinc deficiency is introduced in healthy men. Of course, the mono-folate uptake remains unaltered, but perhaps only 25% of our folate uptake comes from single folates in food. So the inability to divide complex folates could be important, I think. Later on, as a further step, there is an increase of faecal lipid loss, but that's a late sign. Severe steatorrhea is a very late sign. When there is severe steatorrhea there is also a binding of trace elements into these lipid stools. There is a correlation between increase in faecal fat loss and decrease in serum zinc as well as iron and copper. So I think this steatorrhea adds to the imbalance but comes fairly late.

AGGETT: I have just a few comments and I would invite a retort from Dr Jameson. My first comment about coeliac disease: Certainly I think people who look after adults should continue to be on the lookout for it, but our experience with children now is indicative that the incidence of coeliac disease is falling. Whether this is due to altered patterns of breast-feeding or later introduction of solids, including wheat, we don't know. But the other intriguing thing now is that it's becoming more obvious that a lot of enteropathies, especially non-responsive so-called gluten-sensitive enteropathies, could well be sensitivities to soy-protein or cow's milk. So there are other mechanisms which can induce this sort of malabsorption.

My main comment reverts back to what we were talking about earlier about the oral zinc tolerance test versus zinc 65 as a means of measuring absorption.

We certainly found the oral zinc tolerance test to be a very effective detector of abnormal proximal intestinal function, more effective, in fact, than other indicators. But I think, as I said earlier on, when we actually came to test zinc absorption in active coeliac patients, using zinc 65 at very low levels, just labelling 2 mg of zinc incorporated in a meal, the absorption of zinc from that meal was just the same in patients with active coeliac disease as it was in volunteer individuals. This could well be because that zinc is being absorbed in the distal intestine which is less affected in coeliac disease. That, of coure, hasn't been proven. But what we did find was that there was an increased loss of endogenous zinc. Therefore these patients, even though their absolute absorption was the same as the control's or reference group's, had reduced net absorption because of this endogenous loss.

JAMESON: Yes, I agree. Of course it's always dubious when you give a very high zinc dose above the normal levels in food and daily intake. We still think it's a fairly good test to use, but it's difficult to do these tests. It's expensive and we don't often do them today.

We try to take biopsies as fast as possible. That's the best way to diagnose. The other thing is that the very intriguing problem is to find out the extent of mucosal damage and there is today no good method for this measurement. The area damage is, of course, the crucial point. Today we have to rely upon single biopsies and the indirect measurements which are difficult to perform.

ABDULLA: I have a question again to Dr Jameson. Folic acid conjugase is a very interesting zinc-dependent enzyme and I wonder if you could elaborate a little about it, because we have a group in my laboratory working on this particular enzyme. *In vitro* studies do not show any correlation between zinc and the activity of the enzyme. But, if we look at the plasma of pregnant women, for example, you will find that the majority of them at the last stage of their pregnancy have low folic acid levels as well as low zinc levels. I wonder if there is a connection between the enzyme activity and the zinc concentrations.

JAMESON: I don't really know, but if you look for reports from Chuck Halstead's group, you will find several papers in the last years about folate conjugates. The first important one is written by Tamura. We have no new data of our own so I can't answer.

STJERNFELDT: We have not talked much about the role of selenium in coeliac disease, but you showed that the selenium level was low in the coeliac patients. Was that after they were substituted or when they were sick?

JAMESON: We had not given selenium supplementation to this group. All my data are given before any treatment. You gave me a reprint of a new paper that was in the

British Medical Journal in June, 1984, about low selenium levels in coeliac disease. I think that it's another new finding which is important. In proximal intestinal disease there is a good possibility of developing multiple deficiencies of trace elements.

STJERNFELDT: It's very interesting because Hinks and collaborators showed that the selenium in leucocytes, whole blood and plasma, was on a lower level than normal in these patients when they were healthy. I think this is remarkable because coeliac patients have a higher incidence of intestinal lymphomas and other cancers.

JAMESON: That's the interesting association. I could only give you another association: intestinal tumours in New Zealand sheep, which were, formerly, often found. Otherwise, there are very few tumours in that area of the small intestine. Since they were given routine selenium supplementation, this type of tumour has disappeared.

FELLSTRÖM: Dr Weismann, I was surprised by your slide stating that there was an increase in serum zinc by thiazides and loop-diuretics. One would expect the effects by diuretics to be on the renal level. Do you have any information about the excretion of zinc from giving thiazides or loop-diuretics? Is there an increase in the excretion?

WEISMANN: I think you should ask Dr Wester about this, he's an expert.

WESTER: Indeed, there is a large urinary increase of the zinc excretion when you are treating the patients with thiazides and, also to some extent, with loop-diuretics. With regard to the loop-diuretics the urinary zinc increase is an effect of increased urinary volume and not increased urinary zinc concentration. The thiazides cause a raised urinary zinc concentration and the amount excreted is increased by up to 50 per cent. It is then astonishing that the serum zinc is somewhat increased. I found in balance studies, that there was no change in zinc absorption. I also found that, when you are treating the patients with thiazides, the liver zinc is very much reduced and also to some extent muscle zinc. I can't explain why there is a small increase in serum zinc, perhaps it may be related to volume depletion.

Skeletal Effects of Aluminium Accumulation in Chronic Renal Failure

By PER NILSSON and BO G. DANIELSON

INTRODUCTION

The frequent association between chronic renal disease and skeletal problems has been appreciated for over 100 years (Lucas 1883). The introduction of dialysis and transplantation have made possible extended survival of the uraemic patient. At the same time bone disease has gained increasing clinical importance as a long-term complication of renal failure (Coburn & Slatopolsky 1981). During the last ten years major advances have been made regarding the pathogenesis and therapy of renal bone disease and it has become increasingly evident that both long-term dialysis and renal transplantation introduce new pathogenetic factors of importance for the development of skeletal problems in these patients. This paper will be devoted to a presentation of some current views regarding the pathogenesis of renal bone disease, with special emphasis on the possible toxic role of aluminium accumulated into bone.

PATHOGENESIS OF RENAL BONE DISEASE

Renal insufficiency is universally accompanied by disturbances of calcium and phosphorus homeostasis having direct and indirect effects on the skeleton. A short summary of generally accepted interrelationships is presented in Fig. 1.

A tendency towards phosphate retention and at least transient postalimentary episodes of hyperphosphataemia occurs in very early renal failure, causing reciprocal lowering of serum calcium and probably also some inhibition of the renal hydroxylase system responsible for the conversion of vitamin D or cholecalciferol to its most active metabolite, 1,25–dihydroxycholecalciferol. With further reduction of renal function hyperphosphatae-

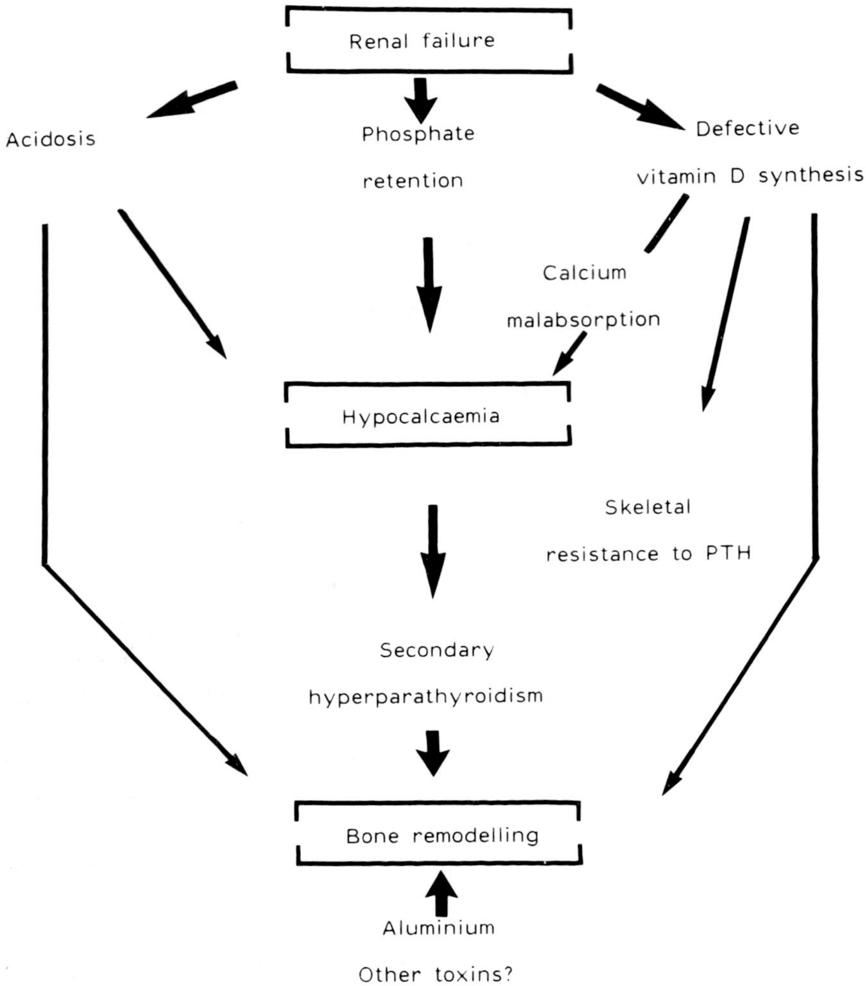

Fig. 1 Suggested interrelationships in the pathogenesis of renal bone disease

mia becomes constant, and vitamin D conversion definitely deficient due to the decrease of functioning renal tissue. Deficiency of the active vitamin D metabolite is of major importance for the defective intestinal absorption of calcium observed when the glomerular filtration rate decreases below approximately 40 ml/min. Calcium deficiency is further enhanced by a frequently low dietary intake of calcium, and possibly by an increased fractional renal excretion of calcium secondary to metabolic acidosis, a frequent accompaniment of renal insufficiency.

Thus, several factors contribute to a lowering of serum calcium, providing a potent stimulus to increased secretion of parathyroid hormone (PTH)

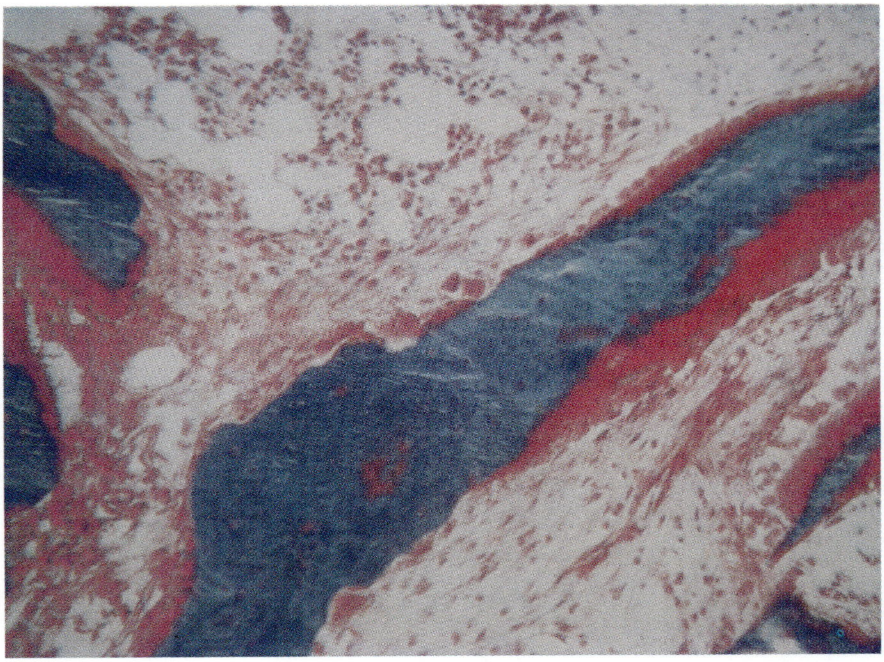

Fig. 2 High turnover state typical of predominant hyperparathyroidism in a haemodialyzed patient

Note moderately widened osteoid seams (red) with lining osteoblasts and intervening resorptive lacunae. Trabecular bone from iliac crest. Goldner trichrome

and to parathyroid gland hyperplasia. This secondary hyperparathyroidism is further promoted by a skeletal resistance to the calcium-raising effects of PTH, which is probably related to vitamin D deficiency and lack of the normal synergism of PTH and vitamin D in mobilizing mineral from the skeleton.

Calcium and vitamin D deficiency and excess parathyroid activity affect the skeleton through their effects on bone remodelling, the life-long process of internal replacement or turnover of bone tissue by orderly, sequential and quantitized events of resorption, formation and mineralization. This turnover of bone is essential for the maintenance of mechanical skeletal integrity, and also continuously provides young bone active in the regulation of extracellular mineral homeostasis (Frost 1973). Calcium deficiency secondary to vitamin D deficiency, and probably vitamin D deficiency *per se*, lead to defective bone matrix mineralization, or osteomalacia. PTH is the major modulator of the rate of bone remodelling or turnover, and massive PTH stimulation leads to a state of excessive bone resorption with replacement by poorly mineralized woven bone, known as osteitis fibrosa.

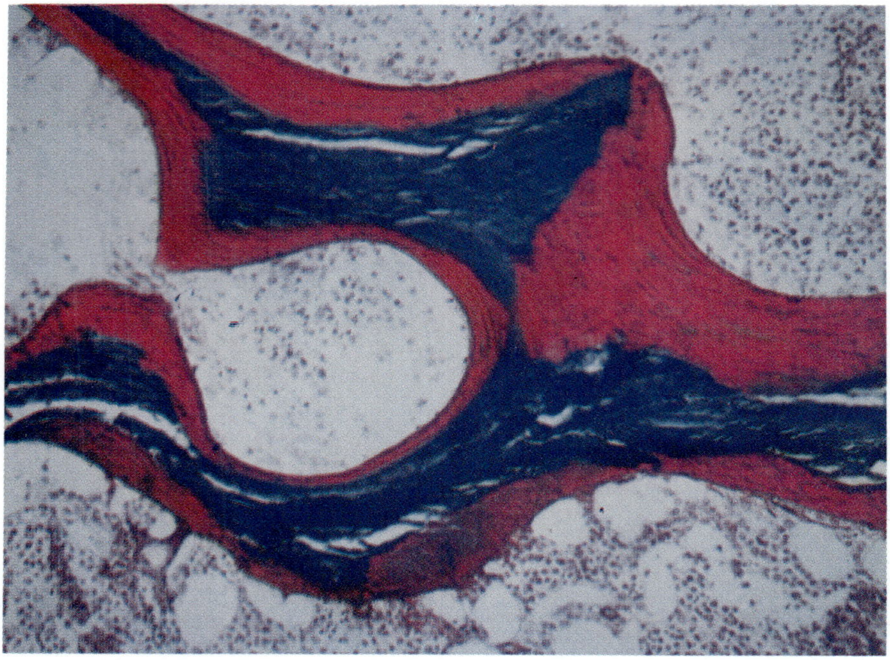

Fig. 3 Typical histological appearance of dialysis osteomalacia

Note massive hyperosteoidosis (red), virtual absence of identifiable osteoblasts and absence of resorptive activity. Trabecular bone from iliac crest. Goldner trichrome

From the above pathogenetic considerations it would be reasonable to expect the bone disease of renal failure to contain components both of osteitis fibrosa of secondary hyperparathyroidism and of defective mineralization or osteomalacia. This is also the usual finding in the non-dialyzed uraemic patient (Ellis & Peart 1973). With careful quantitative histological analysis all patients with advanced uraemia will show evidence of disturbed bone remodelling. The bone turnover rate is usually low due to a predominance of defective mineralization. In patients treated with dialysis against a dialysate with a calcium concentration high enough to allow definite intradialytic calcium accretion, mineralization may become largely normal, but signs of hyperparathyroidism usually persist or progress (Fig. 2).

Recently, however, one further distinct type of skeletal pathology has been described with increasing frequency, so far almost exclusively in patients treated with long-term haemodialysis. The bone disease in these patients is histologically characterized by a severe and isolated or almost isolated mineralization defect with no or very few signs of hyperparathyroidism (Fig. 3). Due to the defective mineralization, bone-remodelling rates are low to unmeasurable. This histological picture has been termed dialysis osteomalacia, and has been shown to carry a high incidence of symptomatic skeletal disease, with bone pain and spontaneous fractures being prominent features. Also by serum-biochemical variables, these patients are usually distinguishable from the ordinary population of haemodialysis patients, showing a tendency towards hypercalcaemia, occurring spontaneously or easily provoked by vitamin D or calcium supplementation, normal or only slightly elevated serum levels of alkaline phosphatases, and normal or only moderately elevated serum levels of PTH. An increasing body of evidence, to be presented below, now connects the appearance of dialysis osteomalacia with bone aluminium accumulation.

ALUMINIUM AND DIALYSIS OSTEOMALACIA

The first literature report of dialysis osteomalacia appeared in 1972 (Posen et al. 1972), where clinical, radiographic and histological osteomalacia was described in 50% of patients in the Ottawa district treated with haemodialysis for more than 18 months against a dialysate prepared with ordinary tap water, while no such problems were noted in patients treated with a dialysate prepared from deionized water. Similar findings were described from across the Atlantic in the Newcastle area (Siddiqui & Kerr 1972) and interestingly, the first report was published on the specific neurological disorder of haemodialysis patients, later termed dialysis encephalopathy (Alfrey et al. 1972). The fact that these problems seemed to be exclusive to patients treated with long-term dialysis led to early investigations into the possible presence of external, water-borne agents of pathogenetic significance. Several trace elements, including tin and fluoride, were discussed at this time. A few years later (Alfrey et al. 1976), results of aluminium determinations in patients with uraemia and on haemodialysis were published. Markedly elevated aluminium levels were found in all tissues, and in dialyzed patients especially in brain gray matter and trabecular bone from patients dying with the syndrome of dialysis encephalopathy. Several later studies have demonstrated a significant correlation between the occurrence of encephalopathy, bone disease of osteomalacic type, and long-term dialysis against untreated or softened water in geographical areas where the aluminium content in the water supply has been high (usually >100 μg/l), due to the use of aluminium as a flocculating agent during water purification (Platts et al. 1977, Parkinson et al. 1979, Walker et al. 1982). Patients with dialysis encephalopathy and osteomalacia have also been found to have a high incidence of microcytic anaemia, and an aluminium intoxication syndrome with these three components has been suggested (Parkinson et al. 1981).

Dialysis patients with clinical and histological dialysis osteomalacia have been shown to have a higher bone aluminium content than patients without these disorders when estimated by atomic absorption photometometry on bone biopsies (Hodsman et al. 1982), by X-ray microanalysis (Boyce et al.

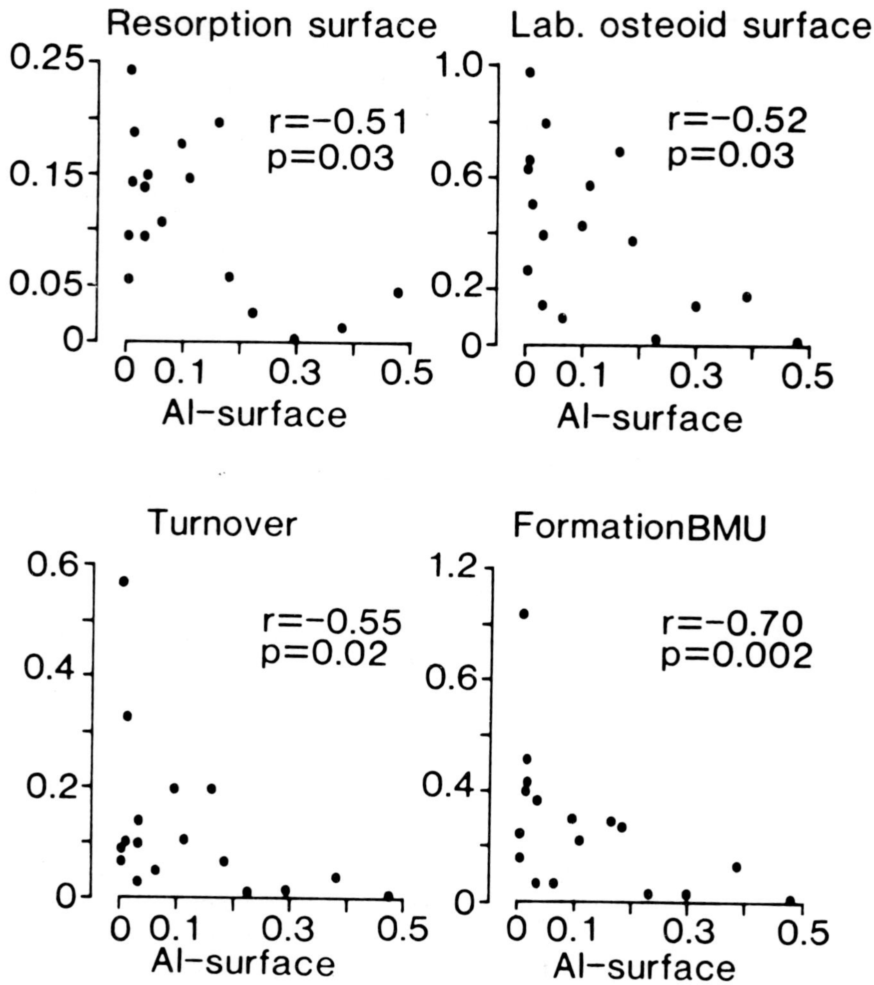

Fig. 4 *Relationships between parameters of trabecular bone-remodelling and fractional extent of trabecular bone surfaces with positive aluminium staining (Al-surface)*

Lab. osteoid surface = Fraction of osteoid surfaces labelled with tetracycline. Turnover = Calculated bone formation rate averaged over the entire trabecular bone surface. Formation BMU = Bone formation rate calculated at the level of the bone-remodelling unit

1982), and by histochemical staining with aurine tricarboxylic acid which is specific for aluminium (Ott et al. 1982). Moreover, an inverse relationship between aluminium and ash content in trabecular bone has been demonstrated (Alfrey et al. 1979).

Animal experimental studies, so far only performed in rats, which lack human-type bone remodelling, also seem to support the connection between aluminium accumulation and deficient bone mineralization (Robertson et al. 1983).

While there, thus, is a large body of data linking symptomatic dialysis osteomalacia to heavy bone aluminium accumulation, the direct pathophysiologic actions of aluminium on bone remodelling remain to be elucidated. Our own studies (Nilsson et al. 1984a), performed in patients on long-term haemodialysis, entirely without symptoms of musculo-skeletal disease, and exposed to only moderate dialysate concentrations of aluminium of about 20 μg/l, indicate that bone aluminium accumulation is of pathophysiological significance also in such patients, and also indicate that other factors than the total amount and time of aluminium exposition govern the tendency of the individual patient to accumulate aluminium in bone.

Thus, out of 17 patients treated with haemodialysis for a mean time of 19 months against a mean dialysate aluminium concentration of 20 μg/l, aluminium deposition was demonstrable in 13 by histochemical staining of trabecular bone obtained at iliac crest biopsy. Although patients with a positive bone stain for aluminium had, on the average, spent a longer time on dialysis than patients without this finding, there was no direct relationship between the time on dialysis or the total amount of aluminium ingested as aluminium-containing phosphate binders and the extent of trabecular bone surfaces stainable for aluminium. Significant relationships were, however, observed between the extent or fraction of trabecular bone surfaces stainable for aluminium and parameters of bone turnover and mineralization (Fig. 4). Especially interesting, there was a clear inverse relationship between aluminium staining and the fraction of osteoid surfaces active in bone mineralization, as estimated by tetracycline labelling. The appositional rate, or linear calcification rate was, however, normal in those areas where active mineralization did occur. This could indicate that aluminium might act as an inhibitor of the initiation of the mineralization process. Such a role for aluminium is also suggested by studies of serial sections of bone biopsies which indicate that mineralization does not occur on most bone surfaces stainable for aluminium (Maloney et al. 1982), and would seem to fit well with the almost selective localization of aluminium along the osteoid-bone interface appearing on histochemical staining (Fig. 5).

PROBLEMS OF ALUMINIUM EXPOSURE

Even if the majority of reports of clinical aluminium toxicity in dialysis patients have emanated from centres where the dialysate aluminium concentration has been 100 μg/l or more, other dialysate-related factors than the absolute aluminium concentration are probably of importance for aluminium kinetics during dialysis. It has, thus, been shown that the dialyzability of aluminium is strongly pH-dependent, increasing sharply at both acid and alkaline pH (Gacek et al. 1979). The pH and bicarbonate content of water

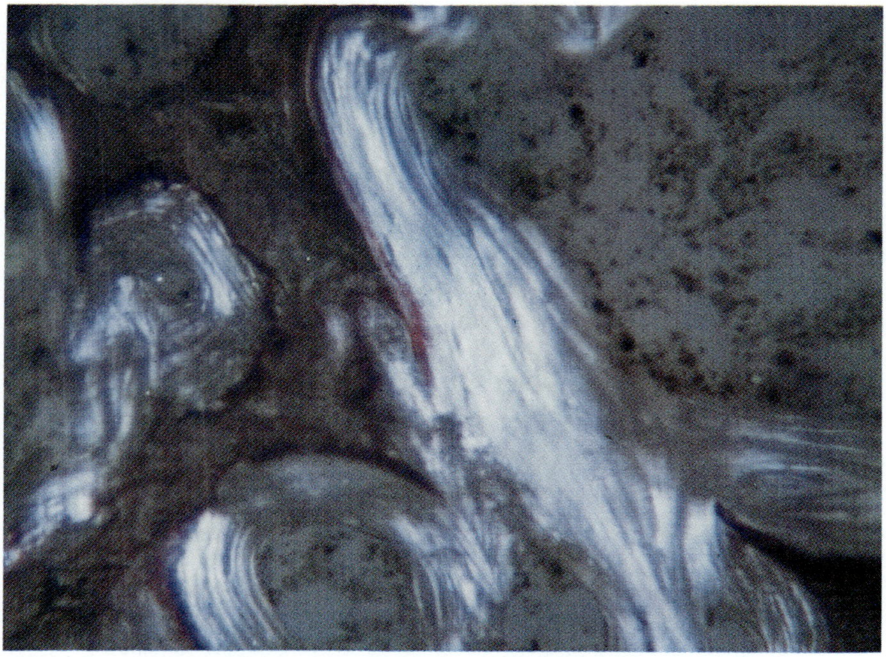

Fig. 5 Positive staining for aluminium (red) in trabecular bone

Note aluminium localization along interface of mineralized bone (dark) and the lighter birefringent osteoid. Trabecular bone from iliac crest. Polarized light

used for the preparation of dialysate varies greatly between different countries and between different dialysis centres in the same country. This could explain the diverging results concerning the possibility of aluminium elimination by dialysis reported in the literature (Kaehny et al. 1977a, Graf et al. 1981), and probably makes it difficult to predict a generally safe dialysate aluminium concentration.

In patients dialyzed against low aluminium concentrations, the ingestion of aluminium-containing phosphate binders in all probability makes an important contribution to the total aluminium burden. Significant aluminium absorption from phosphate binders does occur both in normal and uraemic subjects (Berlyne et al. 1970, Kaehny et al. 1977b), and such absorption in the uraemic patient may lead to plasma aluminium concentrations of well over 100 μg/l, a level suggested to carry a high risk of tissue accumulation and eventual clinical toxicity (Fleming et al. 1982). The importance of aluminium hydroxide ingestion in the production of aluminium-associated disease is also suggested by reports of improvement of dialysis encephalopathy after the cessation of phosphate-binding therapy (McKinney et al. 1982).

As suggested by our own studies, specific patient-related factors in all probability are also of a great importance, at least for the tendency towards bone aluminium accumulation. The parathyroid function seems to be of special importance in this context. As in the normal subject, PTH is the major modulator of bone-remodelling rates in the uraemic patient (Fig. 6). It is our observation, as well as that of others (Hodsman et al. 1982), that dialysis patients with heavy bone aluminium accumulation show lower serum PTH levels than patients without demonstrable bone aluminium. Further, the mineralization defect of dialysis osteomalacia together with signs of aluminium accumulation has been reported to appear after parathyroidectomy in dialysis patients (Ellis 1982). This seems to indicate that PTH has a role in the protection of bone against aluminium deposition. It could be speculated that a low bone-remodelling rate secondary to low PTH facilitates aluminium deposition.

Moreover, abnormal parathyroid function, in the form of a deficient PTH response to an acute hypocalcaemic stimulus, has been demonstrated in haemodialysis patients with osteomalacia and aluminium accumulation (Kraut et al. 1983). This deficiency of parathyroid activity could possibly be explained by aluminium accumulation in the parathyroid glands (Cann et al. 1979), but it is our experience that serum PTH levels remain constant over time in patients on long-term haemodialysis (Nilsson et al. 1984b). It seems more likely that a relative hypoparathyroidism in a situation of increased skeletal resistance to the actions of PTH is the primary event in those patients who accumulate aluminium rapidly when placed on dialysis.

THERAPEUTIC CONSIDERATIONS

As might be expected if aluminium, indeed, directly inhibits the mineralization process, dialysis osteomalacia is generally quite resistant to treatment with the active vitamin D metabolites. Histopathological changes are not favourably affected by such therapy, and in general hypercalcaemia develops rapidly (Pierides et al. 1976). Purification of the water used for dialysis by means of reverse osmosis or deionization has given inconsistent results in the treatment of symptomatic dialysis osteomalacia, but some promising results have been reported when these measures have been combined with attempts at augmented aluminium elimination by use of the chelating agent desferrioxamine in combination with haemodialysis. Such therapy has been documented to give symptomatic and radiographic improvement in some cases (Brown et al. 1982).

SUMMARY

While, thus, the precise factors, governing the tendency of the individual dialysis patient to accumulate aluminium in bone when exposed to aluminium via the dialysate and/or via intestinal absorption from aluminium-

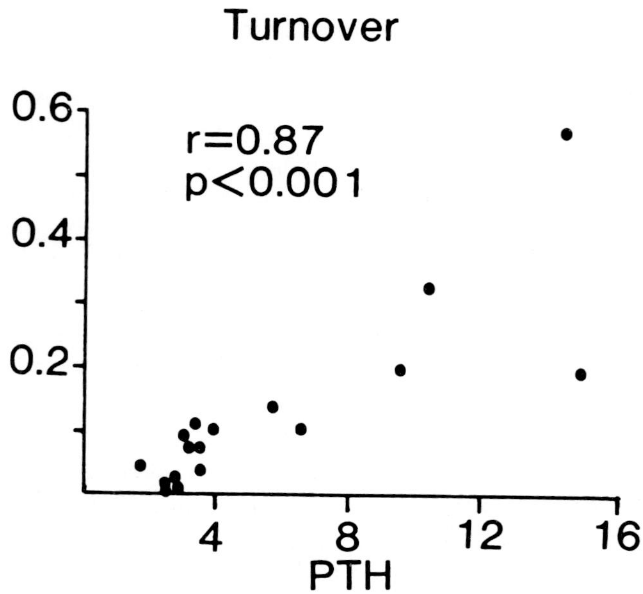

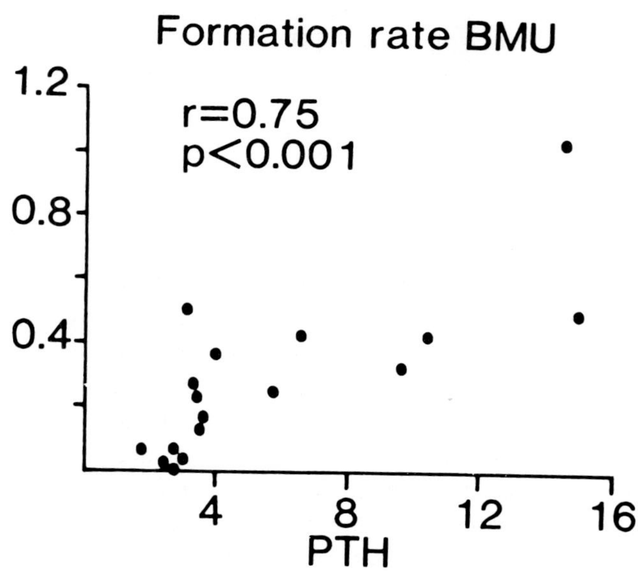

Fig. 6 Relationships between parameters of bone-remodelling and serum PTH in haemodialysis patients

For explanation see Fig. 4

containing phosphate binders, have yeat to be determined, as has the direct pathophysiologic effect of aluminium on bone remodelling, the very large body of epidemiological, clinical and experimental data which have been reported, overwhelmingly support a direct pathogenetic role of aluminium in dialysis bone disease and encephalopathy. Thus, every effort should be made to lessen the aluminium burden of the uraemic patient, by means of optimal purification of the water used for dialysis as well as for preparing the dialysate concentrate, and by attempting to find alternatives to aluminium-containing compounds for intestinal phosphate binding in these patients.

REFERENCES

ALFREY, A. C., LE GENDRE, G. R. & KAEHNY, W. D. (1976). The dialysis encephalopathy syndrome. Possible aluminium intoxication. *New Engl. J. Med.* 294, 184.

ALFREY, A. C., HEGG, A., MILLER, N., BERL, T. & BERNS, H. (1979). Interrelationship between calcium and aluminium metabolism in dialyzed uremic patients. *Mineral Electrolyte Metab.* 2, 81.

ALFREY, A. C., MISHELL, J. M., BURKS, J., CONTIGUGLIA, S. R., RUDOLPH, H., LEWIN, E. & HOLMES, J. G. (1972). Syndrome of dyspraxia and multifocal seizures associated with chronic hemodialysis. *Trans. Amer. Soc. Artif. Intern. Organs* 18, 257.

BERLYNE, G. M., BEN-ARI, J., PEST, D., WEINBERGER, J., STERN, M., GILMORE, G. R. & LEVINE, R. (1970). Hyperaluminiaemia from aluminium resins in renal failure. *Lancet* ii, 494.

BOYCE, B. F., ELDER, H. Y., ELLIOT, H. L., FOGELMAN, J., FELL, G. S., JUNOR, B. J., BEASTALL, G. & BOYLE, G. T. (1982). Hypercalcaemic osteomalacia due to aluminium toxicity. *Lancet* ii, 1009.

BROWN, D. J., DAWBORN, J. K., HAM, K. N. & XIPELL, J. M. (1982). Treatment of dialysis osteomalacia with desferrioxamine. *Lancet* ii, 343.

CANN, C. E., PRUSSIN, S. G. & GORDAN, G. S. (1979). Aluminium uptake by the parathyroid glands. *J. clin. Endocr.* 49, 543.

COBURN, J. W. & SLATOPOLSKY, E. (1981). Vitamin D, parathyroid hormone, and renal osteodystrophy. In *The Kidney*, pp. 2213–2305. Ed. by B. M. Brenner and R. C. Rector. W. B. Saunders Company, Philadelphia.

ELLIS, H. A. (1982). Aluminium and osteomalacia after parathyroidectomy. *Ann. intern. Med.* 96, 533.

ELLIS, H. A. & PEART, K. J. (1973). Azotaemic renal osteodystrophy: a quantitative study on iliac bone. *J. clin. Pathol.* 26, 83.

FLEMING, L. W., STEWART, W. K., FELL, G. S. & HALLS, D. J. (1982). The effect of oral aluminium therapy on plasma aluminium levels in patients with chronic renal failure in centra with low water aluminium. *Clin. Nephrol.* 17, 222.

FROST, H. M. (1973). *Bone Remodeling and Its Relationship to Metabolic Bone Disease*. C. C. Thomas, Springfield, Illinois.

GACEK, E. M., BABB, A. L., UVELLI, D. A., FRY, D. L. & SCRIBNER, B. H. (1979). Dialysis dementia: The role of dialysate pH in altering the dialyzability of aluminium. *Trans. Amer. Soc. Artif. Intern. Organs* 25, 409.

GRAF, H., STUMMVOLL, H. K., MEISINGER, V., KOVARIK, J., WOLF, A. & PINGGERA, W. F. (1981). Aluminium removal by hemodialysis. *Kidney Int.* 19, 587.

HODSMAN, A. B., SHERRARD, D. J., ALFREY, A. C., OTT, S., BRICKMAN, A. S., MILLER, N. L., MALONEY, N. A. & COBURN, J. W. (1982). Bone aluminium and histomorphometric features of renal osteodystrophy. *J. clin. Endocr.* 54, 539.

KAEHNY, W. D., ALFREY, A. C., HOLMAN, R. E. & SHORR, W. J. (1977a). Aluminium transfer during hemodialysis. *Kidney Int.* 12, 361.

KAEHNY, W. D., HEGG, A. P. & ALFREY, A. C. (1977b). Gastrointestinal absorption of aluminium from alumnium-containing antacids. *New Engl. J. Med.* 296, 1389.

KRAUT, J. A., SHINABERGER, J. H., SINGER, F. R., SHERRARD, D. J., SAXTON, J., MILLER, J. H., KUROKAWA, K. & COBURN, J. W. (1983). Parathyroid gland responsiveness to acute hypocalcemia in dialysis osteomalacia. *Kidney Int.* 23, 725.

LUCAS, R. C. (1883). On a form of late rickets associated with albuminuria, rickets of adolescence. *Lancet* i, 993.

MALONEY, N. A., OTT, S. M., ALFREY, A. C., MILLER, N. L., COBURN, J. W. & SHERRARD, D. J. (1982). Histological quantitation of aluminium in iliac bone from patients with renal failure. *J. Lab. clin. Med.* 99, 206.

MCKINNEY, T. D., BASINGER, M., DAWSON, E. & JONES, M. M. (1982). Serum aluminium levels in dialysis dementia. *Nephron* 32, 53.

NILSSON, P., MELSEN, F., MALMAEUS, J., DANIELSON, B. G. & MOSEKILDE, L. (1984a). Relationships between calcium and phosphorus homeostasis, parathyroid hormone levels, bone aluminium, and bone histomorphometry in patients on maintenance hemodialsysis. *Metab. Bone Dis. Rel. Res.* in press.

NILSSON, P., MALMAEUS, J., WIDE, L. & DANIELSON, B. G. (1984b). An investigation of biochemical and radiographic signs of secondary hyperparathyroidism in chronic renal disease. *Scand. J. Urol. Nephrol.* 84, Suppl.

OTT, S. M., MALONEY, N. A., COBURN, J. W., ALFREY, A. C. & SHERRARD, D. J. (1982). The prevalence of bone aluminium deposition in renal osteodystrophy and its relation to the response to calcitriol therapy. *New Engl. J. Med.* 307, 709.

PARKINSON, I. S., FEEST, T. G., WARD, M. K., FAWCETT, R. W. P. & KERR, D. N. S. (1979). Fracturing dialysis osteodystrophy and dialysis encephalopathy. An epidemiological survey. *Lancet* i, 406.

PARKINSON, I. S., WARD, M. K. & KERR, D. N. S. (1981). Dialysis encephalopathy, bone disease and anaemia: the aluminium intoxication syndrome during regular haemodialysis. *J. clin. Pathol.* 34, 1285.

PIERIDES, A. M., SIMPSON, W., WARD, M. K., ELLIS, H. A., DEWAR, J. H. & KERR, D. N. S. (1976). Variable response to long term 1α-hydroxy-cholecalciferol in haemodialysis osteodystrophy. *Lancet* i, 1092.

PLATTS, M. M., GOODE, G. C. & HISLOP, J. S. (1977). Composition of domestic water supply and the incidence of fractures and encephalopathy in patients on home dialysis. *Brit. med. J.* ii, 657.

POSEN, G. A., GRAY, D. G., JAWORSKI, Z. F., COUTURE, C. & RASHID, A. (1972). Comparison of renal osteodystrophy in patients dialyzed with deionized and non-deionized water. *Trans. Amer. Soc. Artif. Intern. Organs* 18, 405.

ROBERTSON, J. A., FELSENFELD, A. J., HAYGOOD, C. C., WILSON, P., CLARKE, C. & LLACH, F. (1983). Animal model of aluminium-induced osteomalacia: Role of chronic renal failure. *Kidney Int.* 23, 327.

SIDDIQUI, J. & KERR, D. N. S. (1972). Complications of renal failure and their response to dialysis. *Brit. med. Bull.* 27, 153.

WALKER, G. S., AARON, J. E., PEACOCK, M., ROBINSON, P. J. A. & DAVISON, A. M. (1982). Dialysate aluminium concentration and renal bone disease. *Kidney Int.* 21, 411.

Renal Failure and Trace Element Metabolism

By Bo G. Danielson, Bengt Fellström, Nils Grefberg, Per Nilsson, Lars Weiss and Björn Wikström

Patients with chronic renal failure on dialysis may *accumulate* or *lose* substantial amounts of trace elements across the peritoneal and hemodialysis membranes. The volume of the dialysis solution used in one patient on hemodialysis in one year is about 15,000–20,000 l. This may result in a disturbed metabolism of trace elements.

The peritoneal cavity of a patient on continuous ambulatory peritoneal dialysis (CAPD) is rinsed with about 3,000 l every year.

The purpose of this investigation was to study the trace element levels in the blood of patients on CAPD and compare these results with those of healthy controls in our region. The comparison with the results from patients on chronic hemodialysis has also been included.

METHODS AND MATERIAL

Since 1979, about 75 patients have been trained on CAPD. This report includes results from 50 patients on CAPD with the mean age of 45 (22–72) years. Twenty-four of the patients were diabetics. The patients had on average been on CAPD for 15 (3–45) months. The results have been compared to those of 30 patients on hemodialysis with the mean age of 50 years, of which two patients were diabetics, and also compared to 50 healthy persons who have served as controls. The controls had an age of 17–67 years, ten of each decade.

Since there was no significant change with age for any trace element analyzed, the results of the controls are given as the average for the whole control population.

For the analysis induced, coupled plasma emission spectrometry, X-ray fluorescence or atomic absorption with heated graphite furnace have been used.

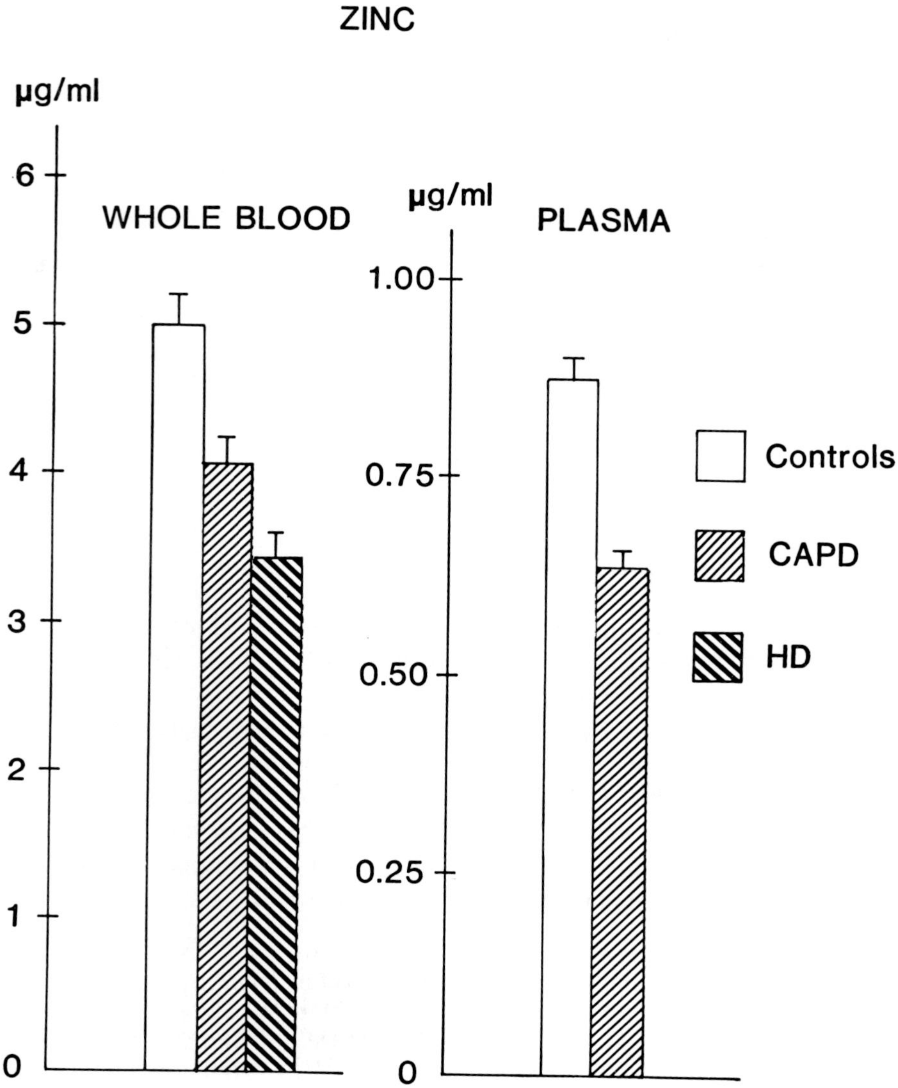

Fig. 1 *Mean concentration + 1 SEM in whole blood for healthy controls, CAPD and hemodialysis patients*

Several elements have been analyzed. Whole blood or plasma have been used for zinc, copper, nickel, aluminium, tin, chromium, manganese, selenium, lead, cadmium, arsenic and mercury.

ZINC IN SKIN BIOPSIES

Shave biopsies weighing 1.5–2.0 mg dry weight were taken from shoulder or gluteal regions from healthy controls and from dialysis patients. Biopsies

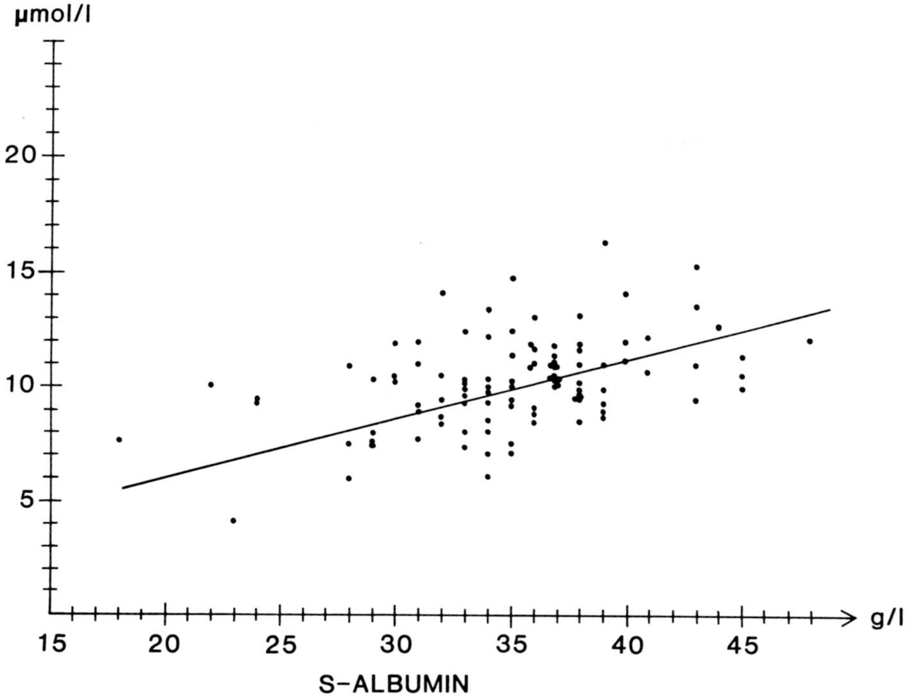

Fig. 2 Plasma zinc related to serum albumin in the CAPD patients

were placed on aluminium foil in a drop of saline, heated for 5 sec to 52°C, whereafter the biopsies were separated into epidermis and dermis with stainless steel tweezers. The biopsies were then dried for two hours, weighed and transferred to acid-washed glass tubes. To each sample 50 µl of millipore-treated water was added and left for 24 hours, followed by the addition of 250 µl of 65% nitric acid left for 96 hours. The zinc content was determined after dilution by atomic absorption spectrophotometry.

RESULTS

Zinc. More than 70 zinc-containing enzymes are known. Zinc depletion in adults has been related to sexual dysfunction, impaired taste and impaired wound healing and skin manifestations. Zinc depletion has been described in some dialysis patients.

Whole-blood zinc was significantly lower in both CAPD and hemodialysis patients than in controls. Plasma zinc levels in the CAPD patients were also significantly lower than in normals (Fig. 1). This may be due to low plasma albumin concentration, since zinc is to about 70% bound to plasma albumin and to about 30% to α_2-macroglobulin. In Fig. 2 the plasma zinc is plotted versus the serum albumin level. The plasma zinc is related to the serum

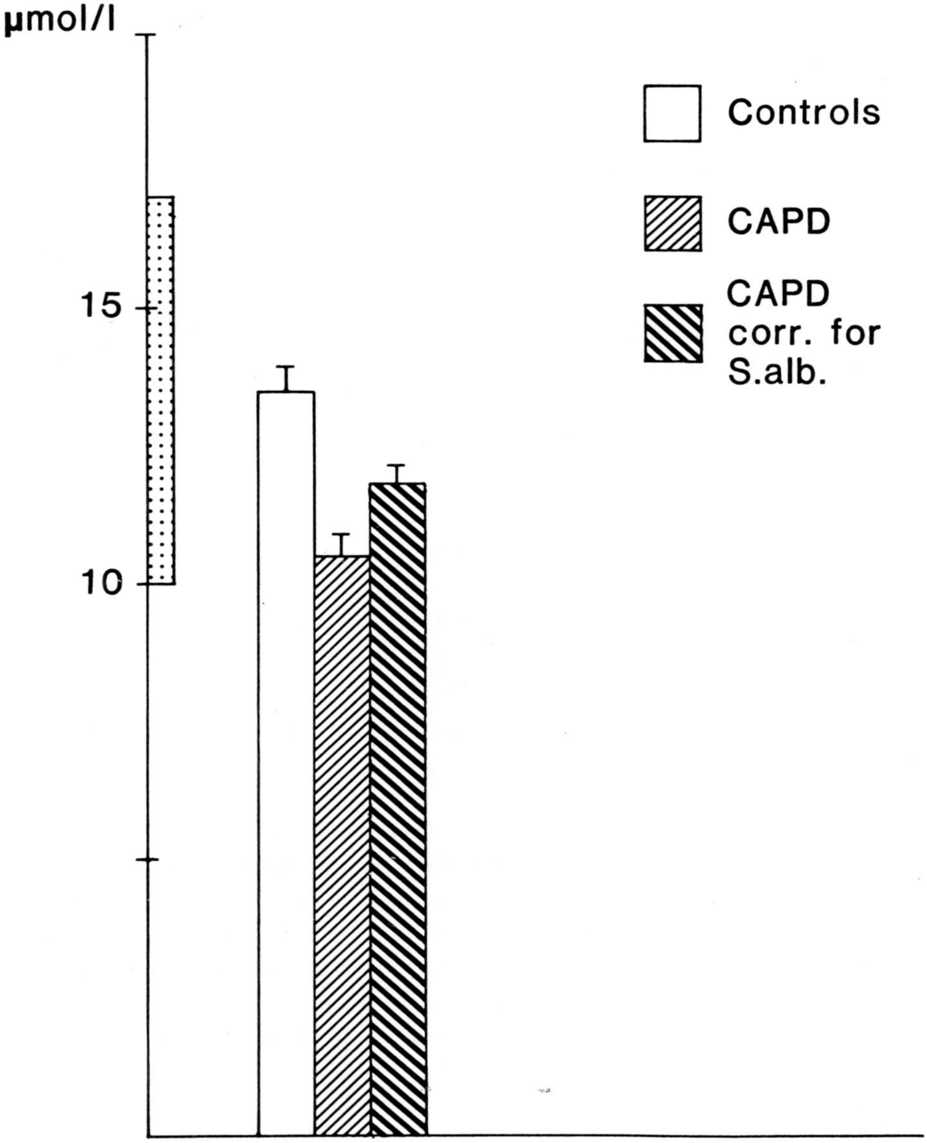

Fig. 3 Plasma zinc levels in CAPD patients corrected for reduced serum albumin

albumin. The relation found was used for correction of plasma zinc level to a normal serum albumin. Figure 3 shows the results. The CAPD patients had lower zinc levels than the controls but within the normal range. One has also to bear in mind that such a correction will not take into account the portion of plasma zinc which is bound to α_2-macroglobulin. The concentration of this protein may vary significantly in uremic patients and may differ from healthy controls.

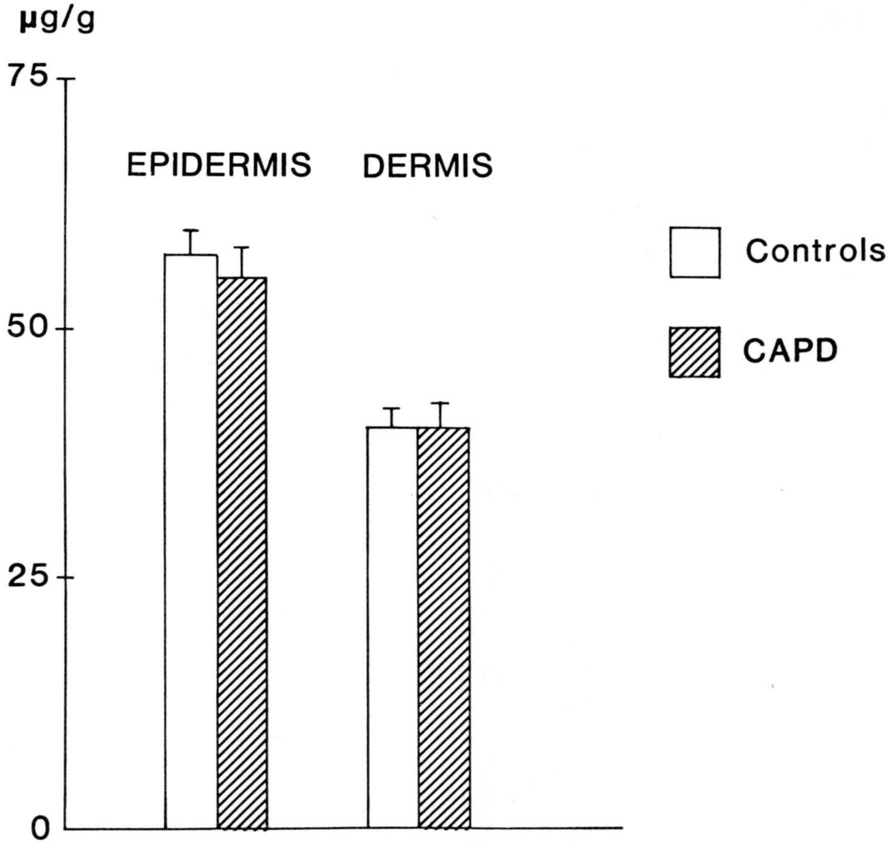

Fig. 4 Zinc content in skin biopsies in controls and CAPD patients

When the plasma zinc was plotted vs time on CAPD no significant change was found with time, indicating that no obvious effect on plasma zinc levels could be seen.

Since the serum level may not reflect the zinc content of the main tissue stores, which are located in the skin, muscle, bone and liver, we also analyzed skin biopsies for zinc in order to get an estimate of the zinc stores. Skin biopsies were obtained from 15 patients and from 40 healthy controls.

Figure 4 shows the zinc content of the biopsies in epidermis and dermis compared to the controls. As can be seen, no difference could be observed. The results are expressed as micrograms zinc per gram dried tissue. Even if the group as a whole did not show any signs of depletion there are always patients who are at special risk, e.g., patients who have a low caloric intake, who have a diet with low animal protein or patients who have inflammatory bowel disease, etc. Besides that observation, time may have been too short in order to detect signs and symptoms of zinc depletion. Corresponding figures were also found in a group of 15 hemodialysis patients who have been treated for various lengths of time.

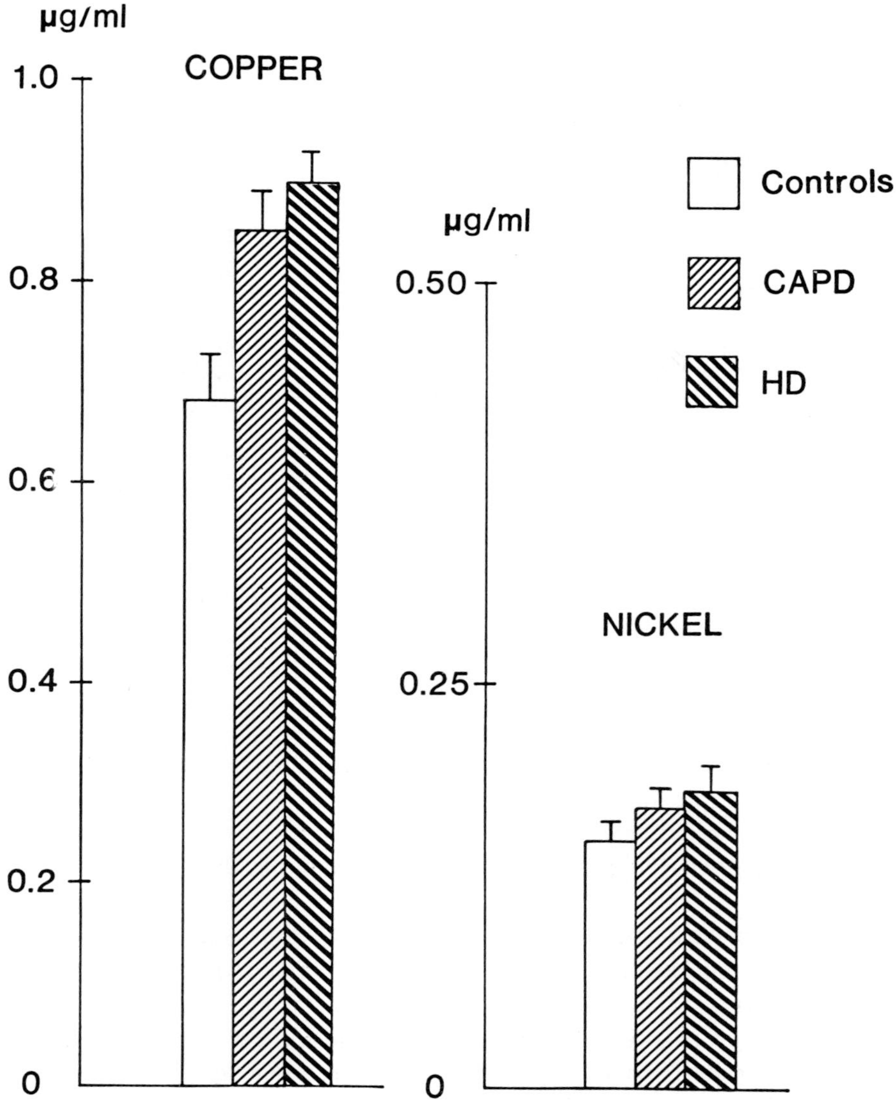

Fig. 5 Mean whole-blood concentration of copper and nickel in controls, CAPD and hemodialysis patients (+ 1 SEM)

In other studies (Thomson et al. 1981, Mahajan et al. 1984) various results have been found. Both low red-blood zinc and elevated erythrocyte zinc levels have been found in uremic patients. Plasma levels of zinc have been found to be low in dialysis patients in several reports (Thomson et al. 1981, Mahajan et al. 1984, Abu-Hamdan et al. 1984). This can be due to several factors, e.g., reduced plasma albumin level, reduced gastrointestinal absorption of zinc, or the use of phosphate binders.

When corrected for plasma albumin, the plasma zinc is not significantly

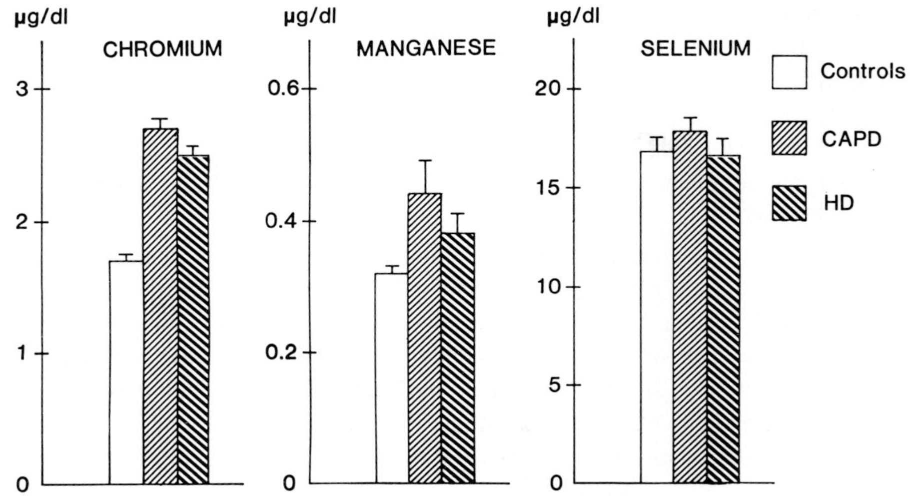

Fig. 6 Mean plasma level + 1 SEM of chromium, manganese and selenium in controls, CAPD and hemodialysis patients

lower than in normals but in the lower part of the normal range. When whole-blood zinc is corrected for the lower haematocrit fraction and the low plasma albumin, the zinc levels in blood were not lower than in normals. Therefore, the results do not indicate any sign of zinc deficiency as measured from blood levels, which was reported by Thomson et al. 1981 and interpreted as zinc deficiency.

Copper is an essential element that takes part in several fundamental enzymes, e.g., in the respiratory oxidation system. Significantly higher levels of whole-blood copper were found in both CAPD and hemodialysis patients compared to normal controls (Fig. 5). From Australia, Thomson and co-workers (1981) have reported unchanged plasma copper and reduced red-cell copper, which may indicate Cu-depletion in CAPD patients, which is not in accordance with these results. Our results do not indicate, however, any copper depletion, as found in the Australian study.

Nickel is also an essential element, the physiological role of which has not been established. In experimental work in rats, nickel deficiency leads to retarded growth and anaemia. Nickel is also a nephrotoxic agent. The nickel levels in our CAPD and hemodialysis patients (Fig. 5) were not significantly different from the controls.

Chromium is an essential element required for the optimal effect of insulin. Chromium deficiency leads to impaired glucose tolerance, hyperlipidemia and probably also arteriosclerotic heart disease.

The average chromium plasma levels (Fig. 6) were significantly higher in both CAPD and hemodialysis patients than in the controls. These results were in accordance with studies from Australia. In a recent study from United Kingdom the chromium levels in uremic patients on hemodialysis and continuous ambulatory peritoneal dialysis were studied. A greater than ten-fold rise in serum chromium level was observed in patients on hemodialysis and CAPD, while no significant changes occurred in patients with chronic renal failure but not on dialysis. The hemodialysis and CAPD dialysate were found to contain a high level of chromium indicating that the high serum levels may have been a result of dialysate contamination (Leung et al. 1984a).

Manganese is a highly essential element for cellular membrane integrity and is essential for growth, the reproductive functions, bone formation and glucose and lipid metabolism. Manganese deficiency is very rare in man. It may result in dermatitis, nausea, changed hair colour etc. Manganese overload leads to bone formation defects and neurologic disturbances such as ataxia. The plasma levels of manganese (Fig. 6) were significantly higher in CAPD and hemodialysis patients than in the controls, and especially pronounced in CAPD patients.

It is well-known that *selenium* is an essential trace element. The most well-known selenium-containing enzyme is glutathione peroxidase. Selenium plays a role for the integrity of the cellular and subcellular membranes. It is also known to be anticarcinogenic. Especially in veterinary medicine, depletion syndromes are known. It is known that selenium depletion may lead to progressive muscle dystrophy. The selenium plasma levels in our CAPD (Fig. 6) patients as well as in the hemodialysis patients were, however, not significantly different from the levels in the controls.

In a recent study from Glasgow (Leung et al. 1984b) a significant decrease in serum selenium was observed in uremic patients before dialysis as well as on hemodialysis and CAPD. The serum glutathione peroxidase activity was below the normal range in both serum and red blood cells. The results indicated a relative selenium deficiency state in patients both on and before dialysis. This was interpreted as due to reduced dietary intake or to an increased loss across the dialysis membrane.

Aluminium is not an essential element for man. It has been shown earlier in several studies that aluminium is accumulated in patients with chronic renal failure. In our study the aluminium levels were significantly higher in both the CAPD patients and the hemodialysis patients than in the controls (Fig. 7). High plasma aluminium may have a number of causes. Probably the intake of aluminium-containing phosphate binders is one important cause, but other sources may also play a role. The dialysate itself may also play a significant role since the solutions may contain aluminium. However, after accidents with aluminium-contaminated dialysis solutions the manufacturers are more aware of the problem and now guarantee a low aluminium content.

During the last couple of years, *tin* has been accepted as an essential trace element. Tin participates in oxidation-reduction reactions but details are not known. From experimental work in rats it has been found that tin deficiency

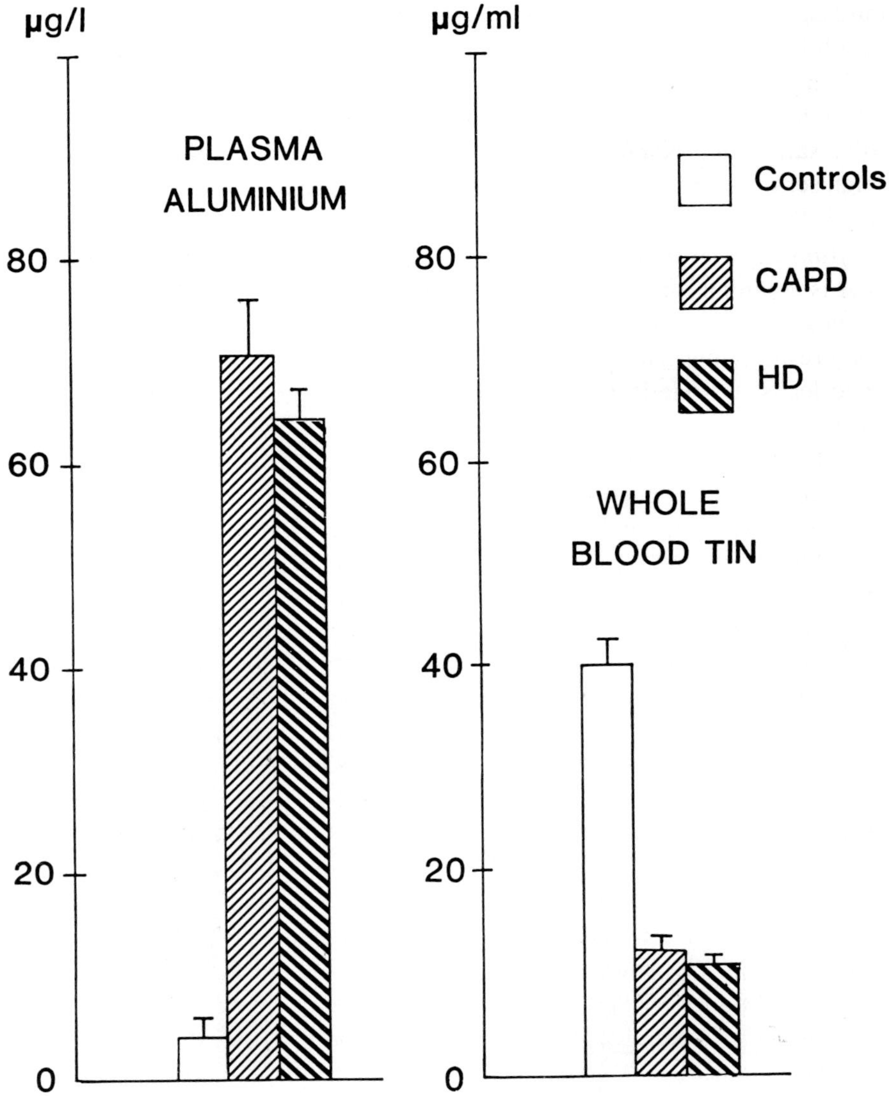

Fig. 7 Mean plasma aluminium and whole-blood levels in controls, CAPD and hemodialysis patients

leads to retarded growth. Very little is known about tin deficiency in man. The tin levels were significantly lower (Fig. 7) in the CAPD patients as well as in the hemodialysis patients than in the controls. The significance of this is so far not obvious.

Cadmium has not been found to have any specific function either in plants or in animals and is therefore regarded as a non-essential element. It is known to give toxic effects on renal tubule and bones. Cadmium is thought to impair the vitamin-D metabolism.

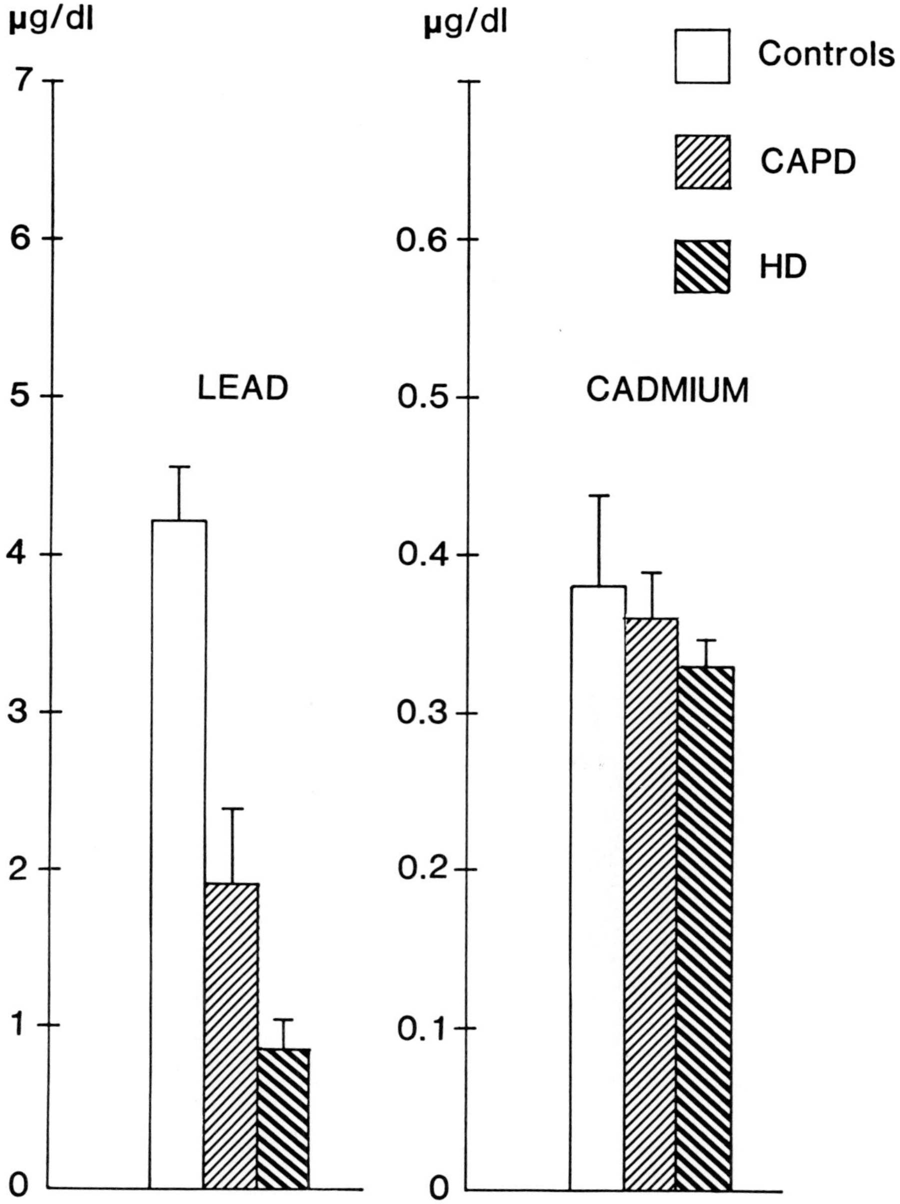

Fig. 8 Mean whole-blood concentration of lead and cadmium in controls, CAPD and hemodialysis patients

It is known that cadmium may accumulate in patients with chronic renal failure. Our CAPD and hemodialysis patients had cadmium levels (Fig. 8) which were not different from the controls.

Lead is a toxic element for man. Significantly lower levels were found (Fig. 8) in CAPD and hemodialysis patients compared to controls.

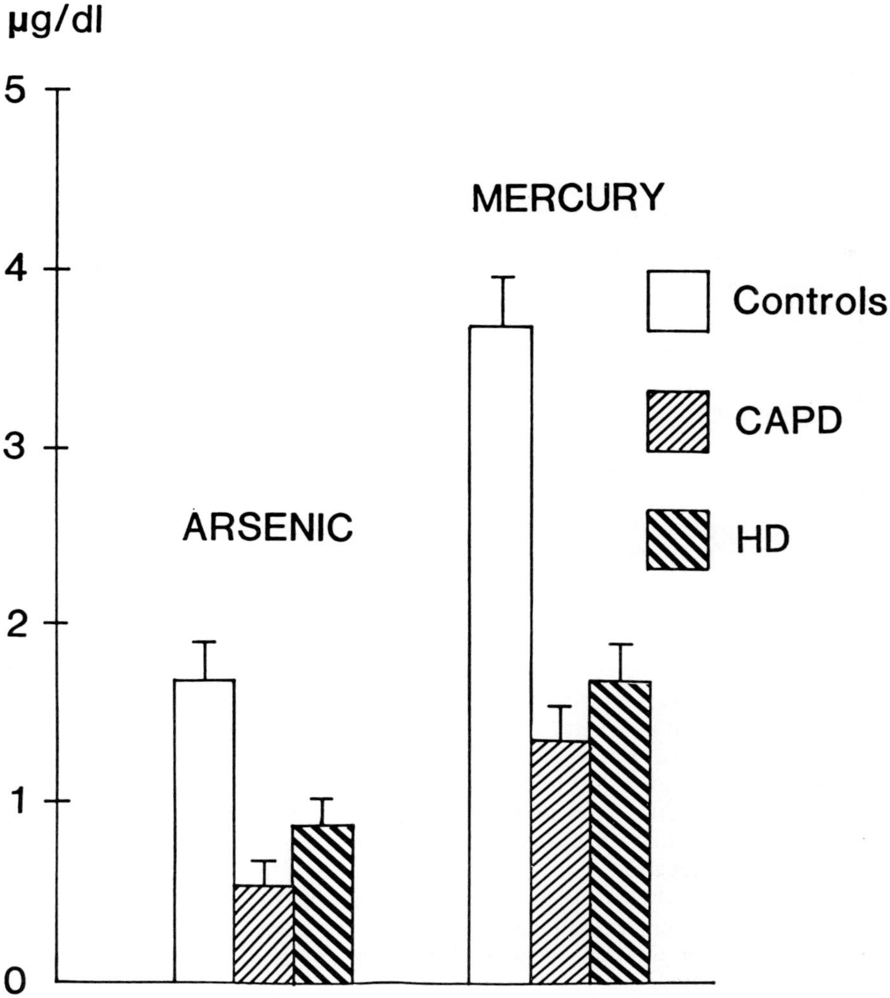

Fig. 9 Mean plasma levels + 1 SEM of arsenic and mercury in controls, CAPD and hemodialysis patients

Arsenic seems to be an antagonist of selenium especially of the cancer-protecting effect of selenium. No arsenic deficiency syndrom is known. Toxic doses of arsenic are known to lead to an increased risk of cancer, especially of the skin, the urinary bladder and the gastrointestinal tract. The plasma levels in CAPD and hemodialysis patients were significantly lower than in controls (Fig. 9).

Mercury is not an essential element and is known to be nephrotoxic. Significantly lower levels were found in both CAPD and hemodialysis patients (Fig. 9).

CONCLUSIONS

Even if more sensitive analytical methods could have been used for some elements, from these results it could be concluded that CAPD patients as well as hemodialysis patients seem to have disturbed metabolism of trace elements, where both accumulation and depletion may occur. A number of causes can be mentioned such as a disturbed absorption in the gut, the use of aluminium phosphate binders, contamination of the dialysate solutions, diet, among others. The findings may also reflect redistribution caused by the disease itself. The results also indicate that further studies and longer follow-ups are necessary.

REFERENCES

Abu-Hamdan, D. K., Mahajan, S. K., Migdal, S. D., Prasad, A. S. & McDonald, F. D. (1984). Zinc absorption in uremia: effect of phosphate binders. In *Abstracts IXth International Congress of Nephrology*, p. 307A, Los Angeles.

Leung, A. C. T., Henderson, I. S., Dobbie, J. W., Halls, D., Fell, G. & Kennedy, A. C. (1984a). Accumulation of chromium in patients on maintenance haemodialysis and CAPD. In *Abstracts IXth International Congress of Nephrology*, p. 173A, Los Angeles.

— (1984b). Selenium deficiency in patients with end-stage chronic renal failure. In *Abstracts IXth International Congress of Nephrology*, p. 314A, Los Angeles.

Mahajan, S., Prasad, A., Rye, D. & McDonald, F. (1984). Plasma zinc, erythrocyte zinc, and serum ammonia in uremia: Effect of zinc supplementation and renal transplantation. In *Abstracts IXth International Congress of Nephrology*, p. 314A, Los Angeles.

Thomson, M. N., Stevens, B. J., Humphery, T. J. & Atkins, R. C. (1981). Trace elements in patients on continuous ambulatory peritoneal dialysis. In *Advances in Peritoneal Dialysis*. Ed. by G. M. Gahl, M. Kessel and K. D. Nolph. Excerpta Medica, Amsterdam.

Discussion (the papers by Nilsson and Danielson)

Chairman: BOSTRÖM

WESTER: I think you showed that some trace elements were higher in the serum in patients on dialysis. It could have two explanations: one, of course, that there are impurities in the water, which you told about, and another that urine is the normal excretion pathway for some elements. I remember from some early studies of mine that patients who had chronic uraemia and were not on dialysis had very high levels of some trace elements, for instance arsenic was ten times higher than in normals. Of course, you have shown now that with hemodialysis you can take away the arsenic. But, perhaps concerning some elements you may not be so effective. So that's another way to explain high levels in your patients. I wonder if you have also analyzed the patients before they were on dialysis? That's one question.

I have one more and that's about aluminium. Do you know anything about aluminium absorption? When we use aluminium vessels for cooking, we have found that we get a lot of aluminium from these cooking vessels, especially, of course, if the pH is low or if it's high. If the pH is in the normal range there was not very much released, but if you cook food at a low pH it rose at least tenfold. Do you know how much is absorbed of the aluminium released from cooking vessels?

DANIELSON: Could I start with the first question? We are just now investigating uraemic patients who have not been put on dialysis because that's a natural consequence of the findings—to see how much actually the dialysis treatment as such means for these findings. We are also analyzing the different solutions.

Switching over to aluminium absorption, I don't know exactly how much aluminium is absorbed. On average, about 0.5% of the intake is absorbed, but I don't know how significant aluminium coming from cooking vessels is. It's quite clear if we take, for instance, aluminium-containing antacids in normal people, they absorb aluminium, you can see it in serum, and it is excreted in the urine. There are probably several factors influencing the absorption, but I think one factor which may be important is, at least in these patients, that vitamin D preparations seem to increase the absorption of aluminium as such. But I think Dr Nilsson has more comments on this.

NILSSON: I agree about the importance of aluminium absorption. I'm not aware of any investigations on the amount of aluminium absorbed from food prepared in aluminium vessels, but those studies that have been performed have been made with aluminium hydroxide-containing antacids. The normal daily urinary excretion of about 15 μg is increased to about 500–700 μg if you give 2 g of aluminium hydroxide a day. That is what happens in a healthy person. It is known, that even though serum levels of aluminium give a rather poor indication of the total body burden of aluminium, they do reflect fairly well recent or current exposure to aluminium. It is quite possible to reach serum aluminium levels in uraemic patients which are probably harmful and which lead to the risk of tissue accumulation just by giving aluminium hydroxide. Thus, there is a definite absorption.

CHRISTOPHERSEN: I have a comment regarding aluminium. I wonder if you have tried to consider the interaction with fluoride, because it has been shown in animal experiments that, if you give high doses of aluminium and if you also give fluoride, the tissue retention is decreased by fluoride. I think one possible, partial explanation is that fluoride may form negatively-charged complexes alone or together with other ligands and that the inside of the plasma membrane in the cell has a negative electric potential. The negatively-charged complexes then go out of the cell. I would also mention, that the fluoride concentrations of drinking water vary very much geographically. So I think one should consider the possibility that some of the geographic differences between cities or nations as regards aluminium retention may be related to different intakes of fluoride.

Secondly, there is another aspect of this. When you have aluminium intoxication, one should not only give chelates but also give fluoride to improve the rate of elimination of aluminium from the body.

I have another question. You have been discussing patients on dialysis and I wonder about the possible importance of geographical differences in aluminium ingestion for bone disease in other patients. I was thinking about the very high prevalence of osteoporosis in Norway, for instance. It is possible that this may, in part, be due to the high aluminium ingestion from cooking vessels. Also, it's possible that because of acid soils we have more aluminium in plant foods than in some other countries, especially when we have a combination of aluminium intake and low intake of fluoride. Could this be one reason for the very high prevalence of osteoporosis?

NILSSON: These are certainly very interesting points. Fluoride is also an element that is accumulated into bone in these patients. On dialysis, they have quite high serum fluoride concentrations and fluoride has, as I said, been discussed as a possible agent of pathogenetic significance in renal osteodystrophy. So far, no conclusive evidence has been presented. I was not aware of this inverse relationship between aluminium and fluoride accumulation and I'm not aware of any human studies of that problem. What you can say concerning fluoride, is that the bones of the uraemic patients or the dialysis patients don't usually show any signs typical of fluorosis even though the fluoride content may be quite high.

As far as the possible significance of aluminium for bone disease in other patient groups, I don't think that the risk of aluminium accumulation would be very great if you have a normal renal function. The only other situation where it has been suggested that aluminium may be toxic is in patients on chronic parenteral nutrition, especially in patients given casein hydrolysate as a source of protein. This casein hydrolysate may contain high levels of aluminium as a contaminant. In such patients skeletal abnormalities similar to those in the dialysis patients have been described. Otherwise I don't think, with normal renal function and normal enteral nutrition, there would be any great risk of aluminium accumulation.

DANIELSON: Could I just ask a short question? Has anyone stained for aluminium in bone biopsies performed on elderly, osteoporotic patients?

NILSSON: No, I don't know that, but those control materials where bone has been analyzed by absorption photometry have contained quite a few elderly patients. There is aluminium detectable in bone in almost all persons but in very low concentrations. I've not seen anything about relationship with age.

BRUCE: There is at the moment a lively Swedish discussion about the environmental effects of aluminium in relation to the increased environmental acidity. There are data indicating that birds like the pied flycatcher and fishes like salmon and trout breed unsuccessfully.

When it comes to aluminium in water and in human foods we know much less, because the analyses have been rather difficult to perform. Our data indicate that the intake of aluminium from contaminating mineral components in vegetables is much more than what comes from the vessels in which the food is prepared. The exceptions may be when very acidic soups are prepared. I do not think that we very often cook basic foods. The toxicologists of the Food Administration a few years ago studied the uptake of aluminium hydroxide and found that citrate increased the absorption quite considerably.

ANDERSON: High levels of aluminium have been associated with Alzheimer's disease. Do you see any increase in Alzheimer's disease in dialysis patients?

DANIELSON: The entity of dialysis encephalopathy maybe bears some resemblance to Alzheimer's disease. I know it has been suggested that there are some common traits in the pathogenesis, but I'm not aware of any increased incidence of typical Alzheimer's disease in uraemic or dialysis patients.

JAMESON: I just want to say that I think we have different criteria for Alzheimer's disease in Scandinavia and in the United States. Many cases of Alzheimer's disease are reported in the ongoing studies in the United States. That's not true here and I suggest that it's a matter of definition.

PLANTIN: I have some questions about the values in your control material. I'm a little puzzled about the magnitude, because if we take Fig. 6 in your paper you have about ten times the values considered normal in people for chromium and manganese. This might be that there is some error in the units on the axis. You say it's μg/dl. If it's μg/l, it would be just about correct.

DANIELSON: ICP was used for this and I think there is a difference, which I don't know, between the atomic absorption and the ICP. So I don't know the reason why. But even with this less sensitive method there is quite a difference between the controls and the dialysis patients. I agree there is a difference, but I don't know for sure the reason for it. We have been discussing this.

PLANTIN: So the magnitude may be wrong but the results may be indicative of a difference?

DANIELSON: Yes.

PLANTIN: Another comment concerns the selenium values, as they are apparently acquired from people in Uppsala, perhaps blood donors. I find them twice as high as those I get from the same group of blood donors from Uppsala. I had just about half the magnitude.

DANIELSON: Yes, we have observed that too. These are not blood donors, they are healthy controls from an investigation of healthy people going on in Uppsala. Also these were measured with ICP and we will compare ICP with atomic absorption just to find out if there is a methodological error in what we did. We are aware of it but, still, what we actually were after in this study was if we could, even with these less sophisticated methods, see if there is a difference between healthy controls and dialysis patients. We are in the process of concentrating on the different elements, where we hope to see more detailed differences.

SHAMBERGER: Has either Dr Danielson or Dr Nilsson looked at the water-soluble vitamins, namely B_1, B_2 and B_6, because some of these severe deficiencies in animals will cause ataxia similar to that seen in dialysis dementia?

NILSSON: We haven't studied that. We have only studied vitamin A and there is an accumulation of that in dialysis patients.

CHRISTOPHERSEN: Dr Bruce was talking about aluminium in minerals. I think that when one considers the intake of aluminium, it may be important to distinguish between the different forms of aluminium in food. It is probable that there is even some dissolution of aluminium from soil minerals going to the stomach. But this would probably not be a very rapid process, so I would expect that aluminium from minerals is much less available than organically-bound aluminium in plant foods and also aluminium from cooking vessels.

Then I'd just like to comment on osteoporosis. I think one should remember that this is a disease which usually develops progressively and probably over many years. In renal dialysis patients I presume you have a much more rapid development of the bone disease. So it is possible that a similar functional disturbance but much milder, nevertheless, would be important when it operates during, for instance, periods of 20 years.

NILSSON: Yes, that is possible. Of course, it has not been excluded that aluminium may be of importance in osteoporosis. On the other hand, the type of changes in bone-remodelling dynamics related to aluminium accumulation are rather specific. You usually don't see anything like that in senile or post-menopausal osteoporosis. That, I guess, would speak against such a connection.

WEISMANN: A few years ago there were several reports on toxic zinc effects during hemodialyses and I want to ask if you have observed such changes in your patients.

Futhermore, I'd like to ask if you have tried to correlate the aluminium concentration in the blood to the zinc concentration of the patients.

DANIELSON: We haven't correlated that, but I didn't get the first part of your question.

WEISMANN: A few years ago, I think it was mostly from England, there were reports on toxic effects of zinc during hemodialysis. This was due to release of zinc from the piping system.

DANIELSON: We haven't seen that. All patients have been on the low side for serum zinc. In CAPD solutions, I don't know the exact levels, but there is an increased zinc concentration because the zinc is coming from the plastic material in the bags.